Glomerular Dysfunction
and
Biopathology of Vascular Wall

Academic Press Rapid Manuscript Reproduction

Glomerular Dysfunction and Biopathology of Vascular Wall

Edited by

Satimaru Seno
Division of Pathology
Shigei Medical Research Institute
Okayama, Japan

Alfred L. Copley
Laboratory of Biorheology
Polytechnic University
New York, New York

Manjeri A. Venkatachalam
Department of Pathology
The University of Texas
Health Science Center at San Antonio
San Antonio, Texas

Yoshihiro Hamashima
Department of Pathology
Faculty of Medicine
Kyoto University
Kyoto, Japan

Tadashi Tsujii
Division of Ultrastructure Research
Shigei Medical Research Institute
Okayama, Japan

1985

ACADEMIC PRESS, INC.
Harcourt Brace Jovanovich, Publishers
Tokyo Orlando San Diego New York
Austin Boston London Sydney Toronto

ACADEMIC PRESS JAPAN, INC.
Hokoku Bldg. 3-11-13, Iidabashi, Chiyoda-ku, Tokyo 102

United States Edition published by
ACADEMIC PRESS, INC.
Orlando, Florida 32887

United Kingdom Edition published by
ACADEMIC PRESS, INC. (LONDON) LTD.
24/28 Oval Road, London NW1 7DX

Library of Congress Cataloging in Publication Data

Glomerular dysfunction and biopathology of vascular wall.

Papers from the Satellite Symposium on Biopathology of Vascular Wall and Glomerular Dysfunction held in Kurashiki, Japan in the fall of 1984, following the Third International Congress on Cell Biology.
Includes index.
1. Glomerulonephritis—Congresses. 2. Capillaries—Diseases—Congresses. 3. Endothelium—Congresses. 4. Kidney glomerulus—Diseases—Congresses. 5. Physiology, Pathological—Congresses. I. Senoo, Sachimaru, Date . II. Satellite Symposium on Biopathology of Vascular Wall and Glomerular Dysfunction (1984 : Kurashiki-shi, Japan) III. International Congress on Cell Biology (3rd : 1984 : Tokyo, Japan) [DNLM: 1. Endothelium—cytology—congresses. 2. Endothelium—Pathology—congresses. 3. Kidney Glomerulus—immunology—congresses. 4. Kidney Glomerulus—pathology—congresses. WJ 301 G562 1984]
RC918.G55G56 1986 616.1'48 86-47725
ISBN 0-12-636775-2 (alk. paper)

PRINTED IN THE UNITED STATES OF AMERICA

85 86 87 88 9 8 7 6 5 4 3 2 1

Contents

Preface

In the fall after the Third International Congress on Cell Biology in Tokyo, we had the Satellite Symposium on "Biopathology of Vascular Wall and Glomerular Dysfunction" at Kurashiki. What pleased us most was that many active researchers working on this topic in Europe, the United States, and Japan came together at this symposium. Twenty-two eminent speakers and more than 200 participants accepted the invitation extended by the Shigei Medical Research Institute, Okayama, to meet at the City Museum and Art Gallery in Kurashiki, an old town near Okayama. We, the staff of the Institute and the Hospital, considered it a great honor to offer our hospitality and provide people engaged in the application of vascular and glomerular research with the opportunity for an intensive exchange of knowledge.

The scientific program of the symposium included morphological observations of capillaries in general and glomeruli in terms of anionic barriers, rheological studies of blood in relation to anionic barrier of endothelial cells, the size and charge barrier of glomerular wall against protein leakage, and the mechanism of immune complex deposition. On the first afternoon we had a special lecture from Dr. G. E. Palade on "The Vascular Endothelium, a Source of Continuous Surprises." Each presentation was followed by active discussions, and all the participants seemed to be very much excited and deeply impressed. After the meeting, we aimed to publish the proceedings and most speakers agreed with our intent to include the recent data obtained after the symposium. Hence, this book covers the most recent data in the research field of vascular endothelium and glomerular dysfunction.

We wish to thank the authors for presenting their valuable scientific contributions. I believe that each title enables us to present an almost complete review of the most recent results in the field concerned.

Grateful acknowledgment is due to Dr. Hiroshi Shigei, Chairman of the Board of Sôwakai Foundation, for financial support for the contributors and the publication of this book.

In particular, we wish to express our thanks to the staff of Academic Press, Tokyo, for their excellent cooperation.

Satimaru Seno
Okayama, Japan

Glomerular Dysfunction
and
Biopathology of Vascular Wall

I. Morphologic and Chemical Bases of Vascular Wall

In the past few decades, a large number of studies on capillary permeability and renal function have been published, resulting in the tremendous expansion of our knowledge on glomerular function. Biochemical, histochemical, and morphological studies together with physiological observations have contributed much to our better understanding of the mechanism of glomerular filtration. These findings give us theoretical bases for the clinical studies and medical care of patients suffering from glomerular dysfunction.

Discussed in this section are regional difference in the density of anionic sites in endothelium, physiologic changes of glomerular function in aging, morphologic changes of glomeruli by simple congestion, and the special contribution of a new method for vascular study, back-scattered electron imaging. These will be helpful for the readers who deal with glomerular nephropathy.

Satimaru Seno

REGIONAL DIFFERENTIATION OF THE SURFACE CHARGE DISTRIBUTION IN THE CONTINUOUS ENDOTHELIUM OF THE MICROVASCULATURE

Maya Simionescu

Institute of Cellular Biology and Pathology, Bucharest

Continuous endothelium lines the great majority of blood vessels including capillaries of major organs such as heart, lung and diaphragm. Like all other epithelial cells, the endothelial cells are provided with a complete set of organelles but have characteristically a large population of plasmalemmal vesicles (Palade, 1960). The interface between endothelial cells (EC) and circulating blood is of major importance for various processes such as transport of macromolecules as well as for the relationship with circulating blood cells. As the plasma membrane of all eukaryotic cells, EC luminal surface has a net negative charge (Danon, 1979; Skutelsky et al., 1975), a condition which insures non-adhesion to endothelium of similarly charged blood cells.

Although most plasma proteins are negatively charged (Blomback and Hanson, 1979), they do cross the endothelium to reach the interstitial fluid. This suggests that along the negatively charged plasma membrane there should be pathways which allow and/or facilitate transport of anionic plasma proteins.

Use of Charged Probes to Investigate EC Surface Charge

To map anionic sites on the surface of continuous endothelium, ferritin molecules cationized to different pIs (6.8, 7.15, 7.6, 8.0, 8.4) were perfused in mice through the aorta or vena cava after washing out the blood and supposedly the attached plasma proteins. At time intervals ranging from 2 to 10 min, excess cationized ferritin (CF) was washed out and heart, diaphragm and lungs were fixed *in situ* and processed for electron microscopy, as described in details elsewhere (Simionescu D. and Simionescu M., 1983; Simionescu M. et al., 1985). Since in the mouse diaphragm, sequential microvascular segments — arterioles, capillaries and venules — could be easily identified (Simionescu M. et al., 1978), comparative qualitative data and quantitative studies were performed along the endothelium of this microvasculature (Simionescu M., 1980; Simionescu M. and Simionescu N., 1984).

To visualize cationic sites, native ferritin pI 4.7 and albumin adsorbed onto 5 nm gold particles pI 5.1 were used in similar conditions as above (Ghitescu et al., 1985).

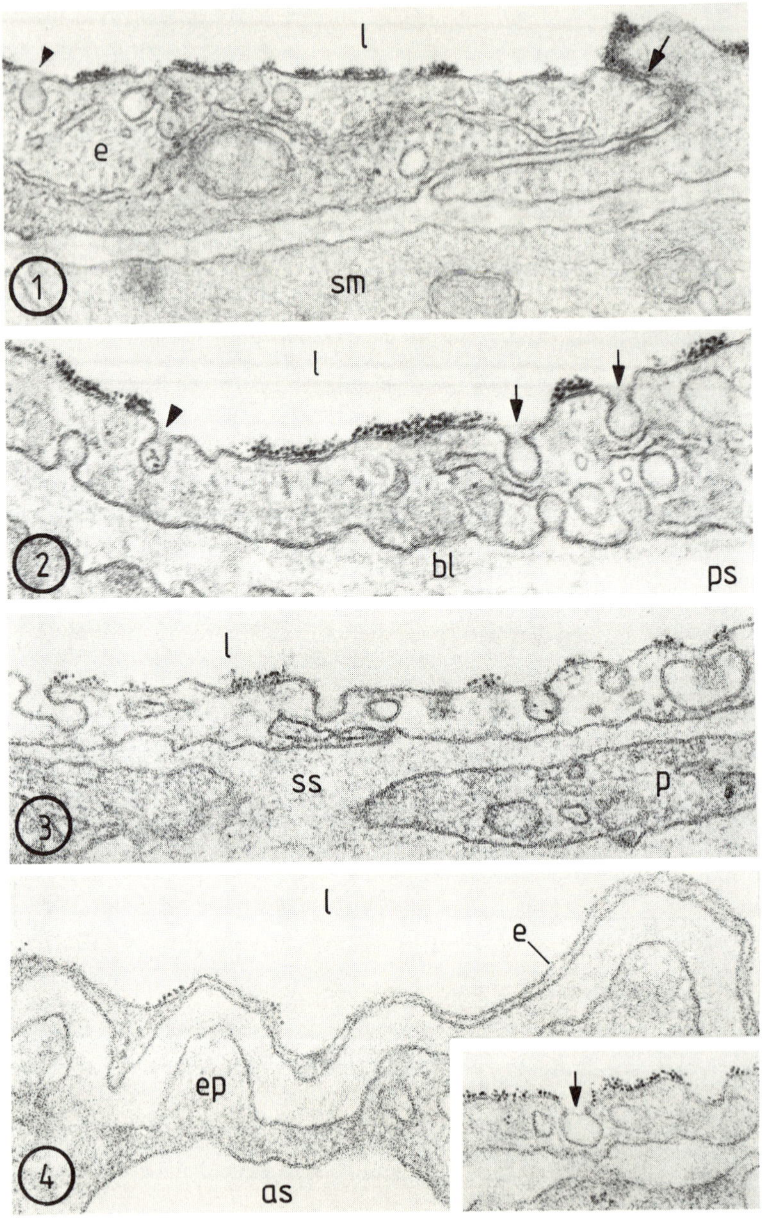

FIG. 1. Terminal arteriole (diaphragm). The luminal surface of the endothelium is discontinuously labeled by cationic ferritin (CF), and the marker penetrates the intercellular space up to the level of the junction (arrow). Plasmalemmal vesicle membrane is not labeled by CF (arrowhead). *sm*, smooth muscle cell; *l*, lumen; *e*, endothelium. x 62,000.

FIG. 2. Capillary endothelium (diaphragm). Plasmalemma proper is decorated by CF particles, whereas plasmalemmal vesicle membranes and their infundibula are not labeled

Surface Charge of Endothelium in Sequential Segments of Microvasculature

In the heart and diaphragm, the EC luminal plasmalemma was in general heavily but discontinuously labeled by CF of pI$\gg$7.6 (Figs. 1, 2). As compared to arterioles and capillaries, less extensive binding was observed in venular endothelium (Fig. 3). The distribution of CF often suggested that the interacting acidic molecules were tightly packed (~ 15 nm apart) and protruded high above the lipid bilayer (~ 20 nm or more). The membrane of plasmalemmal vesicles generally was not labeled by CF, but ~15% of opened vesicles contained some CF molecules probably taken up by fluid phase uptake.

Like the vesicle membrane, in most cases, the introits leading to vesicular opening, the stomal diaphragms of vesicles and transendothelial channels, when present, were not labeled.

TABLE 1

Cationic Ferritin Labeling of the Luminal Endothelial Plasma Membrane in Sequential Segments of the Microvasculature (Mouse Diaphragm): Effects of Various Enzymes and Age of Animals

	Luminal plasmalemma labeled by CF (% ± SD)		
	Arterioles	Capillaries	Venules
YOUNG MICE			
perfusion CF pI 8.4	76±12	81±9	61±7
Neuraminidase/CF	61±7	68±8	43±4
Heparinase/CF	60±8	78±10	55±7
Heparitinase/CF	78±14	76±14	58±9
OLD MICE			
perfusion CF pI 8.4	73±7	79±11	32±5
Neuraminidase/CF	60±6	62±9	18±4

The aggregate perimeters surveyed were: 48 μm for arterioles, 216 μm for capillaries, and 1,428 μm for venules.
For details see Simionescu, M. et al., 1985.
±SD, standard deviation of the mean.

(arrows). One plasmalemmal vesicle has CF molecules as content marker (arrowhead). *l*, lumen; *ps*, pericapillary space; *bl*, basal lamina. x 67,000.

FIG. 3. Pericytic venules (diaphragm). Endothelial surface is decorated by small CF patches, most plasmalemmal vesicles are not decorated by CF except one vesicle which has 2 molecules in the content. *p*, pericyte; *ss*, subendothelial space; *l*, lumen. x 67,000.

FIG. 4. Alveolar capillary (lung). A sector of the thin avesicular zone of endothelium provided with very few CF-detectable anionic sites. Long stretches of plasmalemma are unlabeled. *Inset.* The vesicular zone of the same capillary whose plasmalemma is continuously labeled by CF and vesicle membrane and its diaphragm is not decorated (arrow). *l*, lumen; *as*, air space; *ep*, type I epithelial cell; *e*, endothelium. x 80,000. *Inset*, x 67,000.

Morphometric analysis showed that in young animals, the percentage of luminal perimeter labeled by CF was similarly high in arterioles (~ 76%) and capillaries (~ 81%) but lower in pericytic venules (~ 61%) (Table 1). The percentage of vesicles containing CF molecules (pI 8.4) was higher in venules (~ 17%) than in arterioles (~ 10%) and capillaries (~12%) (Table 2). Vesicular labeling in capillaries was function of marker pI and concentration: it increased with decreasing pI and with higher concentration (Table 2).

TABLE 2

LABELING BY CATIONIZED FERRITIN OF PLASMALEMMAL VESICLES OF THE MICROVASCULAR ENDOTHELIUM (MOUSE DIAPHRAGM) AS A FUNCTION OF TRACER ISOELECTRIC POINT AND CONCENTRATION

CF pI	CF concentration			
	10 mg/ml			50 mg/ml
	Arterioles	Capillaries %±SD	Venules	Capillaries
6.8	n·d	26±5	n·d	34±7
7.4	n·d	17±3	n·d	21±4
8.4	10±4	12±3	17±3	18±5

For each experimental condition the number of counted vesicles was: 410 for arterioles, 2,100 for capillaries, 1,050 for venules. The figures represent percentages of labeled vesicles of the total population of vesicles opened on the luminal front of EC.
For more details see Simionescu M. et al., 1985.
n·d, not determined.
±SD, standard deviation of the mean.

A PARTICULAR SITUATION: LUNG ALVEOLAR CAPILLARIES

Although alveolar capillaries are lined by a continuous endothelium, characteristically they exhibit two zones: an area provided with vesicles (as in any type of continuous endothelium) and an area highly attenuated and devoid of vesicles (avesicular zone); usually, the latter is closely apposed to the type I epithelial cells constituting together the air-blood barrier. In the vesicular zone, the CF-detectable sites on plasmalemma proper and plasmalemmal vesicles exhibit a differentiated distribution (Fig. 4, inset), comparable to that observed in other continuous endothelia, or in the corresponding areas of fenestrated capillaries (Simionescu N. et al., 1981). A characteristic feature of the alveolar capillaries is the paucity of anionic sites over the avesicular zone (Fig. 4), a large domain of this EC particularly involved in O_2/CO_2 exchanges (Pietra et al., 1982; Simionescu D. and Simionescu M., 1983).

The significance of this uneven distribution of anionic sites in the same capillary bed is not clearly understood. It may be speculated that (a) in the vesicular zone, the uncharged plasmalemmal vesicles are involved in the transport of anionic proteins, and (b) in the avesicular zone (with low density of anionic sites), the erythrocytes are not strongly repelled, a condition which may facilitate the exchange of gases.

A Special Segment: Venular Endothelium (Particularly in Old Animals)

In young animals, in the diaphragm microvessels the density of CF-detectable anionic sites on plasma membrane proper was low in pericytic (postcapillary) venules and even lower in muscular venules as compared to arterioles and capillaries. In old animals, as compared to young mice, the density of anionic sites is reduced by $\sim$50% in venules whereas in arterioles and capillaries no major changes were recorded (Simionescu M. et al., 1985). Neuraminidase perfusion prior to CF affected particularly the decoration of venular endothelium and this appeared even more pronounced in old animals where the percent of labeled luminal perimeter dropped from 32% to 18% (Table 1). Fluid phase uptake of CF by plasmalemmal vesicles of venular endothelium was higher than that observed in other vascular segments (Table 2). All these data suggest that venules (pericytic and muscular) constitute a special segment of the microvasculature; the paucity of anionic sites may facilitate the attachment of leukocytes followed by their diapedesis in normal and pathologic conditions (Majno et al., 1961; Ryan and Majno, 1977). The reduction in anionic charge density in old animals may explain the increased frequency with age of venular thrombosis (Sawyer and Srinivasan, 1972).

Partial Chemical Characterization of Acidic Sites of EC Surface

To detect the molecules responsible for the negative charge of EC surface, various enzymes were perfused before the cationic probe. Papain and pronase, enzymes of broad specificity practically prevented completely CF binding to EC plasmalemma. Neuraminidase reduced CF binding to plasmalemma especially in venular endothelium and in particular in old animals. Heparinase and heparitinase reduced slightly CF binding on EC along the entire microvasculature (Table 1). These results indicate that sialoglycoproteins in particular, and to a lesser extent sulfated proteoglycans are major contributors to the acidic sites of the EC surface and that venular endothelium especially in old animals is particularly sensitive to neuraminidase.

In Lung, Heart and Diaphragm Capillaries, Albumin Binds to EC Plasmalemmal Vesicles by Specific Binding Sites

To investigate cationic sites, native ferritin (NF) pI 4.7, and albumin adsorbed to 5 nm gold (Alb-Au_5) pI 5.1, were perfused in blood-free vasculature, and the decoration pattern recorded. Both tracers labeled the vesicle membrane but while NF could be easily removed by a high ionic strength buffer (denoting electrostatic binding), Alb-Au_5 was not detached from vesicle membrane even when very high ionic concentrations (0.45 M NaCl) were used. Perfusion of strongly anionic heparin prior to Alb-Au_5 did not affect the binding of this conjugate. Moreover, binding of Alb-Au_5 to vesicle membrane was saturable and could be competed by excess free albumin (3%) present in the perfusate (Ghitescu et al., 1985). These results indicate that vesicle membrane possesses receptors for albumin molecules; such receptors would provide a specific mechanism for albumin transport across the endothelium. These findings extend and complete earlier immunocytochemical evidence that albumin is transported across the endothelium *via* vesicles (Yokota, 1983). The observations support the previous findings of the role of vesicle in transport of molecules (Bruns and Palade, 1968; Simionescu N. et al., 1975; Wagner and Casley Smith, 1981) and supplement the evidence that some normal plasma constituents are shuttled across the endothelium by receptor-mediated transcytosis (Simionescu N. et al., 1979; Vasile et al., 1983; Jeferris et al., 1984, Soda and Tavassoli, 1984; King and Johnson, 1985). Moreover, only such a specific mechanism, and modulations of the density of receptors may explain the existance and maintenance of different lymph/plasma concentration of albumin in various organs (Taylor and Granger, 1984).

Plasmalemmal Vesicles: Carriers Devised to Shuttle Plasma Proteins by Transcytosis

Vesicles and transendothelial channels in continuous as well as fenestrated capillaries represent chemically differentiated microdomains characterized by very low density of anionic sites on their membranes (Simionescu N. et al., 1981; Simionescu M. et al., 1985). However, a small fraction of vesicle population takes up CF pI 8.4 but this fraction increases when the pI of the tracer decreases close to neutrality. Thus, it can be expected that plasmalemmal vesicles may represent a preferential carrier for anionic proteins. Moreover, the new data on the existance of specific binding sites (receptors) for albumin on vesicle membrane support the idea that vesicles are devised to transport plasma proteins by transcytosis (Simionescu N., 1980); the plasma molecules are probably selected by their size (Renkin, 1977), as well as by their charge and/or specific chemical adsorption.

Factors Possibly Involved in Maintaining the Specificity of Microdomains along the Fluid Lipid Bilayer

The differentiated microdomains of the luminal surface of the endothelium are maintained along the fluid plasma membrane during repeated fusion and fission of vesicles. There are a number of factors which may cooperate to prevent randomization and to secure the segregation of these specialized domains. A fine fibrillar infrastructure is often observed along the cytoplasmic aspect of luminal endothelial plasmalemma. Recent experiments have demonstrated the presence of spectrin in endothelial cells *in situ* (Heltianu et al., 1984), and in culture (Pratt et al., 1984). Spectrin may play an important role in maintaining the integrity and segregation of the microdomains; this function can be accomplished in concert with other cytoskeletal proteins such as actin and band 4.1. Actin is present in all endothelial cells and band 4.1 was recently demonstrated by immunocytochemistry (Constantinescu E., Heltianu C., Simionescu M., manuscript in preparation). These complexes of cytoskeletal components by interaction with integral membrane proteins (or glycoproteins) may be important factors in the restriction and segregation of the differentiated microdomains along the plasmalemma proper. It was also demonstrated in various endothelia that vesicular openings are provided with rings of sterols (Simionescu N. et al., 1983) at the level of which anionic molecule are virtually absent. These peristomal rings of cholesterol may contribute to the phase separation between the cell membrane proper and the vesicle membrane. As such, infrastructural elements of both endothelial plasmalemma and vesicular membrane may function in preventing randomization by restricting lateral diffusion of molecules along the plasma membrane.

REFERENCES

Blomback, B., and Hanson, L.A. (1979). "Plasma Proteins." John Wiley and Sons, New York.

Bruns, R.R., and Palade, G.E. (1968). Studies on blood capillaries. II. Transport of ferritin molecules across the wall of muscle capillaries. *J. Cell Biol.* 37, 277–299.

Danon, D. (1970). Blood vessel surface charge analysis by electron microscopy. *6th Eur. Conf. Microcirculation*, 1970, Aalborg, Denmark. pp. 415–419, Karger, Basel.

Ghitescu, L., Fixman, A., Simionescu, M., and Simionescu, N. (1985). Albumin is transported through capillary endothelium by receptor-mediated transcytosis. (in press)

Heltianu, C., Bogdan, I., Constantinescu, E., and Simionescu, M. (1984). Detection of a spectrin-like protein in endothelial cells. *In* "International Cell Biology 1984" (S. Seno and Y. Okada, eds.), p. 522. Academic Press, Tokyo.

Jefferis, W.A., Brandon, M.R., Hunt, S.V., Williams, A.F., Gater, K.C., and Mason, D.Y. (1984). Transferrin receptor on endothelium of brain capillaries. *Nature* 312, 162–163.

King, G.L., and Johnson, S.M. (1985). Receptor-mediated transport of insulin across endothelial cells. *Science* 227, 1583–1586.

Majno, G., Palade, G.E., and Schoefl, G.I. (1961). Studies on inflammation. II. The site of action of histamine and serotonin along the vascular tree: a topographic study. *J. Biochim. Biophys. Cytol.* 11, 607–626.

Palade, G.E. (1960). Transport in quanta across the endothelium of blood capillaries. *Anat. Rec.* 136, 254.

Pelikan, P., Gimbrone, M.A., and Cotran, R.S. (1979). Distribution and movement of anionic cell surface in cultured human vascular endothelial cells. *Arteriosclerosis* **32**, 69–80.

Pietra, G.G., Fishman, A.P., Lanken, P.N., and Hansen-Flaschen, J. (1982). Permeability of pulmonary endothelium to neutral and charged macromolecules. *Ann. N.Y. Acad. Sci.* **401**, 241–247.

Pratt, B.M., Harris, A.S., Morrow, J.S., and Madri J.A. (1984). *In vitro* substratum modulation of the aortic endothelial cell cytoskeletal component spectrin. *J. Cell. Biol.* **99**, 235a (abstract).

Renkin, E.M. (1977). Multiple pathways of capillary permeability. *Circ. Res.* **41**, 735–743.

Ryan, G.B., and Majno, G. (1977). Acute inflammation. *Am. J. Pathol.* **86**, 184–276.

Sawyer, P.N., and Srinivasan, S. (1972). The role of electrochemical surface properties in thrombosis at vascular interface: cumulative experience of studies in animals and man. *Bull. N.Y. Acad. Med.* **48**, 235–249.

Simionescu, D., and Simionescu, M. (1983). Differentiated distribution of the cell surface charge on the alveolar-capillary unit. Characteristic paucity of anionic sites on the air-blood barrier. *Microvasc. Res.* **25**, 85–109.

Simionescu, M. (1980). Structural and functional differentiation of microvascular endothelium. *In* "Blood Cells and Vessel Walls: Functional Interactions" Ciba Found. Symp. 71 (new series), pp. 39–60, Excerpta Medica,

Simionescu, M., and Simionescu, N. (1984). Ultrastructure of the microvascular wall: functional correlations. *In* "Handbook of Physiology, The Cardiovascular System. Vol. 4, Microcirculation. Part I." (E.M. Renkin and C.C. Michel, eds.), American Physiological Society, Bethesda.

Simionescu, M., Simionescu, N., and Palade, G.E. (1978). Structural basis of permeability in sequential segments of the microvasculature of the diaphragm. I. Bipolar microvascular fields. *Microvasc. Res.* **15**, 1–16.

Simionescu, M., Simionescu, N., Santoro, F., and Palade, G.E. (1985). Differentiated microdomains on the luminal plasmalemma of murine muscle capillaries. Segmental variations in young and old animals. *J. Cell Biol.* **100**, 1396–1407.

Simionescu, M., Simionescu, N., Silbert, J.E., and Palade, G.E. (1981). Differentiated microdomains on the luminal surface of capillary endothelium. II. Partial characterization of their anionic sites. *J. Cell Biol.* **90**, 614–621.

Simionescu, N. (1979). The microvascular endothelium: segmental differentiations, transcytosis, selective distribution of anionic sites. *In* "Advances in Inflammation Research" (G. Weissman, B. Samuelson and R. Paoletti, eds.), pp. 61–70, Raven Press, New York.

Simionescu, N. (1981). Transcytosis and traffic of membranes in the endothelial cells. *In* "International Cell Biology, 1980–1981" (H.G. Schweiger, ed.), pp. 657–672. Springer-Verlag.

Simionescu, N., Simionescu, M., and Palade, G.E. (1975). Permeability of muscle capillaries to small hemepeptides. Evidence for the existence of patent transendothelial channels. *J. Cell Biol.* **64**, 586–607.

Simionescu, N., Simionescu, M., and Palade, G.E. (1981). Differentiated microdomains on the luminal surface of capillary endothelium. I. Preferential distribution of anionic sites. *J. Cell Biol.* **90**, 605–613.

Simionescu, N., Lupu, F., Simionescu, M. (1983). Rings of membrane sterols surround the openings of vesicles and fenestrae, in capillary endothelium. *J. Cell Biol.* **97**, 1592–1600.

Skutelsky, E., Rudich, Z., and Danon, D. (1975). Surface charge properties of the luminal front of blood vessel walls: an electron microscopic analysis. *Thrombos. Res.* **7**, 623–631.

Soda, R., and Tavassoli, M. (1984). Transendothelial transport transcytosis of iron-transferrin complex in the bone marrow. *J. Ultrastruct. Res.* **88**, 18–29.

Vasile, E., Simionescu, M., and Simionescu, N. (1983). Visualization of the binding, endocytosis and transcytosis of low density lipoprotein in the arterial endothelium *in situ*. *J. Cell Biol.* **96**, 1677–1689.

Wagner, R.C., and Casley-Smith, J.R. (1981). Endothelial vesicles. *Microvasc. Res.* **21**, 267–298.

Yokota, S. (1983). Immunocytochemical evidence for transendothelial transport of albumin and fibrinogen in rat heart and diaphragm. *Biomed. Res.* **4**, 577–586.

STRUCTURAL CHANGES OF GLOMERULI IN RENAL CONGESTION

Hiroko Yokota, Kazushige Ogawa, Kazushi Fujimoto and Kazuo Ogawa

Department of Anatomy, Faculty of Medicine, Kyoto University, Kyoto

Information pertaining to the characterized structural alterations of glomerular basement membrane and the associated elements of the glomerular capillary wall, has been accumulated largely from detailed light and electron microscopic analyses of renal biopsy specimens and experimental injury models (Arakawa et al., 1981; Farquhar, 1975; Glassock, 1978; Gubler et al., 1980a, b; Hayashi et al., 1979; Solez et al., 1981).

Optimal hemodynamic conditions of glomerular capillaries are required for optimal ultrafiltration which is important for renal function, and also for the maintenance of the normal structure of the glomeruli (Campanacci et al., 1981; Ryan and Karnovsky, 1976; Westberg and Michael, 1970). We have made observations on an experimental congestive kidney model made by clipping the unilateral renal vein in rabbits.

In the present study, ultrastructural changes as well as cytochemical alterations in glomerular capillary components caused by experimental congestion were studied using transmission and scanning electron microscopy.

MATERIALS AND METHODS

Animals: A total of 50 adult male rabbits, 2.5 — 3.0 kg body weight were used. These rabbits were divided into 4 groups after the clipping procedure. Three animals were sacrificed at 4 — 7 days, 10 animals at 1 — 2 months, 8 animals at 3 — 4 months and 19 animals at 6 — 7 months after the clipping unilateral renal vein. Ten animals were used as control.

Rabbits were anesthetized with sodium pentobarbital (Somnopentyl) intravenously 3.5 mg/100 g body weight. The peritoneal cavity was opened and an Olive Krona aneurysm clip of a 2 mm diameter ring by using 16 gauge transfusion needle was then fixed into the left renal vein.

Transmission electron microscopy (TEM): A midline incision was performed therefore exposing the abdominal cavity and the ventral aspect of each kidney. The renal capsule was gently stripped from the surface using fine forceps. A mixture of 2 % paraformaldehyde and 1.25 % glutaraldehyde in 0.1 M phosphate buffer, pH 7.4, at room temperature, was continually dripped onto the renal surface *in situ* for 20 — 30 min. The superficial rim of fixed cortical tissue, approximately 1 mm deep, was diced with razor blades. After immersion fixation in the same solution for 2 hr, the tissue blocks were washed in 0.1 M phosphate buffer, pH 7.4, 0 − 4 ℃, overnight, and postfixed in 1 % OsO_4 in 0.1 M phosphate buffer, pH 7.4, 0 − 4 ℃, for 1 hr. The tissue blocks were routinely dehydrated in alcohol and embedded in Epon.

Ruthenium red (RR) staining: The abdomen was opened and abdominal aorta was catheterized with a 21 gauge polyethylene tube, which was held in position by two ligatures; one above and one below the origin of the left renal artery. A small opening was made in the left renal vein and retrograde aortic perfusion was started. Initially, Hanks' balanced salt solution was perfused at a pressure of 100 − 120 cm H_2O with a flow rate of 5 − 6 ml/min to wash out the blood, followed by perfusion with 1 % paraformaldehyde in 0.1 M cacodylate buffer, pH 7.4, for 5 min at room temperature, and perfusion with RR fixative solution for 10 min at room temperature. The RR fixative solution was 1 % paraformaldehyde and 3 % glutaraldehyde in 0.1 M cacodylate buffer, pH 7.4, with 4.4 mM $CaCl_2$, and was passed through a millipore filter (0.22 μm) before use to remove large dye particles. Small pieces of kidney cortex were excised and immersed in RR fixative for 3 hr at room temperature. The tissue blocks were then placed for 1 hr in 0.15 M cacodylate buffer, pH 7.4, containing 0.1 % RR at room temperature and postfixed in 1 % OsO_4 in 0.1 M cacodylate buffer, pH 7.4, containing 0.05 % RR for 3 hr at room temperature. They were routinely dehydrated in alcohol and embedded in Epon (Kanwar and Farquhar, 1979; Luft, 1971).

Tannic acid fixation: Small pieces of kidney cortex were excised and immersed in the fixative containing 2 % glutaraldehyde in 0.1 M phosphate buffer, pH 7.0, with 1 − 2 % tannic acid, for 2 hr at room temperature. The tissue blocks were then washed in 0.1 M phosphate buffer, pH 7.0, 0 − 4 ℃, overnight, postfixed in 1 % OsO_4 in 0.1 M phosphate buffer, pH 7.4, 0 − 4 ℃, for 1 hr, dehydrated in alcohol and embedded in Epon (Fujiwara and Linck, 1982).

Ultrathin sections described above were all cut by an LKB ultrotome and doubly stained with uranyle acetate and lead citrate.

Periodic acid-silver methenamine (PAM) staining: Ultrathin sections of Epon-embedded tissue were mounted on gold grids, floated on aqueous 1 % periodic acid, which was freshly prepared each time, for 10 min at room temperature, and washed in distilled water (d.w.). The sections were then floated in silver methenamine solution for 40 − 60 min at 60 ℃, in a dark room, before being rinsed with d.w. This solution was freshly prepared daily by slowly adding 5 ml of 5 % silver nitrate to 50 ml of 3 % hexamethylenetetramine, followed by adding 5 ml of 2 % solution borate and 45 ml of d.w. After several rinses with d.w., the sections were washed in 5 % sodium thiosulfate for 10 min and again rapidly rinsed with d.w. (Rambourg and Leblond, 1967).

Performic acid-phosphotungstic acid (PFP) reaction: Ultrathin sections of Epon-embedded tissue were mounted on gold glids. They were oxidized or bleached with 4.7 % performic acid, which was freshly prepared each time, for 30 min at 0 − 4 ℃, and rinsed thoroughly with d.w. The sections were then stained with 1 % phosphotungstic acid in 0.5 N HCl for 30 min at room temperature and rinsed with d.w. Poststaining with uranyl acetate and/or lead citrate was usually omitted (Fujioka and Ogawa, 1979; Ogawa et al., 1971).

The ultrathin sections were observed by transmission electron microscopy (TEM) using either a Hitachi H-500 or a JEOL JEM-100S electron microscope operated at 75 kV and 80 kV.

Scanning electron microscopy (SEM): A midline incision was made to expose the abdominal cavity. The abdominal aorta was catheterized with a 21 gauge polyethylene tube, and two ligatures were placed on it, one above and the other below the origin of the left renal artery. A small opening was made in the left renal vein and retrograde aortic perfusion was performed. First, Hanks' balanced salt solution was perfused at 100 – 120 cm H_2O pressure, 0 – 4 ℃ at a rate of 5 – 6 ml/min, followed by perfusion with 2 % glutaraldehyde in 0.1 M phosphate buffer, pH 7.4, 0 – 4 ℃ for about 30 min. These blocks were removed from the kidney, further fixed in the same fixative solution for 2 hr, washed overnight in 0.1 M phosphate buffer, pH 7.4, 0 – 4 ℃, and postfixed in 1 % OsO_4 in 0.1 M phosphate buffer, pH 7.4, 0 – 4 ℃, for about 90 min. The tissue blocks were then washed in 0.1 M phosphate buffer, pH 7.4, 0 – 4 ℃, for about 30 min and sufficiently dehydrated using a graded alcohol series. Some tissue blocks were fractured in frozen absolute alcohol with a cracking instrument (Eiko TF-1) at approximately –115 ℃. All tissue blocks were transferred to isoamyl acetate, dried in a Hitachi HCP-1 critical-point dryer, and coated with gold in an ion coater (Eiko IB-3). Observation was made with either a Hitachi S-450 or a Hitachi HFS-2S field-emission scanning electron microscope operated at 20 kV or 25 kV with a 10 – 15 ℃ specimen tilt angle.

Results

Morphological changes: TEM revealed that the glomerular basement membrane (GBM) of the control kidney was divided into *lamina rara interna*, *lamina densa* and *lamina rara externa*. These three layers were almost uniform thickness.

In the GBM of the congestive kidney, localized and/or widespread thickening and some polypoid changes of 2 – 3 μm length were seen in the peripheral regions of the glomerular capillaries (Figs. 1, 2). In the GBM near the mesangium, some complicated wrinklings were observed (Fig. 3). These changes were especially marked in the kidneys 6 – 7 months after the renal vein clipping. Occasionally the changed areas of GBM were less uniform than the controls in the routine double staining (Fig. 2).

SEM of the control kidney revealed the characteristic interdigitation pattern among the pedicles of epithelial cells or podocytes, although the podocytes and their processes differed in shape from cell to cell (Fig. 4). The epithelial cell body had a smooth surface. Their processes, which tapered gradually, had end feet or pedicles that lined the capillary walls (Fig. 4).

In the congestive kidney, the surface of the epithelial cell body was markedly irregular and rugged (Fig. 5). The cell processes unsystematically rapidly tapered (Fig. 5).

In the control kidney, the surface of the endothelial cell body and the attenuated areas between the cytofolds (ridge-like structures) were rather smooth (Fig. 6). The surface of the cytofolds was not rugged (Fig. 6). The cell body and attenuated cell sheets were observed to contain a finely fenestrated mesh with multiple pores (Figs. 6, 7).

In the congestive kidney observed by SEM, the endothelial cell body, the radiating cytofolds and the attenuated areas, divided by them, all showed extremely irregular surfaces (Fig. 8). The different-sized verrucous protrusions were found in such numbers that there was no visible distinction between the fenestrae in the cell body and the attenuated cell sheet (Fig. 8). The verrucous protrusions, which were rarely encountered in the attenuated cytoplasm between the cytofolds in the control kidney, were increased. Numerous microvillus-like structures were also observed in some areas of the capillary lumen as well (Fig. 9). In spite of these various alterations, the gross structure of the endothelium remained unchanged and it was impressive that there was no significant change in the number or size of the fenestrae.

TEM revealed an increase in the mesangial matrix size in the congestive

---

FIG. 1. Transmission electron microscope (TEM) image of glomerular capillaries from a kidney 6 months after experimental procedure. Widespread thickening are observed (arrows).

FIG. 2. TEM image of glomerular capillary wall from a kidney 2 months after experimental procedure. Several polypoid changes are observed (arrows).

FIG. 3. TEM image of glomerular capillaries from a kidney 6 months after experimental procedure. Lipid droplet-like structures are visible in the mesangial cell. In the basement membrane near the mesangium, complicated wrinklings are visible (arrows).

FIG. 4. Scanning electron microscope (SEM) view of glomerular epithelial cell in a control kidney. Surface of the cell body is smooth. The pattern of the interdigitation of cell processes differs from podocyte to podocyte.

FIG. 5. SEM view of glomerular epithelial cell from a kidney 6 months after experimental procedure. Surface of the cell body is irregular in comparison with the control. Thinning and irregularity in the cell processes is noticeable.

FIG. 6. SEM view of glomerular capillary endothelium in a control kidney. Surface of the endothelial cell body is smooth. Fenestrations are observed not only in the peripheral cytoplasm, but also on the surface of the cell body.

FIG. 7. SEM view of fenestrated capillary endothelium from a control kidney.

FIG. 8. SEM view of glomerular capillary endothelium from a kidney 6 months after experimental procedure. Numerous and different-sized verrucous protrusions are seen.

FIG. 9. SEM view of capillary endothelium from a kidney 6 months after experimental procedure. A large number of microvillus-like structures and verrucous protrusions are visible on the endothelial surface.

ABBREVIATIONS: *BM*, glomerular basement membrane; *C*, glomerular capillary lumen; *US*, urinary space; *MS*, mesangium; *MM*, mesangial matrix; *D*, lipid droplet-like structure; *EP*, epithelium; *EN*, endothelium; *F*, foot processes; *FM*, filamentous matrix; scale bar: 1μm

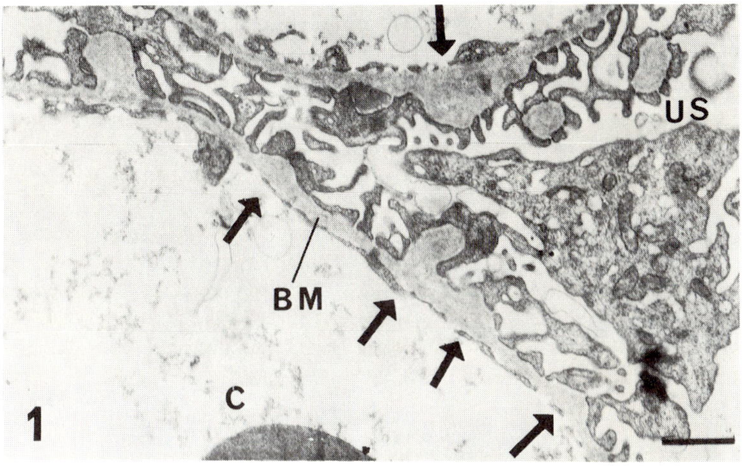
US
BM
C
1

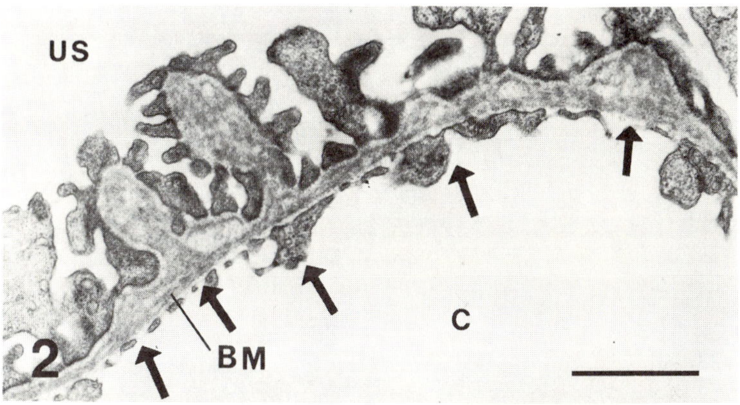
US
C
BM
2

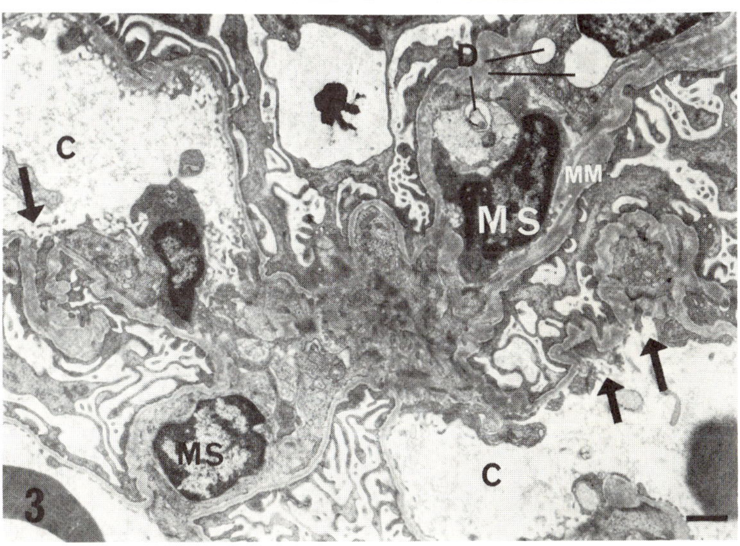
D
C
MM
MS
MS
C
3

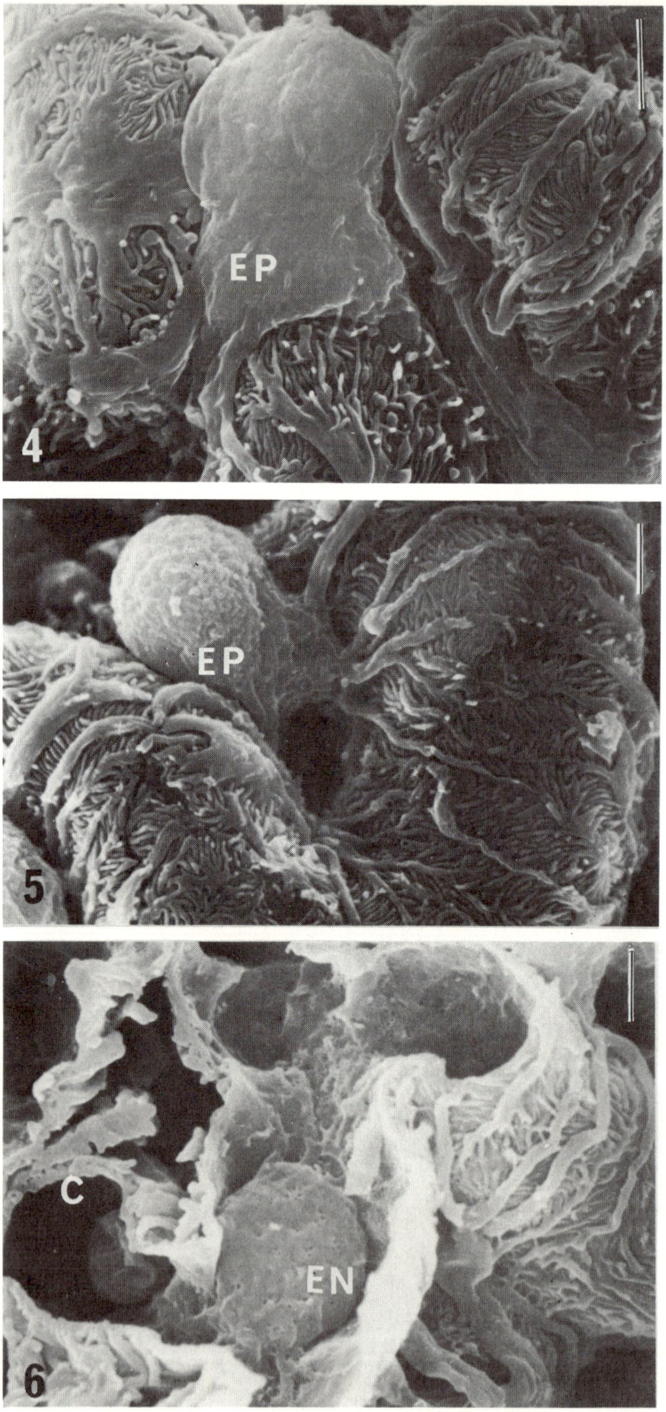
EP
4
EP
5
C
EN
6

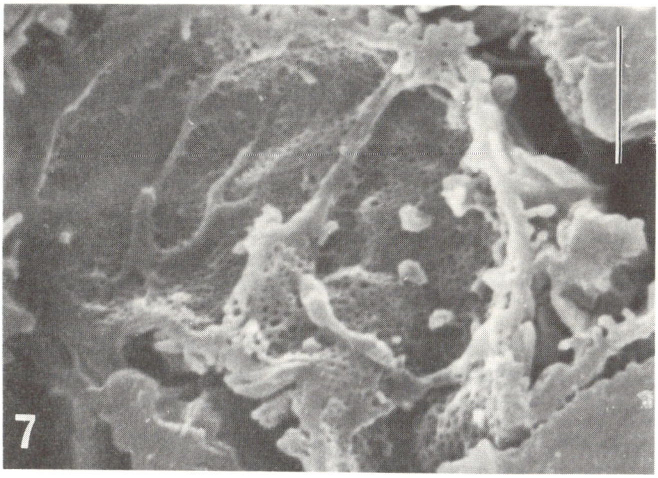
7

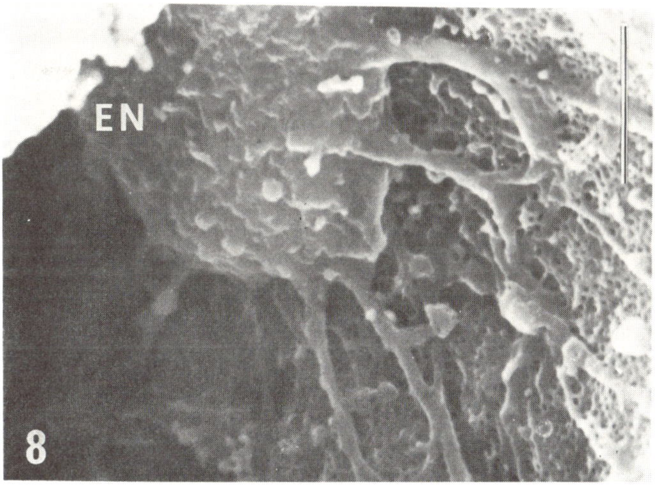
EN
8

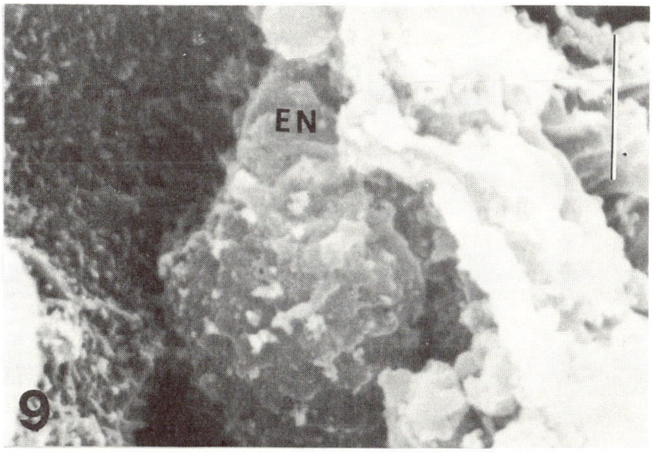
EN
9

kidney (Figs. 10, 11). The mesangial matrix was observed to have an irregular appearance, and even in the cross-section of the capillary walls, islands of mesangial cytoplasm were apparent (Fig. 11). Lipid droplet-like structures were frequently observable in the mesangial cell of the congestive kidney than in that of the control kidney (Fig. 3).

It is of importance that although a certain amount of variation in the above mentioned changes of the renal glomerular components is seen between individual animals and from glomerulus to glomerulus of the same animal, the morphological changes are, in general, reproducible for a given period of time after the clipping procedure.

Cytochemical observations: Ruthenium red (RR) staining of the control kidney revealed small RR-stained particles distributed throughout the *lamina rara interna*, *lamina rara externa* and mesangial matrix at quasi-regular intervals of about 40 – 60 nm (Fig. 12). In the congestive kidney, a similar quasi-regular interval pattern of about 40 – 60 nm was observed in the altered basement membrane and mesangial matrix (Figs. 12, 13).

Periodic acid-silver methenamine (PAM) staining of the control kidney revealed intensely stained basement membrane and mesangial matrix. In the congestive kidney, the staining findings from the altered basement membrane and mesangial matrix were similar to those from the control kidney (Figs. 14, 15).

Performic acid-phosphotungstic acid (PFP) reaction of the control kidney revealed a slightly positive reaction of the basement membrane and mesangial matrix (Fig. 16). In the congestive kidney, reaction findings for the altered basement membrane and mesangial matrix were showed a similar reaction to those in the control kidney (Figs. 17, 18).

Tannic acid fixation of the control glomerular epithelial cell gave clear pictures of the three kinds of cytoskeletal elements, which were microtubules, intermediate filaments and microfilaments (Figs. 19A, B). Numerous microfilaments in the foot processes made up the matrix of filaments (Fig. 19A). In the congestive kidney, no distinct difference in microfilamentous pattern in comparison with the controls was found (Figs. 20A, B).

Discussion

The present observations indicated that renal vein congestion induces structural changes in cellular as well as acellular components of rabbit glomeruli.

Ultracytochemical findings of the altered portions of the acellular components were similar to the control acellular component (Yokota and Ogawa,

---

FIG. 10. TEM image of glomerular mesangium from a control kidney.

FIG. 11. TEM image of glomerular mesangium from a kidney 6 months after experimental procedure. Increase in the size of the mesangial matrix is observed.

FIG. 12. TEM image of glomerular capillary wall from a kidney 6 months after experimental procedure. RR-stained particles are seen as a quasi-regular pattern in the basement membrane and also in the altered basement membrane (arrows).

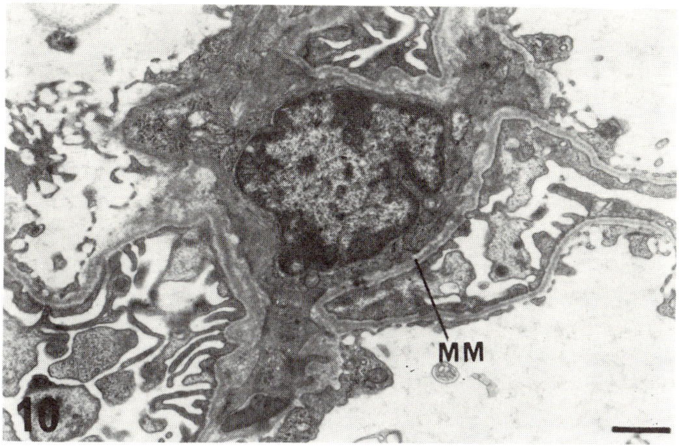
MM
10

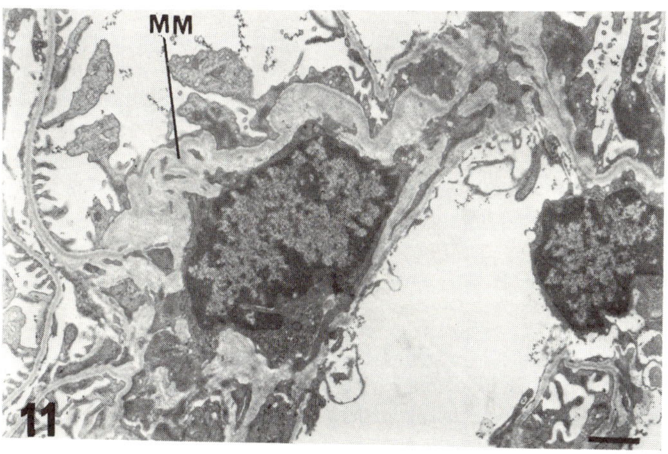
MM
11

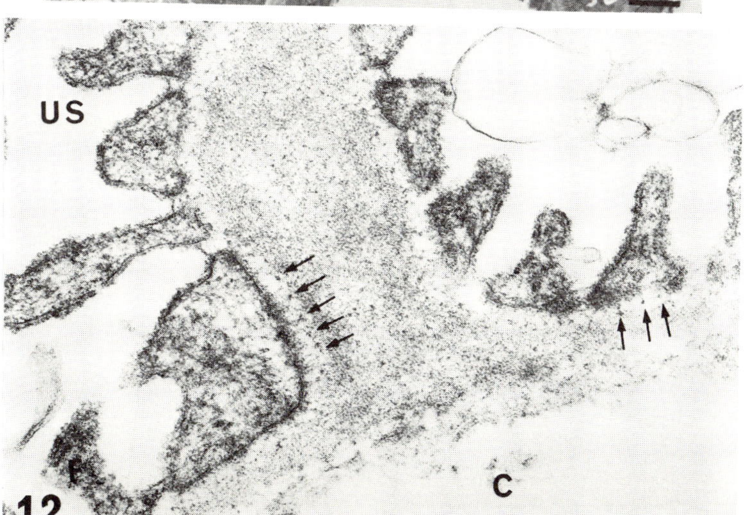
US
C
12

1982). The cytoskeletal element of the epithelial cell was preserved as far as the microfilament is concerned.

As known clinically, the glomerular basement membrane (GBM) shows specific pathological changes in various nephropathies with proteinuria or circulatory disturbances. Some of the well characterized structural alterations of the GBM in these nephropathies have already been summarized as the following: diffuse and nodular thickening with hyalinization in diabetes mellitus, deposition in nephritis, amyloidosis and nail-patella syndrome, gaps in nephritis, localized thinning in Alport's syndrome, wrinkling in nephrosclerosis and ischemia, and polypoid changes in congenital heart disease (Glassock, 1978; Gubler et al., 1980a, b; Hayashi et al., 1979).

In the present congestive kidney, it is of interest to know that the altered GBM is cytochemically similar to the control GBM proper. Concerning the complicated wrinklings of the GBM observed in our experiment, it is unclear whether or not these changed reflect a contraction of glomerular capillary wall.

The morphologic pictures of glomerular epithelium in the congestive kidney are quite different from the so-called fusion of foot processes which is observed in nephropathies with massive proteinuria (Seiler et al., 1977). The irregular thinning of the epithelial processes, which was found to occur in the congestive kidney, has been encountered in reports on glomerular diseases.

Capillary endothelial alterations, such as verrucous protrusions found by SEM have also been reported in experimental aortic coarctation (Gerrity and Naito, 1980). The microvillus structures found in the endothelium of the present study are similar to those observed in the experimentally microsurgically anastomosized carotid endothelial cells (Tomasello et al., 1981). These changes are related to circulatory disturbances.

An increase of the mesangial matrix material is comparable with the mesangial alterations in diabetic nephropathy (Glassock, 1978). In our study, it is impressive that the increased area of mesangial matrix is almost uniform as control as observed by cytochemical staining.

Recently, it has been emphasized that the intracellular cytoskeletal elements in the renal glomerulus play an important role in the regulation of glomerular filtration (Accini et al., 1975; Andrews, 1981; Andrews and Coffey, 1983; Kreisberg, 1983). Many investigators have shown the evidence that among the cytoskeletal elements, microfilaments are especially significant

---

FIG. 13. TEM image of glomerular mesangium stained with RR staining from a kidney 6 months after experimental procedure. RR-stained particles are seen as a quasi-regular pattern also in the altered mesangium (arrows).

FIG. 14. TEM image of glomerular basement membrane stained with PAM staining from a kidney 6 months after experimental procedure. The basement membrane is intensely stained with PAM staining. The staining findings from the altered basement membrane are also same (arrows).

FIG. 15. TEM image of glomerular mesangium stained with PAM staining from a kidney 6 months after experimental procedure. The mesangial matrix is intensely stained with PAM staining. The staining findings from the increased mesangial matrix are also same. (arrows).

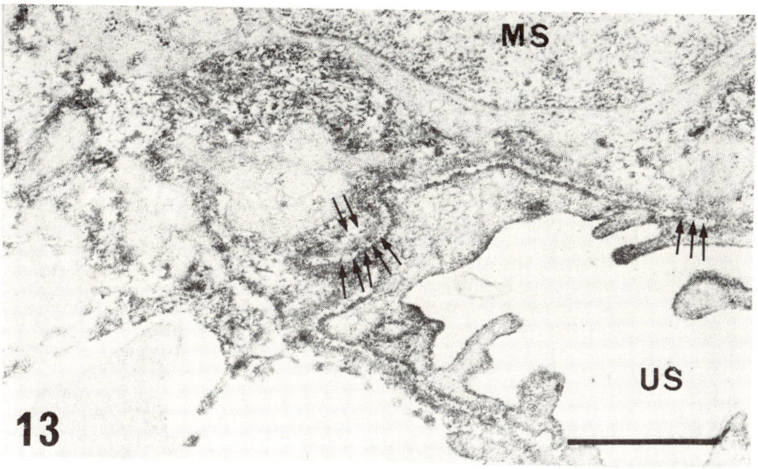
MS
US
13

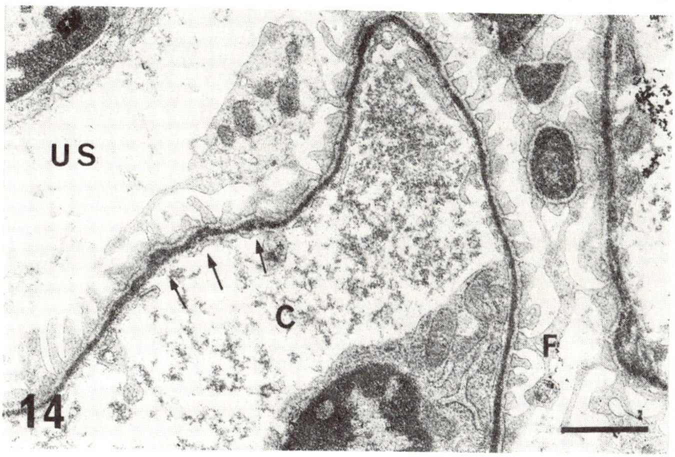
US
C
F
14

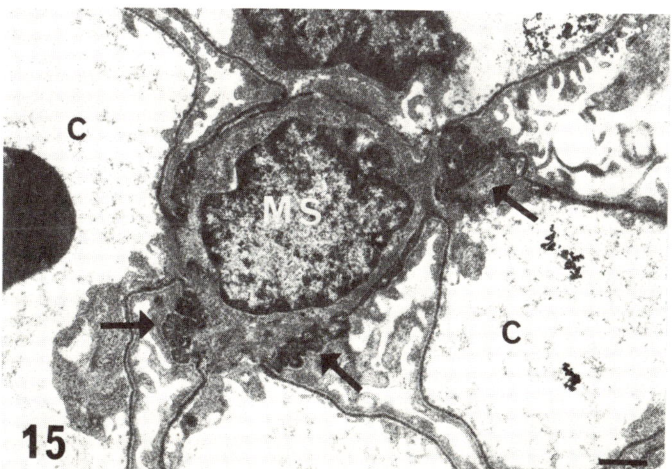
C
MS
C
15

(Andrews and Coffey, 1983). It is of interest that in the congestive kidney, though the tapering and irregularity in the podocyte are severe, intracellular microfilaments are well preserved even in the pedicles.

In conclusion, it should be stressed that mild congestion of the kidney induces morphological changes in the acellular components and also in the cellular components, though cytochemically detectable changes are not observed.

It is suggested that the ultrafiltration is assisted by cytoskeletal elements, especially by the microfilaments, though the optimal hemodynamic conditions are disturbed by mild congestion of the kidney.

Abstract

In order to reveal possible changes in glomeruli caused by a disturbance of the optimal hemodynamic state of glomerular capillaries, observations were made on a new experimental congestive kidney model, which was made by unilateral clipping of the renal vein of rabbits. The basement membrane, epithelium, capillary endothelium and mesangium of glomeruli were morphologically and cytochemically observed at various time intervals after renal vein clipping.

The glomerular basement membrane in the congestive kidney showed localized and/or widespread thickening, polypoid changes and complicated wrinklings. Irregularities appeared on the surface of podocytes and endothelial cells. In the podocytic pedicles, tapering and irregularity were marked. The mesangial matrix showed an increase in size. In the mesangial cells, lipid droplet-like structures were often found.

Cytochemical observations were made with ruthenium red (RR) staining, periodic acid-silver methenamine (PAM) staining, performic acid-phosphotungstic acid (PFP) reaction and tannic acid fixation. In both the control and congestive kidney, the basement membrane and mesangial matrix were intensely stained with RR and PAM, and slightly with PFP. The morphologically altered acellular components in the congestive kidney were cytochemically similar to those of the control acellular components. Intracellular cytoskeletal elements of the podocytes investigated in tannic acid fixed specimens showed the well preserved intracellular microfillaments also in the congestive kidney.

FIG. 16. TEM image of glomerular basement membrane stained with PFP reaction of a control kidney. The basement membrane is slightly stained with PFP reaction.

FIG. 17. TEM image of glomerular basement membrane stained with PFP reaction from a kidney 6 months after experimental procedure. The staining findings of the thickened basement membrane are similar to those of the control kidney.

FIG. 18. TEM image of glomerular mesangium stained with PFP reaction from a kidney 6 months after experimental procedure. This is a section with 1 % tannic acid added to the aldehyde fixative. The mesangial matrix is moderately stained with PFP reaction. The staining findings from the increased mesangial matrix are also same.

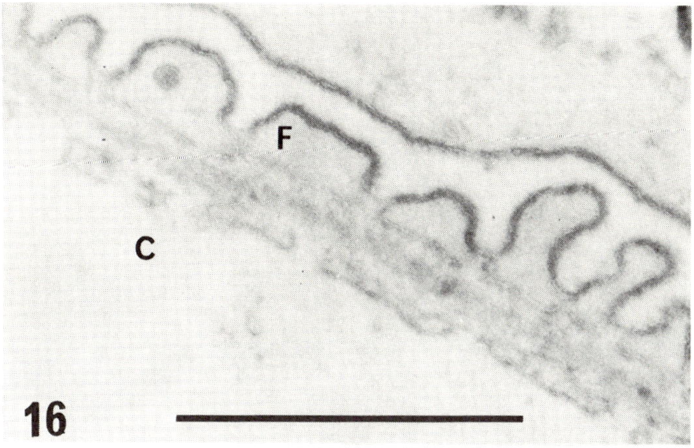
F
C
16

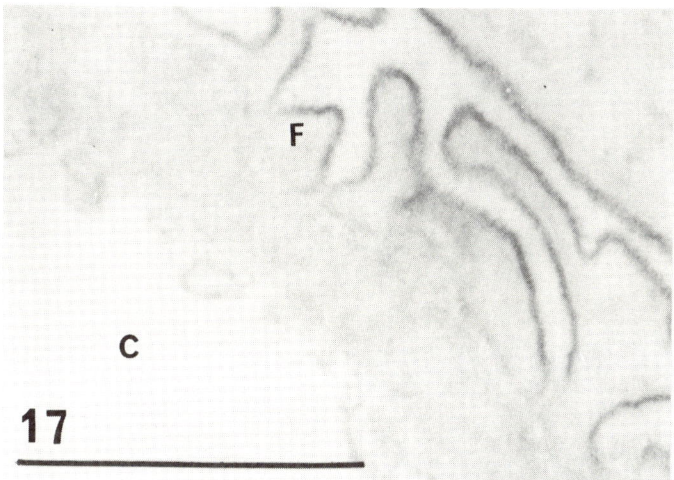
F
C
17

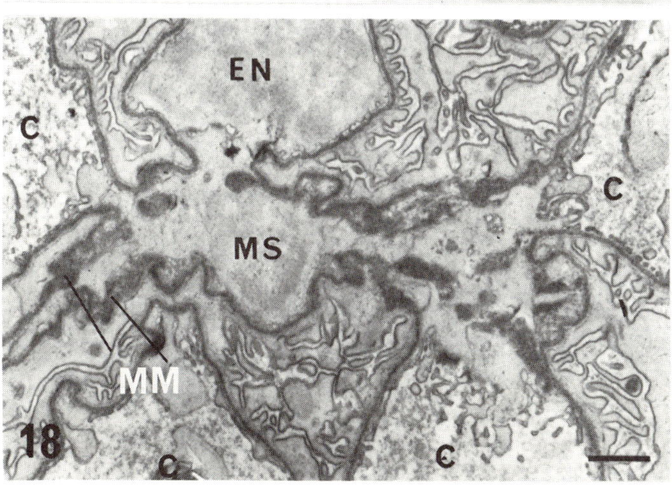
EN
C
C
MS
MM
18
C
C

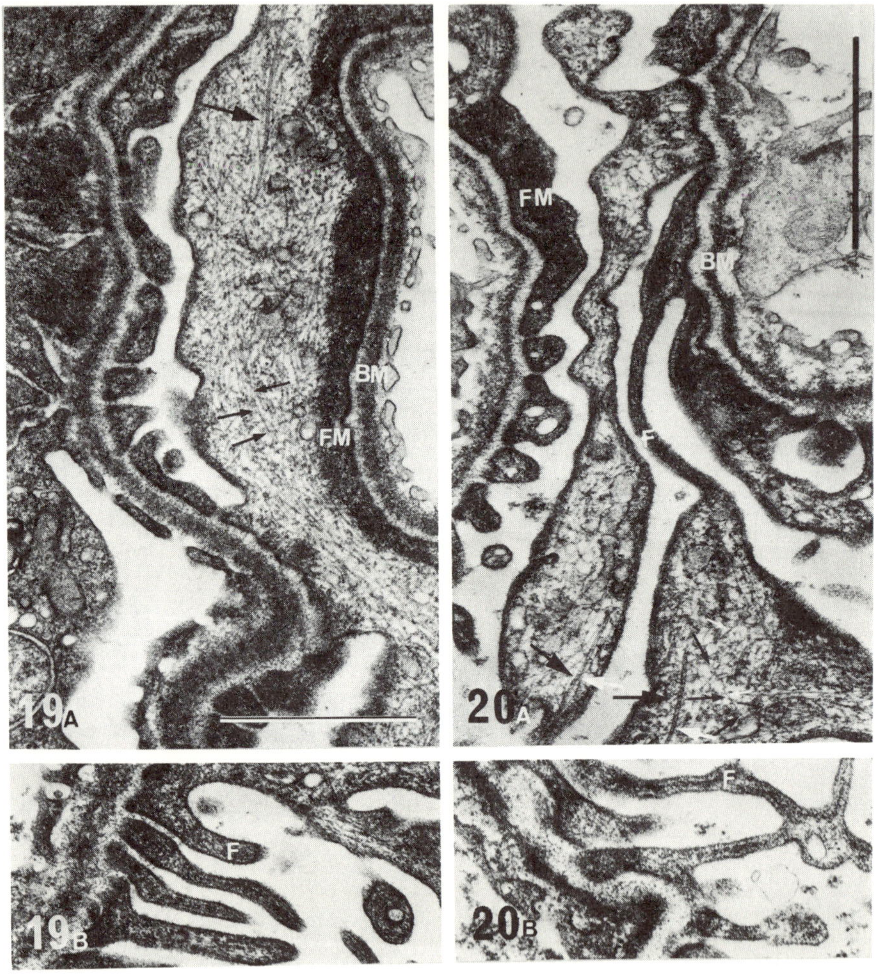

FIGS. 19A, B. TEM images of glomerular epithelium fixed in tannic acid of a control kidney. Fig. 19A shows a transitional section and Fig. 19B a longitudinal one. Three kinds of cytoskeletal elements are observed. The thickest element is a microtubule (large arrow), second, an intermediate filament (small arrows), and the thinnest element is a microfilament (FM). Foot processes are filled with the filamentous matrix.

FIGS. 20A, B. TEM images of glomerular epithelium fixed in tannic acid from a kidney 7 months after experimental procedure. Fig. 20A shows a transitional section and Fig. 20B a longitudinal one. The filamentous matrix is preserved in the thinning podocytic pedicle. A large arrow indicates a microtubule. Small arrows indicate intermediate filaments.

References

Accini, L., Natali, P.G., Vassallo, L., Hsu, K.S., and De Martino, C. (1975). Immunoelectron microscopic evidence of contractile proteins in the cellular and acellular components of mouse kidney glomeruli. *Cell Tissue Res.* **162**, 297–312.

Andrews, P.M. (1981). Investigations of cytoplasmic contractile and cytoskeletal elements in the kidney glomerulus. *Kidney Int.* **20**, 549–562.

Andrews, P.M., and Coffey, A.K. (1983). Cytoplasmic contractile elements in glomerular cells. *Fed. Proc., Fed. Am. Soc. Exp. Biol.* **42**, 3046–3052.

Arakawa, M., Edanaga, M., and Tokunaga, J. (1981). Renal glomerulus. A new findings of its normal and pathological structure. *Biomed. Res. Suppl.* 2, 306–310.

Campanacci, L., Faccini, L., Englaro, E., Rustia, R., Guarnieri, G.F., Barat, R., Carraro, M., De Zotti, R., and Micheli, W. (1981). Exercise-induced proteinuria. *In* "Contributions to Nephrology" (G.M. Berlyne and N.Y. Brooklyn, ed.), pp. 31–41. S. Karger, Basel.

Farquhar, M.G. (1975). The primary glomerular filtration barrier-basement membrane or epithelial slits? *Kidney Int.* **8**, 197–211.

Fujioka, A., and Ogawa, K. (1979). Ultracytochemistry of cell membrane. II. The application of phosphotungstic acid staining to microvillus membranes of the cat small intestine. *Acta Histochem. Cytochem.* **12**, 97–119.

Fujiwara, K., and Linck, R.W. (1982). The use of tannic acid in microtuble research. *In* "Methods in Cell Biology" (L. Wilson, ed.), Vol. 24, pp. 217–233. Academic Press, New York.

Gerrity, R.G., and Naito, K. (1980). Alteration of endothelial cell surface morphology after experimental aortic coartation. *Artery* **8**, 267–274.

Glassock, R.J. (1978). Change of glomerular basement membrane in disease. *In* "Biology and Chemistry of Basement Membranes" (N.A. Kefalides, ed.), pp. 421–441. Academic Press, New York.

Gubler, M.C., Levy, M., Neizot, C., and Habib, R. (1980a). Glomerular basement membrane changes in nonhereditary glomerular diseases. *Renal Physiol.* 3, 395–404.

Gubler, M.C., Levy, M., Neizot, C., and Habib, R. (1980b). Glomerular basement membrane changes in hereditary glomerular diseases. *Renal Physiol.* 3, 405–413.

Hayashi, M., Fukushige, M., Nihira, H., and Itoh, K. (1979). Clinical studies of renal angiography in patients with unexplained renal hematuria. *Jap. J. Urol.* **70**, 634–647. (In Japanese)

Kanwar, Y.S., and Farquhar, M.G. (1979). Anionic sites in the glomerular basement membrane. *In vivo* and *in vitro* localization to the laminae rarae by cationic probes. *J. Cell Biol.* **81**, 137–153.

Kreisberg, J.I. (1983). Contractile properties of the glomerular mesangium. *Fed. Proc., Fed. Am. Soc. Exp. Biol.* **42**, 3053–3057.

Luft, J.H. (1971). Ruthenium red and violet. II. Fine structural localization in animal tissues. *Anat. Res.* **171**, 369–416.

Ogawa, K., Tanaka, T., and Tsuchiya, A. (1977). Electron microscopic cytochemistry of functional groups in the plasma membrane. *Acta Histochem. Cytochem.* **10**, 387–403.

Rambourg, A., and Leblond, C.P. (1967). Electron microscope observations on the carbohydrate-rich cell coat present at the surface of cells in the rat. *J. Cell Biol.* **32**, 27–53.

Ryan, G.B., and Karnovsky, M.J. (1976). Distribution of endogenous albumin in the rat glomerulus: Role of hemodynamic factors in glomerular barrier function. *Kidney Int.* **9**, 36–45.

Seiler, M.W., Rennke, H.G., Venkatachalam, M.A., and Cotran, R.S. (1977). Pathogenesis of polycation-induced alterations ("fusion") of glomerular epithelium. *Lab. Invest.* **36**, 48–61.

Solez, K., Racusen, L.C., and Whelton, A. (1981). Glomerular epithelial cell changes in early postischemic acute renal failure in rabbits and man. *Am. J. Pathol.* **103**, 163–173.

Tomasello, F., Spadaro, A., Albanese, V., and Conforti, P. (1981). SEM evaluation of endothelial changes following end-to-side microvascular anastomoses in rats. *J. Neurosurg.* **54**, 525–531.

Yokota, H., and Ogawa, K. (1982). Effect of hemodynamic factors in renal glomerulus. II. Cytochemistry of glomerular basement membrane and mesangium in the experimental congestive kidney. *Acta Histochem. Cytochem.* **15**, 313–324.

Westberg, N.G., and Michael, A.F. (1970). Human glomerular basement membrane. Preparation and composition. *Biochemistry* **9**, 3837–3846.

ANALYSES OF THE GLYCOSAMINOGLYCANS IN AGING DOG KIDNEY

Nagaswami S. Vasan and John V. Tesoriero[1]

Department of Anatomy, New Jersey Medical School
and Graduate School of Biomedical Sciences, Newark, New Jersey

Seshaiyer Saraswathi

Department of Biotechnology, Owens-Illinois, Toledo, Ohio

Renal cortex and medulla were separated from 1, 3, 6 and 10 year old dogs. Subsequent to delipidation and dehydration, the material was subjected to protease digestion to isolate glycosaminoglycans. Various glycosaminoglycans were further separated on a Dowex 1-X2 column using sodium chloride buffers of increasing ionic strength. Individual glycosaminoglycan components from each sodium chloride fraction were quantitated by digestion with specific enzymes. The results indicate that the glycosaminoglycan content of renal medulla was 25% higher than that of cortex in younger animals and this difference becomes more pronounced with age. The proportion of hyaluronic acid, chondroitin- and dermatan-sulfate in the cortex remained the same in all age groups studied with the exception of a typical decrease at 6 years. However, heparan sulfate, which formed 55% of the total at age 6, decreased to 30% at age 10. In the medulla, hyaluronic acid made up 30% of the total glycosaminoglycans in ages 1 and 3 and increased to more than 50% in 6 and 10 year old dogs. As in the cortex, chondroitin- and dermatan-sulfate remained the same throughout with the exception of a decrease at 6 years. The heparan sulfate level in medulla showed a significant decrease in 10 year olds, forming only 14% of the total glycosaminoglycans. Sepharose CL-6B chromatography of the 0.5 M NaCl fractions (containing only hyaluronic acid) indicated that the size of cortical hyaluronic acid was small and was not altered in aging. A considerable amount of large-size hyaluronate was observed in the medulla of the younger age group and the size decreased with age. Radiolabelled proteoglycans from isolated glomeruli showed a bimodal pattern with the proportion of large-sized molecules decreasing with age. Chemical analyses also showed that the amount of heparan sulfate decreased in aging glomeruli.

[1]Supported by NIH grant 5-S07 PR05393 and HD16147 to NSV and Howard University-Rockefeller Foundation Grant.

Age-related changes in renal function have been attributed to alterations in the size, morphology and chemical composition of kidney tissue (Dunnill and Halley, 1973; Griffiths et al., 1976; Murata and Horiuchi, 1978; Murata, 1978; Sato et al., 1975). Chemical analyses of either whole kidneys or those separated into cortex and medulla has shown that kidney tissue contains an abundance of acid mucopolysaccharide with the proportion being much higher in the medulla (Castor and Greene, 1968; Dicker and Franklin, 1966; Farber and Van Praag, 1970; Inoue et al., 1970).

Physiological studies have shown that the glomerular capillaries function as a size- and charge-selective barrier in the production of the glomerular filtrate and serve to retain plasma protein in circulation (Brenner et al., 1977; Brenner et al., 1978; Rennke et al., 1978). The predominant glycosaminoglycan in glomerular basement membrane (GBM) is heparan sulfate and other glycosaminoglycans such as chondroitin sulfate, dermatan sulfate and hyaluronic acid exist in smaller amounts. Enzymatic removal of GBM glycosaminoglycans (Kanwar et al., 1980) or neutralization with high molality buffer (Kanwar and Rosenzweig, 1982) resulted in the increased leakage of anionic ferritin. In addition to their charge properties, glycosaminoglycans have been shown to exert a steric exclusion effect on proteins in solution (Comper and Laurent, 1978; Farquhar, 1981; Lindahl and Hook, 1978) and facilitate tubular transport of water and electrolytes (Dicker and Franklin, 1966; Pinter, 1967).

In the present study, we have analyzed in detail the glycosaminoglycan composition of renal cortex and medulla from normal dogs of 1, 3, 6 and 10 years of age. In addition, we have isolated the renal glomeruli from these dogs to study the synthesis of radiolabelled sulfated glycosaminoglycans. The results indicate a significant reduction in the heparan sulfate content in aging animals. Our results suggest that age-related proteinuria may be due to this reduction in the anionic barrier.

Materials and Methods

Standard glycosaminoglycans were generously supplied by Dr. M.B. Mathews, University of Chicago, IL, USA. *Streptomyces* hyaluronidase (EC 3.2.1.35) chondroitinase AC (EC 4.2.2.5) and chondroitinase ABC (EC 4.2.2.4) were obtained from Miles Laboratories, Elkhart, IN, USA.

Isolation of glycosaminoglycans: Normal male dogs, ages 1, 3, 6 and 10 years (3 in each age group) were sacrificed and the kidneys removed and immediately decapsulated. Cortex and medulla were manually separated with the aid of a dissecting microscope to ensure pure tissue isolation. The tissues were briefly washed with cold physiological saline, delipidated by chloroform-methanol (2:1) extraction (Folch et al., 1957) and acetone dried. The glycosaminoglycans were released from the dried tissues by sequential digestion with collagenase and pronase (Spiro, 1967). Small amounts of insoluble materials were removed and the digests were treated with cold trichloroacetic acid (TCA) to obtain a final concentration of 8%. After standing overnight at 5 ℃, the TCA precipitate was removed by centrifugation and the supernatant containing the glycosaminoglycans was dialyzed in a Spectrapor 3 membrane (m_r cut-off 3500) against distilled water for 48 hr with six changes. The dialyzed solution was partially concentrated by lyophilization and the glycosaminoglycans were precipitated by adding ethanol to 80% (v/v) in the presence of acetate. The precipitate was collected, after standing overnight at 5 ℃, and dissolved in 0.1 M sodium chloride. The glycosaminoglycan preparation was further fractionated by chromatography on a Dowex 1-X2 column (1.6 x 30 cm; Cl' form, 200—400 mesh). The elution pattern and recovery samples was standardized using a mixture of standard glycosaminoglycans. Stepwise elution of the column was performed using sodium chloride solution: 120 ml each of 0.5 M, 0.75 M. 1.25 M, 1.75 M and 3.0 M. The fractions were assayed for uronic acid by the borate-carbazole method (Bitter and Muir, 1962). The uronic acid containing fractions were pooled separately for each concentration of NaCl, dialyzed, and lyophilized. The glycosaminoglycan composition of these fractions was determined after enzymatic digestions as described below.

Hyaluronic acid estimation: Hyaluronic acid in the above fractions was estimated by digestion with *strep.* hyaluronidase (Orkin and Toole, 1978). The incubation mixture contained 0.1 M formate and 0.15 M NaCl, pH 4.3. Incubation time was 16 hr at 37 ℃ with additional enzyme added after 6 hr. Enzymatic digestion was stopped by immersing the reaction tubes in a boiling water bath for 3 min. Since the 1.25 M, 1.75 M and 3.0 M NaCl eluted fractions did not show the presence of hyaluronate on cellulose acetate electrophoresis they were not subjected to hyaluronidase treatment. Primarily, the 0.5 M and 0.75 M eluted fractions of all samples were analyzed for hyaluronate content. Following hyaluronidase digestion, the undigested glycosaminoglycans were precipitated by the addition of 500 μl of a 10% solution of cetylpyridinium chloride (CPC) in 0.1 M NaCl. This was proceeded by the addition of 25 mg of dry celite, which facilitated sedimentation of the glycosaminoglycan-CPC complex. The samples were incubated at 37 ℃ for 2 hr, then centrifuged at room temperature for 20 min. at 10,000 rpm. The precipitates were resuspended in 1 ml of 0.5 M NaCl, stirred for 1 hr and centrifuged as before. The resultant supernatant was assayed for uronic acid (Bitter and Muir, 1962) using glucouronolactone as a standard. An untreated control run in parallel was used to calculate the digested (hyaluronate) and undigested glycosaminoglycan concentrations.

Estimation of sulfated glycosaminoglycans: Sulfated glycosaminoglycans were estimated by digestion with chondroitinase AC and ABC as described by Saito et al. (1968). These enzymes degrade chondroitin sulfates A and C to unsaturated 4-sulfated and 6-sulfated disaccharides, respectively. In addition, chondroitinase ABC also digests dermatan sulfate to a 4-sulfated unsaturated disaccharide. Heparan sulfate is not affected by these enzymes.

After incubation with the above enzymes, the disaccharide products were separated from the undigested material by descending chromatography on Whatman No. 1 paper in the solvent system butanol/acetic acid/1 M ammonia (2:3:1), for 24 hr (Saito et al., 1968). The disaccharides were visualized with an ultraviolet mineral light at 230 μm. Undigested materials remained at the origin along with the disaccharides and were eluted separately with water following which the uronic acid content was determined. The ABC-resistant glycosaminoglycans isolated by this procedure were further characterized as heparan sulfate by nitrous acid degradation (Cifonelli and King, 1972) followed by cellulose acetate electrophoresis.

Glycosaminoglycans were separated and identified by cellulose acetate electrophoresis in 0.1 M calcium acetate buffer. Electrophoresis was performed on fractions isolated from Dowex chromatography before and after digestion with specific enzymes. The glycosaminoglycans were stained with 1.0% Alcian blue in 1.0 M sodium acetate buffer, pH 6.0.

Molecular weight determination of the 0.5 M Dowex fraction: The material that eluted with 0.5 M NaCl during ion-exchange chromatography was identified as hyaluronic acid due to its complete digestion by protease-free *Strep.* hyaluronidase. The medullary and cortical 0.5 M NaCl fractions were subjected to molecular weight determination on a Sepharose CL-6B column (0.8cm x 75cm). The column was eluted with 0.5 M sodium acetate buffer, pH 5.8. Fractions were collected in 1 ml volumes and an aliquot was used for the uronic acid assay.

Preparation of glomeruli: Kidneys from dogs of various ages were rapidly removed and placed on ice. They were then decapsulated and bisected longitudinally and the cortex isolated. The renal cortex was thinly sliced, thawed, and disrupted by pushing through a 250μm pore stainless steel sieve with a spatula. The sieved material was collected in ice-cold MEM (Minimum Essential Medium — GIBCO, Grand Island, NY, USA) then passed through a second sieve (150μm pore size). The material retained on the sieve was washed several times and inspected under a phase contrast microscope. Isolated glomeruli were incubated in the presence of medium containing 100μCi/ml ^{35}S sulfate. The incubation was carried out at 38 ℃ for 12 hr in a humidified atmosphere of 95% air/5% CO_2.

Extraction of radiolabelled proteoglycans: Radiolabelled proteoglycans were extracted from pellets of intact glomeruli with 5 ml of 4.0 M guanidine hydrochloride (GuHCl) in 0.05 M sodium acetate (pH 5.8) containing proteolytic inhibitors (Oegema et al., 1975). The extraction was carried out at 4 ℃ for 24 hr with gentle rotary shaking. The extract was separated from the tissue residue then dialyzed to remove the unincorporated radioactive sulfate before lyophilization.

Column chromatography: Prior to chromatography, the lyophilized proteoglycan material was resuspended in 0.5 ml of 4.0 M GuHCl then dialyzed against elution buffer (0.5 M sodium acetate, pH 5.8, containing 0.02% sodium azide). The sample, in 0.7 ml of elution buffer, was applied to a Sepharose CL-2B gel column (0.8cm x 100cm). The eluate was collected in 0.7 ml fractions and 100μl aliquots of each fraction were counted in a Beckman LS-8000 liquid scintillation counter using Ultrafluor, (National Diagnostics,

Somerville, NJ, USA) as the scintillant. The peaks were pooled, dialyzed, lyophilized and the proportions of chondroitin- and heparan-sulfate determined.

Results

TABLE 1

DISTRIBUTION OF GLYCOSAMINOGLYCANS IN RENAL TISSUE

Age of Animal	Total Glycosaminoglycans (μg/g Dry Tissue, N=3) Cortex	Medulla	Cortex/Medulla
1	1169±102	1538±138	0.77
3	1486±164	1808±192	0.79
6	1263± 82	2307±186	0.53
10	998± 64	1656±143	0.61

Cortex and medullary glycosaminoglycans were isolated as described in 'Methods.' Uronic acid was assayed by the Carbazole method to calculate total glycosaminoglycans per gram dry, defatted tissue.
N = number of experiments in each group.

The level of glycosaminoglycans (Table 1) in the cortex increased 1.3 times from one year to three year old animals. A peak level was reached at age six and then the concentration declined, reaching only 66% of the peak at age 10. The glycosaminoglycan level in medulla increased until 6 years and subsequently decreased by age 10. It is worth nothing that the glycosaminoglycan content of the medulla was consistently higher than the cortex with this difference being more obvious at age 6 when the cortical level started to decline while the medullary level was at a peak. In an earlier publication it was reported that the medulla contains a significantly higher amount of glycosaminoglycan than does the cortex (Castor and Greene, 1968).

Concentration of various glycosaminoglycans

Cortex: Sodium chloride buffers of various molarities eluted more than one type of glycosaminoglycan. The results of enzymatic or chemical digestions of different glycosaminoglycans are shown in Table 2. The level of hyaluronic acid increased slightly up to three years of age then declined in older animals. However, the proportion of hyaluronic acid to the total glycosaminoglycan content in the cortex showed an increase with age. Hyaluronic acid was identified only in the 0.5 M NaCl fraction and was completely susceptible to *Strep.* hyaluronidase.

TABLE 2

CONCENTRATION OF VARIOUS GLYCOSAMINOGLYCANS IN THE CORTEX AND MEDULLA AT VARIOUS AGE INTERVALS

	Tissue	1 Yr.	% of Total	3 Yr.	% of Total	6 Yr.	% of Total	10 Yr.	% of Total
Hyaluronic Acid	Cortex	316	34.0	424	35.3	287	23.8	251	40.0
	Medulla	366	33.8	494	34.4	982	53.5	911	54.6
Chondroitin Sulfate	Cortex	118	12.7	146	9.8	133	11.0	99	15.8
	Medulla	126	11.6	118	8.2	105	5.7	169	10.1
Heparan Sulfate	Cortex	317	34.1	584	32.6	665	55.1	189	30.1
	Medulla	381	35.2	456	31.8	394	21.5	231	13.9
Dermatan Sulfate	Cortex	108	11.6	153	10.4	53	4.5	65	10.4
	Medulla	114	10.5	120	8.4	195	10.6	217	13.0
Resistant Material	Cortex	71	7.6	176	11.9	68	5.6	23	3.7
	Medulla	96	8.9	247	17.2	160	8.7	140	8.4

Glycosaminoglycans were isolated from the pronase digests of dry, defatted kidney tissues as described in the text and fractionated on Dowex 1-X2 Cl. The individual glycosaminoglycans were characterized by digestion with specific hydrolases. The undigested glycosaminoglycans, after each enzymatic digestion, were separated chromatographically and quantified by uronic acid estimation. The chondroitinase ABC-resistant fraction was further characterized by nitrous acid oxidation and cellulose acetate electrophoresis. Values are quoted as μg uronic acid/g dry tissue.

The materials that eluted in other NaCl fractions were not digested by *Strep.* hyaluronidase. All of the material eluted in the 0.75 M NaCl and 15 – 18% of the material in the 1.25 M NaCl fractions was digested by chondroitinase ABC. The level of chondroitin sulfate was not significantly altered in aging. Heparan sulfate, which is the predominant glycosaminoglycan of the renal cortex, gradually increased until the sixth year of age and then sharply declined. In the renal cortex of ten year old dogs, heparan sulfate formed only 30% of the total glycosaminoglycans. This reduction in heparan sulfate may explain the frequently observed proteinuria associated with aging.

Medulla: As observed in Table 1, the glycosaminoglycan content is much higher in the medulla than in the cortex. Analysis of individual glycosaminoglycans showed that hyaluronate increased steadily with age and formed over 50% of the total glycosaminoglycans in 10 year old animals. Chondroitin sulfate, with the exception of a slight decrease at 6 years of age, was not significantly altered. Heparan sulfate, which formed 34% of the total in one year old renal tissue, steadily decreased in aging and formed only 14% of the total in 10 year old. The proportion of dermatan sulfate was not altered in any of the samples analyzed.

The material that eluted in 0.5 M NaCl contained only hyaluronate. Renal tubules are involved in sodium transport, and the fact that highly polymerized hyaluronate has a pronounced retarding effect on sodium efflux (Castor and Greene, 1968) prompted us to further investigate the unusually high levels of hyaluronate in the medulla. The 0.5 M NaCl eluted material was applied to a Sepharose CL-6B column (Figure not given, see Ref. Vasan et al., 1983). Material from the cortex in all age groups was included in the column and showed heterogeneity. However, the hyaluronate from the three year old medulla contained a large proportion of material that was excluded from the column, and 30% of this eluted with a Kav. of 0.15. Interestingly, the hyaluronate from other age groups was included on the gel and eluted with a Kav. between 0.66 and 0.80. The increased presence of small-size hyaluronate and the loss of excluded material suggests that, in aging, the metabolism of this glycosaminoglycan is severely affected.

Sepharose CL-2B chromatography of the newly synthesized proteoglycan extracted from the glomeruli is shown in Fig. 1. The proteoglycan was eluted in the inner volume of the column and resolved into two fairly homogeneous populations. The size of the proteoglycan that eluted in peak 1 steadily increased up to 6 years of age from Kav. 0.36 to 0.24. The proteoglycan synthesized by the glomeruli obtained from 10 year old dogs was considerably smaller (Kav. 0.43), and the proportion also decreased when compared to young renal tissues. Chemical analysis for sulfated glycosaminoglycan showed that heparan sulfate was the predominant molecule in peak 1 and the level decreased with age. Chondroitin sulfate, however, was not affected. The proteoglycan in peak 2 also showed a steady increase in size until 6 years. The peak 2 proteoglycan synthesized by the glomeruli obtained from 10 year old animals was considerably smaller (Kav. 0.80). Chemical analysis for sulfated glycosaminoglycans showed that up to 60% were heparan sulfate. The level of chondroitin sulfate was much higher in peak 2 when compared to peak 1, and there were increased amounts of materials resistant to nitrous acid and chondroitinase ABC treatment.

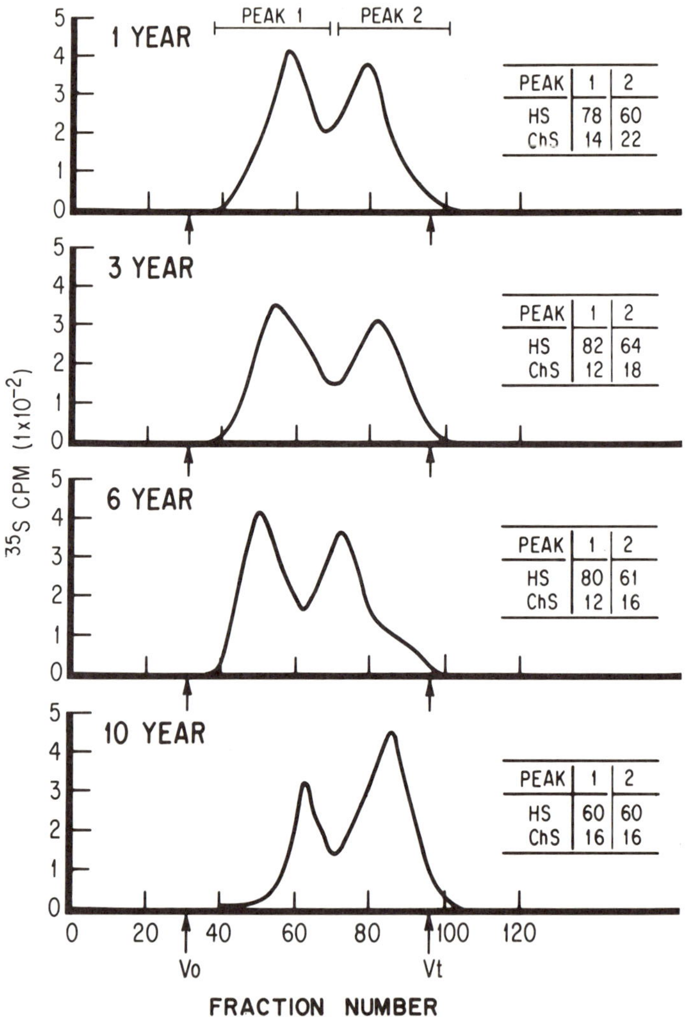

FIG. 1. Sepharose CL-2B elution profile of sulfated proteoglycans synthesized by glomeruli isolated from renal tissues. Peaks 1 and 2 were pooled separately and subjected to analyses as described in 'Methods'. Void volume (V_o) and total volume (V_t) of the column are as marked on the figure. Heparan sulfate (HS) and chondroitin sulfate (ChS) are percent of total, and the material resistant to both enzyme and chemical digestion were not analyzed further.

DISCUSSION

The results of this study show that there is an age related decrease in the total glycosaminoglycans, specifically heparan sulfate, in both cortex and medulla of the dog kidney. The distribution of various glycosaminoglycans shows an increase up to a certain point in life followed by a decline. This observation closely resembles those from human kidneys as previously described (Inoue et al., 1970). In addition to glycosaminoglycans, both in cortex and medulla, we observed the presence of material that was resistant to *strep.* hyaluronidase, chondroitinase AC and ABC, and nitrous acid treatment. It is possible that this material, which also increases at three years of age, is sulfated glycoprotein of renal epithelial origin similar to corneal epithelium (Yonekura et al., 1982). Synthesis and accumulation of sulfated glycoprotein in renal tissue has been previously observed (Kobayashi et al., 1982; Lemkin and Farquhar, 1981; Stow et al., 1983). The level of this glycoprotein in the medulla was significantly higher when compared to the cortex. The function of these glycoproteins is not clear, but their presence in significant amounts during the adult years suggests a role in either cell-to-cell or cell-to-matrix interactions and possibly in the organization of a stable extracellular matrix.

The amount of hyaluronic acid in the cortex, which decreased at middle age and again increased in aging, is consistant with earlier biochemical (Murata, 1978) and histological observations in humans (Rosenquist and Bernick, 1971). Our data, in which hyaluronic acid in the medulla formed 50% of the total glycosaminoglycans, agrees with other reports (Castor and Greene, 1968; Dicker and Franklin, 1966; Farber and Van Praag, 1970). High concentrations of hyaluronic acid in the extratubular stroma of the medulla possibly contributes a resilient, gelatinous support for delicate tubular structures as is seen in Wharton's jelly of the umbilical cord. It seems more appropriate that this diffusely distributed anionic molecule might serve as a retention lattice for the sodium gradient known to be present in this portion of the kidney. Previous reports (Ullrich et al., 1955) also support the concept that hyaluronate slows the translocation of sodium, presumably by virtue of its gel-like consistency rather than its anionic charge. The reason for the hyaluronic enrichment in medulla, especially in aging, is not clear. Molecular weight determination on a Sepharose CL-2B gel column showed that the size of cortical hyaluronic acid was not altered with age. On the other hand, medullary hyaluronic acid showed a loss of the large-size material (seen in three year old dog) due to aging. This reduction in size indicates the probable presence of localized hyaluronidase activity. In an earlier study (Castor and Greene, 1968) it was observed that hyaluronic acid of low molecular weight had no retarding effect on sodium efflux while moderately polymerized hyaluronic acid slowed sodium loss.

Sulfated glycosaminoglycans in the cortex (Tables 2 and 3) formed a major proportion (55%) of the total in all age groups studied and rose to 70% of the total in the 6 year tissue sample. However, in the medulla, the amount of sulfated glycosaminoglycans decreased steadily and formed only 37% of the total in the 10 year old dog. Chondroitin sulfate in both medulla and cortex constituted between 15 – 20% of the total, increasing slightly in the 10 year old animals. On the contrary, heparan sulfate showed significant decrease in aging, while chondroitin sulfate increased. A recent study (Kanwar et al., 1981) provided evidence to show that heparan sulfate and chondroitin sulfate are present on two different protein cores. Hence, it is possible that synthesis and degradation of these two sulfated glycosaminoglycans in aging renal tissues is taking place *via* different mechanisms.

TABLE 3

PERCENT COMPOSITION OF SULFATED GLYCOSAMINOGLYCANS

Glycosaminoglycans	Tissue	1 Year	3 Year	6 Year	10 Year
Chondroitin Sulfate	Cortex	22	19	16	28
	Medulla	20	17	15	27
Heparan Sulfate	Cortex	58	62	78	53
	Medulla	61	66	57	38
Dermatan Sulfate	Cortex	20	19	6	19
	Medulla	19	17	28	35

The sulfated glycosaminoglycan values from Table 2 were used to calculate the various percent levels. This table highlights the changes in the proportion of the different sulfated glycosaminoglycans.

Heparan sulfate in the cortex (Table 2 and 3) increased until 6 years of age forming 78% of the total sulfated glycosaminoglycans then decreased at 10 years. In the medulla, heparan sulfate formed less than 40% of the total sulfated glycosaminoglycans in 10 year old animals (Table 3). This decrease in heparan sulfate may be responsible for the urinary loss of protein in aged humans. Experimentally, removal of heparan sulfate by enzymatic perfusion of the kidney resulted in an increased permeability of the GBM to ferritin (Kanwar et al., 1980) and iodinated albumin (Rosenzweig and Kanwar, 1982). Similarly, in renal diseases and diabetes, clinical proteinuria has been attributed to the loss of anionic macromolecules. The proportion of dermatan sulfate in the cortex did not show any significant changes with age while the medullary dermatan sulfate showed a steady increase and formed 34% of the total sulfated glycosaminoglycans in the renal tissue of 10 year old dogs. It has been suggested (Murata, 1978) that the age-related increase in the renal dermatan sulfate could be due to fibrous deposition in the tissue. A recent study (Oguri et al., 1984) reported that dermatan sulfate is synthesized by the mesangial cells. However, it is not known whether there is any increase in the mesangial cell population with age. The increase of dermatan sulfate in the medulla may be a mechanism to provide support to the delicate tubules in the medulla by interacting with other matrix macromolecules such as collagen (Obrink, 1973). A strong link between sulfated proteoglycans and collagenous components in renal tissues has been reported (Parthasarathy and Spiro, 1981).

Since the kidney is a heterogenous organ, we isolated glomeruli from the cortex and studied the newly synthesized sulfated proteoglycans. Nearly 90% of the labelled proteoglycan was extracted with 4.0 M GuHCl. The glomeruli obtained from younger animals (1 – 6 years) synthesized predominantly heparan sulfate proteoglycan, while in older animals incorporation into heparan sulfate was decreased. Since this type of incorporation pattern was observed in short-term pulse experiments we believe that the loss of heparan sulfate seen in aging is associated with reduced synthesis rather than increased degradation.

In summary, the results described above demonstrate that, in aging, there is loss of glycosaminoglycans in both cortex and medulla. The content and distribution of glycosaminoglycans in cortex is different from the medulla and age-related changes seen in these two tissues are also different. Also, the loss of sulfated glycosaminoglycans may cause age-related proteinuria.

Acknowledgements

The authors wish to acknowledge the technical assistance of Mr. Steve Manley and Mr. Bob Saporito (supported by Howard University-Rockefeller Foundation Grant), Ms. Marge Pascavage, Ms. Karen Lamb and Ms. Alison Heick for preparation of the manuscript.

References

Bitter, T., and Muir, H.M. (1962). A modified uronic acid carbozol reaction. *Anal. Biochem.* **4**, 330–334.

Brenner, B.M., Bohrer, M.P., Bayliss, C., and Deen, W.M. (1977). Determinants of glomerular permselectivity: Insights derived from observations *in vivo*. *Kidney Int.* **12**, 229–237.

Brenner, B.M., Hostetter, T.H., and Humes, H.D. (1978). Molecular basis of proteinuria of glomerular origin. *N. Engl. J. Med.* **298**, 826–833.

Castor, C.W., and Greene, J.A. (1968). Regional distribution of acid mucopolysaccharides in the kidney. *J. Clin. Invest.* **47**, 2125–2132.

Cifonelli, J.A., and King, J. (1972). The distribution of 2-acetamido-2-deoxy-D-glucose residues in mammalian heparius. *Carbohydr. Res.* **21**, 173–186.

Comper, W.D., and Laurent, T.C. (1978). Physiological function of connective tissue polysaccharides. *Physiol. Rev.* **58**, 255–315.

Dicker, S.E., and Franklin, C.S. (1966). The isolation of hyaluronic and chondroitin sulfate from kidneys and their reaction with urinary hyaluronidase. *J. Physiol.* **186**, 110–120.

Dunnill, M.S., and Halley, W.J. (1973). Some observation on the quantitative anatomy of the kidney. *J. Pathol.* **110**, 113–121.

Farber, S.J., and Van Praag, D. (1970). Composition of glycosaminoglycans (mucopolysaccharides) in rabbit renal papillea. *Biochem. Biophys. Acta* **208**, 219–226.

Farquhar, M.G. (1981). The glomerular basement membrane: A selective macromolecular filter. *In* "Cell Biology of Extracellular Matrix" (E.D. Hay, ed.), pp. 335–379. Plenum Press, New York.

Folch, J.M., Lee, M., and Sloan-Stanley, A.H. (1957). A simple method for the isolation and purification of total lipids from animal tissues. *J. Biol. Chem.* **226**, 497–509.

Griffiths, F.J., Robinson, K.B., Cartwright, G.O., and McLachlan, M.S.F. (1976). Loss of renal tissue in the elderly. *Br. J. Radiolo.* **49**, 111–117.

Inoue, G., Sawada, T., Fukunaga, Y., and Yoshikawa, M. (1970). Levels of acid mucopolysaccharides in aging human kidneys. *Gerontologia* **16**, 261–265.

Kanwar, Y.S., Linker, A., and Farquhar, M.G. (1980). Increased permeability of the glomerular basement membrane to ferritin after removal of glycosaminoglycans (heparan sulfate) by enzyme digestion. *J. Cell Biol.* **86**, 688–693.

Kanwar, Y.S., and Rosenzweig, L.J. (1982). Clogging of the glomerular basement membrane. *J. Cell Biol.* **93**, 489–494.

Kanwar, Y.S., Hascall, V.C., and Farquhar, M.G. (1981). Partial characterization of newly synthesized proteoglycans isolated from the glomerular basement membrane. *J. Cell Biol.* **90**, 527–532.

Kobayashi, S., Oguri, K., Asada, H., Kobayashi, K., Kimura, K., and Okayama, M. (1983). Isolation and characterization of proteoheparan sulfate synthesized *in vitro* by rat glomeruli. *J. Biol. Chem.* **258**, 12051–12057.

Lemkin, M.C., and Farquhar, M.G. (1981). Sulfated and non-sulfated glycosaminoglycans and glycopeptides are synthesized by kidney *in vivo* and incorporated into glomerular basement membrane. *Proc. Natl. Acad. Sci. U.S.A.* **78**, 1726–1730.

Lindahl, U., and Hook, M. (1978). Glycosaminoglycans and their binding to biological macromolecules. *Annu. Rev. Biochem.* **47**, 385–417.

Murata, K., and Horiuchi, Y. (1978). Age-dependent distribution of acidic glycosaminoglycans in human kidney tissue. *Nephron* **20**, 111–118.

Murata, K. (1978). Structural sub units of chondroitin sulfate isomers isolated from different aged human kidneys. *Biochem. Med.* **19**, 395–404.

Obrink, B. (1973). The influence of glycosaminoglycans on the formation of fibers from monomeric tropocollagen *in vitro*. *Eur. J. Biochem.* **34**, 129–137.

Oegema, T.R., Hascall, V.C., and Dziewiatkowski, D.D. (1975). Isolation and characterization of proteoglycans from the Swarm rat chondrosarcoma. *J. Biol. Chem.* **250**, 6151–6159.

Oguri, K., Yaoita, E., Kobayashi, S., Kihara, I., and Okayama, M. (1984). Over sulfated proteodermatan sulfates produced by the rat glomerulus. Abstract presented at 'Extracellular matrix macromolecules-structure and function', Tateshina, Japan. Sept..

Orkin, R.W., and Toole, B.P. (1978). Hyaluronidase activity and hyaluronate content of the developing chick embryonic heart. *Dev. Biol.* **66**, 308–320.

Parthasarathy, N., and Spiro, R.G. (1981). Characterization of the glycosaminoglycan component of the renal glomerular basement membrane and its relationship to peptide portion. *J. Biol. Chem.* **256**, 507–513.

Pinter, G.G. (1967). A possible role of acid mucopolysaccharides in the urine concentrating process. *Experientia* **23**, 100–101.

Rennke, H.G., Patel, Y., and Venkatachalam, M.A. (1978). Glomerular filtration of proteins: Clearance of anionic, neutral, and cationic horseradish peroxidase in the rat. *Kidney Int.* **13**, 278–288.

Rosenquist, T.H., and Bernick, S. (1971). Histochemistry of renal basal laminae. Adolescent compared with senescent rats. *J. Gerontol.* **26**, 176–185.

Rosenzweig, L.J., and Kanwar, Y.S. (1982). Removal of sulfated (heparan sulfate) or nonsulfated (hyaluronic acid) glycosaminoglycans results in increased permeability of the glomerular basement membrane to ^{125}I-bovine serum albumin. *Lab. Invest.* **47**, 177–184.

Sato, F., Tsuchihashi, S., and Kawashima, N. (1975). Age changes in number and size of the murine renal glomeruli. *Exp. Gerontol.* **10**, 325–331.

Saito, H., Yamagata, T.S., and Suzuki, S. (1968). Enzymatic methods for the determination of small quantities of isomeric chondroitin sulfates. *J. Biol. Chem.* **243**, 1536–1542.

Spiro, R.G. (1967). Studies on the renal glomerular basement membrane. *J. Biol. Chem.* **242**, 1923–1932.

Stow, J.L., Glasgow, E.F., Handley, C.J., and Hascall, V.C. (1983). Biosynthesis of proteoglycans by isolated rabbit glomeruli. *Arch. Biochem. Biophys.* **225**, 950–957.

Ullrich, K.J., Drenchkahn, F.D., and Jarausch, K.H. (1955). Untersuchungen zum Problem der Hornkonzentrierung underverdunnung. Uber das osmotische Verhalten von Nierenzellen und die beglentende Elektrolytanhaufung im Nierengewede bei versheidenen Diuresezustanden. *Arch. Ges. Physiol.* **261**, 62–75.

Vasan, N.S., Saporito, R.A., Saraswathi, S., Tesoriero, J.V., and Manely, S. (1983). Alterations of renal cortex and medullary glycosaminoglycans in aging dog kidney. *Biochem. Biophys. Acta.* **760**, 197–205.

Yonekura, H., Oguri, K., Nakazawa, K., Shimizu, S., Nakanishi, Y., and Okayama, M. (1982). Isolation and partial characterization of sulfated glycoproteins synthesized by corneal epithelium. *J. Biol. Chem.* **257**, 11166–11175.

APPLICATION OF BACKSCATTERED ELECTRON IMAGING FOR VASCULAR RESEARCH

Paul K. Nakane[1] and Shinichi Izumi

Department of Cell Biology, Tokai University School of Medicine
Isehara

Anthony L. Hartman

Department of Pathology, University of Cincinnati School of Medicine
Cincinnati, Ohio

In many of the routine histology laboratories, surgical biopsy specimens are not examined at the ultrastructural level even when it is known that such observation may yield more precise diagnosis. The more time, more effort, and more expense required for the electron microscopic examination are the usual reasons mentioned by surgical pathologists. One other reason is the fact that usual diagnosis of histological specimens are based upon the long accumulated experience of pathologists with light microscopic preparations and a new set of experience is required when electron microscopic observations are used. Thus in order to make ultrastructural observation practical, it is necessary to develop a method which requires the time, effort and expenses similar to that of light microscopic preparation and capitalizes maximally the vast experience accumulated by pathologist with light microscopic preparations. One way to accomplish this is to examine light microscopic preparation directly with an inexpensive electron microscope. To this end, we have been probing to establish such method for the past several years (Hartman and Nakane, 1981, 1983; Nakane and Hartman, 1980; Nakane et al., 1982).

Because the thickness of light microscopic glass slide is excessive for conventional transmission electron microscopic observation, we have opted for the observation by scanning electron microscopes. Usually scanning electron microscopes are used to obtain high resolution topographical views of the surface of specimen through the use of secondary electrons generated when the incident electron beam strikes the specimens. However, the surfaces of tissue sections mounted on light microscopic glass slide (without the cover glass) are usually flat and the topographic information is of little use in describing the structures of cells and tissues. Consequently we have decided to capitalized on the elastic collisions between electrons of the primary beam and the atomic nuclei of the specimens as the primary electron beam strikes the specimen. This type of interaction results in deflection of primary electrons at large angles and generates back scattered electrons without much reduction with energy. Because of this, back scattered electrons generated deep within specimen (over several μm below the surface) can exit from the specimen and be detected. In addition, the number of back scattered electron

[1]Supported in part by research grant (59870018, 60015094 and 60480156) from Ministry of Education of Japan.

generated is dependent upon the atomic number of the electron impacted material. These physical nature of back scattered electron, then, can be used to form images of sub-surface structures based upon their atomic numbers. The back scattered electron image, however, is expected to have less resolution than the secondary electron image, since the primary electrons as penetrate the specimen are diffused considerably before generating the back scattered electrons.

In order to make the back scattered electron imaging for the observation of tissue sections mounted on glass slide practical, several technical problems associated with both for instruments and for methods of specimen preparation should be solved. Some of expected problems with specimen preparations are; 1) some of fixation methods of tissues and cells used for the light microscopic observation may be inappropriate for the ultrastructural observation, 2) embedding medium such as paraffin may not withstand the electron bombardment, 3) the molecular organization of embedding medium may interfere with the back scattered electron image formation, 4) the electron insulating nature of glass slide may result in electron charging of the specimen, 5) electron contrasting counter-staining methods for the back scattered electron imaging need to be developed, and 6) special staining techniques including immunohistochemical staining may require modifications, etc. In our previous investigation (Hartman and Nakane, 1981, 1983; Nakane and Hartman, 1980; Nakane et al., 1982), some of the above problems were dealt with, and in this report we dealt with the problem of charging.

There are currently two methods in use for coating the glass slide. The first is the evaporation of indium oxide onto the slide (Ogura and Laudate, 1980), and the second is the evaporation of carbon onto the substrate (Hartman and Nakane, 1981). The former has the advantage that it leaves the glass transparent for light microscopic examination and the latter, while being slightly opaque, but not enough to be visible under a light microscope has the advantage of not interfering with the *in vitro* growth of cells directly on the coated slide. When section of paraffin or plastic embedded tissues are mounted on either indium coated or carbon coated slides, no further grounding is necessary. However, the electrical evaporation onto the glass slide requires a special equipment and was found to be time consuming, expensive and impractical for a mass production in the routine histology laboratories. Consequently, we have looked for a more simple method of grounding tissue section mounted on the glass slide.

Materials and Methods

Light microscopic glass slides were cleaned by 1N HCl and acetone. Some of the cleaned slides were then coated with fresh egg albumin (Nakane, 1982). The slides were dipped into solutions containing various organic and inorganic compounds, and were dried at 58 ℃. The glass slides were examined first with a light microscope as to their color and the state of the compound (smooth or crystalline). The slides were then placed on a specially designed stage in a JEOL T200 scanning electron microscope and were scanned with an accelerating voltage of 25 K with a spot size of 500 Å in diameter. The build up of electron at the scanned area was examined by actually electron scanning the surface of slide.

Kidneys from adult mice were removed and were sliced into about 1 mm in thickness. The pieces of tissues were fixed in periodate-lysine-paraformaldehyde fixative (McLean and Nakane, 1974) by immersion for 3 hr at 4 ℃ and were washed in phosphate buffered saline (PBS) at 4 ℃. The fixed tissues were then dehydrated and embedded in methacrylate, JB4, or Immuno-Bed with routine procedure. Some tissues were post fixed in osmium tetroxide, dehydrated and embedded in Epon. The embedded tissues were sectioned into 1—2 μm in thickness using LKB ultramicrotome and were mounted on light microscopic glass slide and were treated with various organic and inorganic materials.

Some sections of kidney embedded in Immuno-Bed and mounted on the slide were processed for immunohistochemistry. Specifically, rabbit antibody against mouse basement membrane was reacted with the section for 2 hr, then reacted with peroxidase labeled anti-rabbit IgG (Nakane and Pierce, 1966) for 2 hr. The antibody reacted sections were developed for peroxidase using 3,3'-diaminobenzidine (Graham and Karnovsky, 1966) as hydrogen donor. The reaction products were then chelated with osmium tetroxide first, then with thiocarbohydrazide and with osmium tetroxide (Aoki and Tavassoli, 1981). The last two steps were repeated once more times. These immunostained sections were then again coated with egg albumin and treated with an electron grounding material. These slides were then examined with the scanning electron microscope.

Results and Discussion

When the surface of slide was scanned with a spot of electron beam, if there was an electron build up, the adjacent area surrounding the scanned area became white (with light/dark reversed); and if there was no build up, the scanned area remained black (with light/dark reversed). The results were summarized in Table 1. The compounds which prevented the electron build up at the area scanned were, in addition to the previously used indium and carbon films, ferric ammonium sulfate, indium sulfate and indium chloride. Electron conducting plastic, poly-9-vinyl carbazole prevented the electron build up for few seconds, but eventually failed. Cupric sulfate and mercuric chloride also prevented the build up partially. The indium sulfate and indium chloride treatments were sufficient to block the electron charging, however because of their rough surface texture, they were not suited for the light microscopic observations. The ferric ammonium sulfate treated slide was clear and did not charge even after a prolonged examination under the electron beam. When, however, the ferric ammonium sulfate coated slides were left standing for more than one week, it oxidized to pale brown color gradually. The oxidized slide may be recoated with the solution of ferric ammonium sulfate for the proper grounding, however the texture became rough and was not satisfactory for the light microscopic observation.

In our previous investigations, the antigenecity proteins such as rabbit IgG was lost when tissues were embedded in JB4 or in Epon. In the present

TABLE 1

COMPOUND	SOLVENT	COLOR	SURFACE*	CHARGE**
None	N.A.	Transparent	N.A.	Yes.
Egg albumin	Ammonium hydroxide	Transparent	Smooth	Yes.
Carbon film	N.A.	Light brown	Smooth	No.
Indium film	N.A.	Transparent	Smooth	No.
Eleguard TM.	Ethanol	Transparent	Smooth	Yes.
Poly-9-vinyl carbazole	Pyridine	Transparent	Smooth	Yes.
Poly-9-vinyl carbazole	Benzene	Transparent	Smooth	Yes.
Poly-9-vinyl carbazole	Tetrahydrofuran	Transparent	Smooth	Yes.
JB4 section	N.A.	Transparent	Smooth	Yes.
Paraffin section	N.A.	White	Rough	Yes.
Epon section	N.A.	Transparent	Smooth	Yes.
Acrytron section	N.A.	Transparent	Smooth	Yes.
Immuno-Bed section	N.A.	Transparent	Smooth	Yes.
10% Cupric chloride	D.W.	Light yellow	Rough	Yes.
10% Cupric acetate	D.W.	Greenish blue	Rough	Yes.
10% Cupric sulfate	D.W.	Light blue	Smooth/rough	Yes.
10% Ferric nitrate	D.W.	Light orange	Smooth/rough	Yes.
10% Ferric ammonium sulfate	D.W.	Transparent	Smooth	No.
10% Ferric chloride	D.W.	Yellow/orange	Smooth/rough	Yes.
10% Ferric sulfate	D.W.	Light orange	Smooth	Yes.
10% Potassium ferricianide	D.W.	Yellow	Rough	Yes.
10% Potassium ferrocianide	D.W.	White	Rough	Yes.
10% Silver nitrate	D.W.	Transparent	Rough	Yes.
40% Indium sulfate	D.W.	Transparent	Smooth/rough	No.
40% Indium chloride	D.W.	Transparent	Smooth/rough	No.
10% Mercuric chloride	D.W.	Transparent	Smooth	Yes.
10% Mercuric oxide	D.W.	Transparent	Smooth	Yes.

* condition of slide surface as examined by light microscope.
** accumulation of electrical charge viewed by scanning electron microscope.
N.A. = not applicable, D.W. = distilled water

study, the antigenicity of mouse epithelial basement membrane which is usually weaker than that of rabbit IgG was well retained when the mouse kidney fixed with PLP was embedded in Immuno-Bed. This embedding medium is not suited for the routine electron microscopic observation, but was found to be satisfactory for observation by scanning electron microscope equipped with a back scattered detector (Fig. 1). One deficiency found with this embedding medium was its tendency to crack when left in vacuum for a long time. The preservation of morphology of tissues embedded in Immuno-Bed was excellent and the tissue processing was easier than that of methacrylate, the another embedding medium which retains antigenicity relatively well (Kawarai and Nakane, 1970). Although we have not yet perfected the best way to stain the sections of tissues embedded in Immuno-Bed for light and scanning electron microscopic observation, among currently available plastic embedding medium, Immuno-Bed appears to be best suited as the embedding medium for the tissue observation for back scattered electron imaging.

This investigation provided one simple way to prevent the electron charging in the area of tissue sections scanned by electron beam. This phenomenon has hindered for the past several years for the mass preparation of histological specimens suitable for the observation by both the light and electron microscopes. With this problem behind us, the remaining major problems are the unavailability of adequate heavy metal containing stains which are visible by both the light and scanning electron microscopes and the lack of resolution with the back scattered electron imaging. With the former problem, we are currently using heavy metal stains used with the routine transmission electron microscopy, however the stains are usually not visible with the light microscope, and when tissue sections stained with routine light microscopic stains such as hematoxylin and eosin are counterstained with the heavy metals, they tend to breach the light microscopic stains. With the latter problem, one obvious solution is to increase the electron density in the beam (to increase the beam current) and to reduce the spot diameter. This may require somewhat more sophisticated lens system than those used with routine scanning electron microscopes. With the instrument used in our investigation, for most times we were able to visualize the pathological changes associated with surgical specimens with one order higher resolution than the light microscopic studies, the resolution attainable with the routine transmission electronmicroscope could not be achieved.

We are now convinced that the approach we have taken has made the ultrastructural examination of bio-medical specimens easier, less time consuming and cheaper, and may become a standard equipment in most routine histology laboratories.

Abstract

At the point of electron impact, in addition to secondary electron, cathodoluminescence and X-ray, back scattered electron are emitted. Since the back scattered electron is generated in an amount proportional to the atomic number of the electron impacted elements, a scanning electron microscope equipped

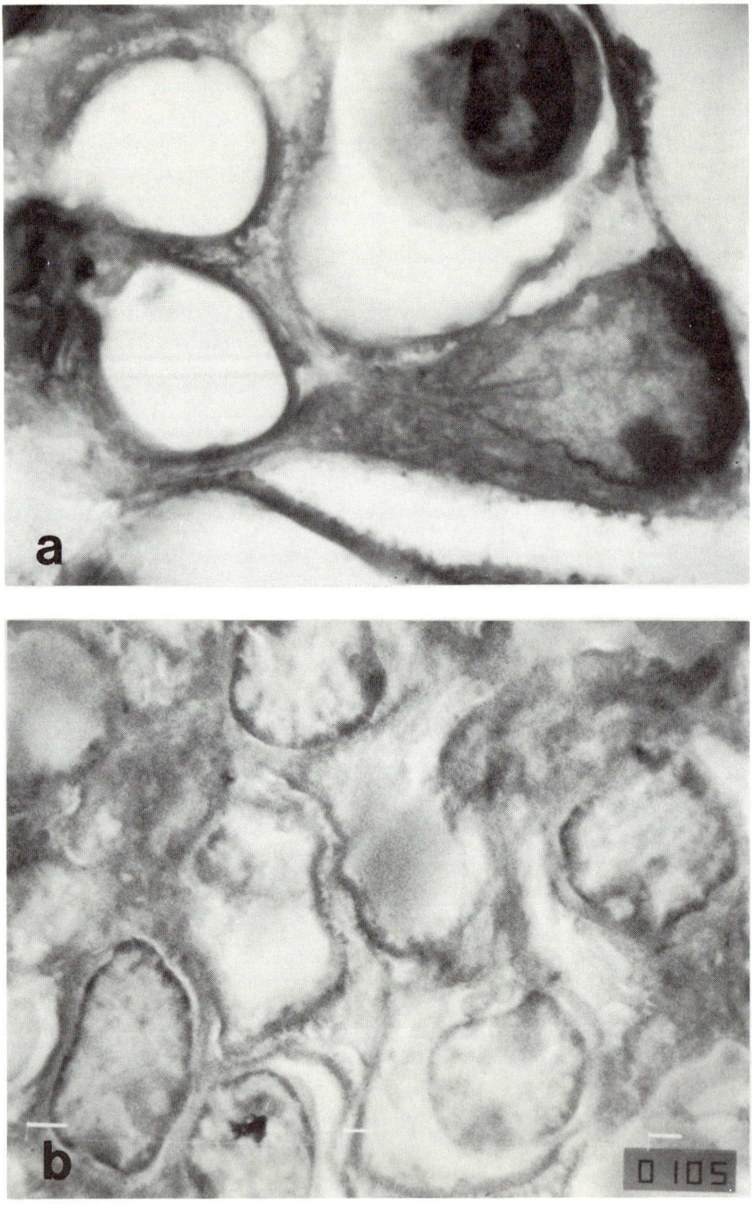

FIG. 1. (a) A section of mouse kidney embedded in JB4 was reacted with first sodium periodate then with 3,3'-diaminobenzidine and osmium tetroxide. The carbohydrates moiety was stained. (b) A section of mouse kidney embedded in Immuno-Bed was stained immunohistochemically for the basement membrane. The basement membrane was stained enhanced with O-T-O reaction.

with a back scattered electron detector may be used to detect heavy metals. By staining the samples with the heavy metals selectively, specific matters and antigens may be localized in cells and tissues. Thus sections of fixed tissues embedded in supporting media, i.e. paraffin, Immuno-Bed, JB4, and Epon, may be placed on the ordinary light microscopic glass slides and examined either by the back scattered electron imaging or by the light microscope. To do this, a proper electrical grounding of the section and slide is required. In this report the method for the grounding was investigated. It was found that ferric ammonium sulfate was the best for the prevention of electron build up at the point of electron scanning. With these methods and instruments, the examination of same tissue section will be made both at the light and electron microscopic-levels.

ACKNOWLEDGMENT

Authors wish to express our thanks to Ms. S. Harada for her help in preparation of this manuscript.

REFERENCES

Aoki, M., and Tavassoli, M. (1981). OTO method for preservation of actin filaments in electron microscopy. *J. Histochem. Cytochem.* **29**, 682–683.

Graham, Jr., R.C., and Karnovsky, M.J. (1966). The bearly stages of injected horseradish peroxidase in the proximal tubules of mouse kidney: Ultrastructural cytochemistry by a new technique. *J. Histochem. Cytochem.* **14**, 291–302.

Hartman, A.L., and Nakane, P.K. (1981). Intracellular localization of antigens with backscatter mode of SEM using peroxidase-labeled antibodies. *Scanning Electron Microsc.* **II**, 33–44.

Hartman, A.L., and Nakane, P.K. (1983). Immunological methods in scanning electron microscopy using peroxidase. *In* "Immunocytochemistry" (P. Petrusz, ed.), pp. 103–116. Academic Press, New York.

Kawarai, Y., and Nakane, P.K. (1970). Localization of tissue antigens on the ultrathin sections with peroxidase-labeled antibody. *J. Histochem. Cytochem.* **18**, 161–166.

McLean, I.W., and Nakane, P.K. (1974). Periodate-lysine-paraformaldehyde fixative. A new fixative for immunoelectron microscopy. *J. Histochem. Cytochem.* **22**, 1077–1083.

Nakane, P.K. (1982). Immunoelectron microscopy. *In* "Methods in Cancer Research, XX" (H. Busch and L.C. Yeoman, eds.), pp. 206–207. Academic Press, New York.

Nakane, P.K., and Hartman, A.L. (1980). Immunohistochemical localization of intracellular antigens with SEM. *Histochem. J.* **12**, 435–447.

Nakane, P.K., Hartman A.L., and Hosoi, J. (1982). SEM for immunoelectron microscopy. *J. Clin. Electron Microscopy* **15**, 383–392.

Nakane, P.K., and Pierce, G.B. (1966). Enzyme-labeled antibodies: Preparation and application for the localization of antigens. *J. Histochem. Cytochem.* **14**, 929–931.

Ogura, K., and Laudate, A. (1980). Comparative observation with a light microscope and an SEM in backscattered electron mode. *Scanning Electron Microsc.* **I**, 233–238.

II. Interface between Blood and Endothelium

This section deals with studies on the interface between blood and the endothelium. The latter is considered to be composed of the endothelial cells and the interendothelial junctions. Although the physiological roles of both the endothelial cells and their junctions have not yet been fully established and considerable conceptual differences continue to exist, their significance is paramount in the exchanges between the blood and the tissues via these two parts of the endothelium.

S. Oka deals with electrical aspects, E. Vasile and N. Simonescu discuss low density lipoprotein transcytosis in capillary blood vessels, whereas T. Murakami *et al.* limit their studies to the structure of human kidney glomeruli. A. L. Copley considers the blood and all layers of the capillary vessel wall as an entity, which he names the "vessel–blood organ." He proposes that in the microstructure of the vessel wall, the endoendothelial fibrin and/or fibrinogenin lining is the crucial barrier between the blood and the tissues. Thrombin-induced fibrin and/or fibrinogenin are contained not merely in the endoendothelial lining, but also in the interendothelial junction and the basement membrane for which certain experimental evidence is presented. *Fibrinogenin* is a new term for experimentally well-established clotting of fibrinogen without thrombin action. Fibrin and fibrinogenin may also be contained in free and stalked endothelial vesicles since J.H.Luft found them to be stained with ruthenium red. The latter is not a specific stain for proteoglycans, but it stains fibrin and fibrinogen as well.

This section is of particular significance for the understanding of mechanisms pertaining to the barriers in blood–tissue exchanges in general and in the glomeruli in particular.

A. L. Copley

ELECTRIC ASPECT OF INTERFACE BETWEEN BLOOD AND ENDOTHELIUM

Syoten Oka

National Cardiovascular Center Research Institute
Suita

The importance of the interface between blood and endothelium has been emphasized more and more in recent years. Among the clinical problems concerning with the interface between blood and endothelium thrombus formation and atherosclerosis may be mentioned. We shall consider the electric aspect of the interface in the following. It is well known that the electric potential of a normal intima is negative to that of the adventitia, while that of an injured intima is positive. The electron micrographs of an injured intima show the coming off of the endothelial cells. Since the isoelectric point of collagen under the endothelium is 7.8, it must be positively charged in contact with blood whose pH is 7.4.

The distribution of negative charges on blood vessel walls has been demonstrated by several investigators. The distribution of the surface charge on the cells which constitute the air-blood barrier was investigated by Simionescu et al. (1983) by perfusing cationized ferritin into the vasculature. Binding of cationized ferritin was shown to be selective and defined highly differentiated domains. Seno et al. (1983a, 1983b) observed on rat kidney tissues that an iron colloid solution was promissing for the detection of anionic sites of cell surfaces in place of cationic ferritin. Ruthenium red, a cationic dye, was used by Charonis and Wissig (1983) to detect at the electron microscopic level the presence of anionic sites in various murine basement membranes.

Another group of investigators has been interested, from rheological standpoint, in the effect of the electric charge on glass capillary tubes upon the blood flow within the tube. A remarkable decrease in the apparent viscosity of blood in negatively charged capillaries has been observed by several investigators. Copley and his collaborators (1958a, 1958b, 1960, 1961) were the first to observe from 1958 to 1961 the so-called Copley-Scott Blair phenomenon, namely, the decrease in the apparent viscosity of blood of $15-30$ per cent in fibrin-coated glass capillaries. Since the isoelectric point of fibrin is 5.5, it must be negatively charged in contact with blood. The result of Copley et al. was reexamined by Koyama et al. (1967, 1970, 1971), but only a slight decrease of 0.7 per cent was observed in the apparent viscosity of blood in fibrin-coated glass capillaries. According to Copley, the difference may be attributed to the difference in the technique of coating fibrin on glass capillaries. Ossoff and Charm (1974) reported that negatively charged substances on a glass capillary caused a decrease of 18 per cent in the apparent viscosity of blood. Fenton et al. (1982) observed a decrease of 4 per cent in the apparent viscosity of blood in a glass capillary coated with endothelial cells.

It is clear that endothelial cells in contact with blood are negatively charged.

The mechanism of the decrease in the apparent viscosity of blood in negatively charged capillaries has not yet been clarified theoretically. The apparent viscosity of blood may be decreased, if the thickness of a plasma layer is increased. However, the present author (1983a) has shown recently that the remarkable decrease in the apparent viscosity of blood cannot be explained by a reasonable increase in the thickness of a plasma layer. An electric double layer may be formed on the surface of negatively charged capillaries, since electrolytes are contained in blood. The present author (1983b, 1984) has recently shown theoretically that an electric double layer causes an increase in the apparent viscosity of blood instead of a decrease.

A New Theory — Electrostatic Entrance Effect upon Hematocrit

A new theory is presented here to explain the decrease in the apparent viscosity of blood in negatively charged capillaries. Let us pay special attention to a red blood cell entering a negatively charged capillary. The red blood cell will receive an electrostatic repulsive force from the negative charge on the capillary, since the red blood cell is also negatively charged. This means that the hematocrit in a negatively charged capillary must be less than that in a neutral capillary. It is clear that the lowering of the hematocrit results in the decrease in the apparent viscosity of blood in the negatively charged capillary. If we denote the hematocrit, or strictly speaking, the volume fraction of red blood cells in a feeding reservoir or in a neutral capillary by H, then the hematocrit in a negatively charged capillary can be written as $H\alpha$, where α is a dimensionless reduction factor less than unity.

The apparent viscosity of blood decreases, of course, with decrease in hematocrit. Chien et al. (1966) investigated a quantitative relation between viscosity and hematocrit. According to Puccini et al. (1977) this relation can be expressed analytically in the form

$$\eta = \eta_p A \frac{H^2}{(1-H)^b} \tag{1}$$

at shear rates $\dot{\gamma}$ = 0.052, 0.52 and 5.2 s^{-1}. Here η_p is the plasma viscosity, A is a constant depending on the shear rate, and b is a constant nearly equal to 0.4.

If we denote the apparent viscosity of blood observed in a negatively charged capillary by η_{ch}, then we have

$$\eta_{ch} = \eta_p A \frac{H^2 \alpha^2}{(1-H\alpha)^b} \tag{2}$$

Consequently, the relative decrease $\triangle$ in the apparent viscosity of blood is given by

$$\triangle = \frac{\eta - \eta_{ch}}{\eta} = 1-(1-H)^b \frac{\alpha^2}{(1-H\alpha)^b} \tag{3}$$

If we take H = 0.3 and b = 0.4 for simplicity, we get

$$\alpha^5 = \frac{(1-\triangle)^{2.5}}{0.7}(1-0.3\alpha) \tag{4}$$

For a given value of $\triangle$, α is obtained as the root of the above equation of fifth degrees. The result is tabulated as follows:

TABLE 1. RELATION BETWEEN $\triangle$ AND α

$\triangle$ %	0	0.5	1	5	10	15	20	30
α	1.000	0.998	0.995	0.977	0.953	0.928	0.902	0.847

It is apparent that the factor α is related to the repulsive electrostatic field E acting on a red blood cell at the entrance of a capillary. The field E depends, of course, not only upon the negative surface charge density σ on the inner surface of the capillary, but also upon the inner radius R of the capillary as well as upon the distance d from the entrance. It seems difficult, however, to find an exact functional form of E (σ, R, d).

As for the relation between α and E, following equation can be derived:

$$\alpha = 1 - 3.19\text{x}10^5 \frac{E}{U} \tag{5}$$

where U is the blood velocity at the entrance of a capillary. For a given value of α, 3.19 x 10^5E/U can easily be obtained from Eq. (5) as shown in the following table:

TABLE 2. RELATION BETWEEN α AND 3.19 x 10^5E/U

α	1.000	0.998	0.995	0.977	0.953	0.928	0.902	0.847
3.19 x 10^5E/U%	0	0.2	0.5	2.3	4.7	7.2	9.5	15.3

Table 1 and 2 show that a relative decrease of 1 per cent in the apparent viscosity of blood corresponds to a 0.5 per cent reduction of hematocrit, and to a 0.5 per cent of 3.19 x 10^5E/U. Similarly, $\triangle$ of 20 per cent corresponds to a 9.8 per cent reduction of hematocrit, and to a 9.5 per cent of 3.19 x 10^5E/U.

RESULT

A new theory is presented to explain the remarkable decrease in the apparent viscosity of blood in negatively charged capillaries. This phenomenon has been first investigated by Copley et al. in 1958 in fibrin-coated glass capillaries. It is pointed out that the red blood cells bearing negative charge receives a repulsive electrostatic force at the entrance of the capillary from the negative charge of the capillary. The repulsive force causes a reduction in the hematocrit in the capillary, resulting in a decrease in the apparent viscosity of blood flowing in the capillary. This electrostatic effect becomes the more remarkable, the smaller the capillary becomes.

The reduction factor α in the hematocrit in the negatively charged capillary is correlated with the relative decrease $\triangle$ in the apparent viscosity of blood based on an analytical expression due to Chien and Puccini et al. For example, $\triangle$ of 1% corresponds to $\alpha = 0.995$, that is, to a reduction of hematocrit of 0.5%. Similarly, $\triangle$ of 20% corresponds to $\alpha = 0.902$, that is, to a reduction of hematocrit of 9.8%. The reduction factor α depends, of course, on the repulsive electrostatic field E at the entrance. It is shown that α decreases linealy with E, while $\alpha = 1$ when $E = 0$. The quantitative relation between α and E is a theoretical problem left for future.

Discussion

It is expected that our new electrostatic entrance effect becomes the more pronounced, the smaller the capillary becomes. It is hoped to measure the hematocrit in the negatively charged capillary tube to test our new electrostatic theory.

Copley and his collaborators also found a remarkable decrease in the viscosity of plasma and serum in fibrin-coated capillaries. This phenomenon can also be explained reasonably by our new theory. Protein molecules in plasma and serum are negatively charged so that they receive an electrostatic repulsive force from the charge on the inner surface of the tube.

The cells and tissues in biological systems are generally charged, so that our electrostatic entrance effect may well be applied to microvessels and to the permeability of charged substances into tissues.

Abstract

A remarkable decrease in the apparent viscosity of blood in negatively charged capillaries has been observed by several investigators including Copley. It is pointed out that the red blood cells receive electrostatic repulsive forces at the entrance of a capillary. Consequently, the hematocrit in the capillary tube becomes less than that in the reservoir, resulting in a decrease in the aparent viscosity of blood. Using the quantitative relationship between viscosity and hematocrit obtained by Chien et al., the relative decrease in the apparent viscosity of blood is quantitatively related to the reduction factor α of the hematocrit. On the other hand, the factor α decreases linearly with the electrostatic field E, namely, $\alpha = 1 - 3.19 \times 10^5 E/U$, where U is the blood velocity at the entrance of a capillary. For a given value of $\triangle$, α can be obtained under some assumptions. Thus, $\triangle$ of 1% corresponds to a 0.5% reduction of hematocrit, and $\triangle$ of 20% corresponds to a 9.8% reduction of hematocrit. Copley and his collaborators also found a remarkable decrease in the viscosity of plasma and serum in fibrin-coated glass tubes. This phenomenon can also be explained reasonable by our new theory, since all protein molecules in plasma and serum are negatively charged and receive electrostatic repulsive forces from the charge on the inner surface of the tube. The cells and tissues in biological systems are generally charged, so that our electrostatic entrance effect may well be applied to microvessels and to the permeability of charged substances into tissues.

References

Charonis, A.S., and Wissig, S.L. (1983). Anionic sites in basement membranes. Differences in their electrostatic properties in continuous and fenestrated capillaries. *Microvasc. Res.* **25**, 265–285.

Chien, S., Usami, S., Taylor, H.M., Lundberg, J.L., and Gregersen, M.I. (1966). Effect of hematocrit and plasma proteins on human blood rheology at low shear rates. *J. Appl. Physiol.* **21**, 81–87.

Copley, A.L. (1958a). Adherence and viscosity of blood contacting foreign surfaces and the plasmatic zone in blood circulation. *Nature* **181**, 551–552.

Copley, A.L., and Scott Blair, G.W. (1958b). Comparative observations on adherence and consistency of various blood systems in living and artificial capillaries. *Rheol. Acta* **1**, 170–176.

Copley, A.L., and Scott Blair, G.W. (1961). Comparative observations on adherence and consistency of various blood systems in living and artificial capillaries. *Rheol. Acta* **1**, 665–668.

Copley, A.L., Scott Blair, G.W., Glover, F.A., and Thorley, R.S. (1960). Capillary flow and wall adherence of bovine blood, plasma and serum in contact with glass and fibrin surfaces. *Kolloid-Z.* **168**, 101–107.

Fenton, B.M., Cokelet, G.R., and La Celle, P.L. (1982). Influence of wall surface on the flow of blood through endothelial-lined glass tubes. *Int. J. Microcirc. Clin. Exp.* **1**, 157–162.

Koyama, K., Kitahara, R., Kanamaru, K., and Wada, E. (1967). *Zairyo* **16**, 525–527 (in Japanese).

Koyama, K., Oki, N., Kanamaru, K., and Wada, E. (1970). Effect of wall surface on capillary flow. *Reports Prog. Polymer Phys. Japan* **13**, 95–98.

Koyama, K., Ooi, E., Wada, E., and Kanamaru, K. (1971). Effect of wall surface on capillary flow III. Effect of fibrin coating. *Reports Prog. Polymer Phys. Japan* **14**, 635–638.

Oka, S. (1983a). Physical theory of some interface phenomena in hemorheology. *Ann. N.Y. Acad. Sci.* **416**, 115–127.

Oka, S. (1983b). Rheological aspect in relation to endothelial fibrin lining. *Thrombosis Res.* **32**, 649–653.

Oka, S. (1984). Copley-Scott Blair phenomenon and electric double layer. *Biorheology* **21**, 417.

Ossoff, R., and Charm, S.E. (1974). Blood viscosity reduction in negative charged capillary tubes. *Biorheology* **11**, 293–299.

Puccini, C., Stasiw, D.M., and Cerny, L.C. (1977). The erythrocyte sedimentation curve: a semi-empirical approach. *Biorheology* **14**, 43–49.

Seno, S., Ono, T., and Tsujii, T. (1983a). Macromolecular charge and cellular surface charge in adhesion, ingestion, and blood vessel leakage. *Ann. N.Y. Acad. Sci.* **416**, 410–425.

Seno, S., Tsujii, T., Ono, T., and Ukita, S. (1983b). Cationic cacodylate iron colloid for the detection of anionic sites on cell surface and the histochemical stain of acid mucopolysaccharides. *Histochemistry* **78**, 27–31.

Simionescu, D., and Simionescu, M. (1983). Differentiated distribution of the cell surface charge on the alveolar-capillary unit. *Microvasc. Res.* **25**, 85–100.

ENDOENDOTHELIAL FIBRIN(OGENIN) LINING: THE INTERFACE BETWEEN THE TWO PORTIONS OF THE "VESSEL-BLOOD ORGAN"

Alfred L. Copley

Laboratory of Biorheology
Polytechnic Institute of New York
Brooklyn, New York

THE VESSEL-BLOOD ORGAN AND THE ENDO-ENDOTHELIAL FIBRIN(OGENIN) LINING (EEFL)

It was in Tokyo when, in 1960, the author first introduced the concept that the circulating blood and the vessel wall are one entity (Copley, 1982). This was in a special lecture on the endoendothelial fibrin lining at the 8th International Congress of Hematology. It was also in Tokyo that three years ago in a plenary lecture before the 4th International Congress of Biorheology he considered this entity as an organ and named it "vessel-blood organ" (Copley 1982). He believes that the concept of the vessel-blood organ will contribute to a reassessment of the roles of the two portions of this unique entity. The vessel-blood organ will have to be related to other organs, which it penetrates, as well as to the entire organism.

The great advances in the past decades in the sciences of cell biology and of molecular biology have often obscured the need for studies at the level of organ systems. Any advances in cell biology and molecular biology will have to be coordinated ultimately with organ systems and the entire organism. This need is especially manifest with regard to cellular and non-cellular studies involving transcapillary transport and its physiological and pathophysiological significance.

In this presentation the author does not dwell on the perspectives which the concept of the vessel-blood organ might invite, but limits his presentation to what he stated to be the interface and crucial barrier between the two portions of this organ. This crucial barrier is not the endothelium, as is generally believed, but the endoendothelial fibrin(ogenin) lining (EEFL).

As it appears probable that the endoendothelial fibrin lining may as well contain fibrinogenin, a new term for fibrinogen clotting without thrombin participation (Copley, 1983), such a probability is identified as follows: Fibrin(ogenin) means fibrin and/or fibrinogenin. The abbreviation EEFL is thus extended to fibrin(ogenin). It is not possible within a short period of time to present most of the evidence available for the existence of the EEFL, and its importance in the pathogenesis of different pathological conditions and disease processes. Such information can be found in several recent publications (Copley, 1981, 1983a, b, c, d, 1984a, b; Copley and Seaman, 1983; Silberberg, 1984).

The Immobile Portion of the Plasmatic Zone

About one hundred-fifty years ago, Poiseuille made the first *in vivo* hemorheological studies of the microcirculation (Poiseuille, 1839; Copley and Staple, 1962; Copley, 1974). He differentiated between an immobile portion, which he postulated, and a mobile portion of the plasmatic zone, which he observed. This is shown diagrammatically in Fig. 1. In 1959 Copley

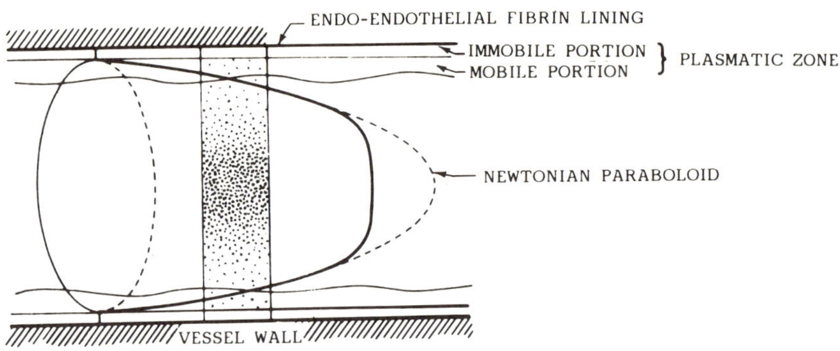

FIG. 1. Diagrammatic figure of extrusion of blood. See: Copley (1983).

and Staple (1962) found suggestive evidence for the existence of such an immobile portion in close proximity to the vessel wall. We postulated that many processes can occur in this more or less immobile layer, undisturbed by the flow of blood. This is of particular significance, because of the homeostatic equilibrium between fibrin formation and fibrinolysis, advanced by Nolf, 1908 (see also Copley, 1983) and other investigators in the beginning of this century, which the author postulated to occur in this 'immobile' portion of the plasmatic zone (Copley and Staple, 1962; Copley, 1983).

The Significance of Extracellular Structures in the Capillary Wall

During the past three decades, the important roles and functions which biological intracellular and extracellular structures play fundamentally in life processes are more and more recognized. This is also the case with regard to the structures comprising the capillary wall.

The interendothelial cement substance, proposed by Julius Cohnheim in 1873 was studied with regard to capillary permeability by Herbst (1900) and Overton (1904) in the beginning of the century (see also Copley, 1983). In 1940 and 1947, Chambers and Zweifach reported their findings on the capillary cement in relation to capillary permeability. They found that with solutions lacking calcium a softening of the cement occurred, which was indicated by its increased stickiness to carbon particles and its being washed away. They concluded from these and other observations that the interendothelial cement controls the permeability of the capillary blood vessel. In 1960, the author proposed the fibrin component of the interendothelial cement substance as an extension of the EEFL which surrounds the endothelial cells (Copley, 1983).

The Endoendothelial Fibrin(ogenin) Lining (EEFL)

Danielli reported in 1940 studies on perfused hind-legs in frogs and offered indirect evidence for an adsorbed protein on the walls of the capillary pores. He based his hypothesis of an endovascular layer on differences in the porosity of the capillary wall, occurring with variations in the colloidal content of the perfusion fluid. Similar experimental findings were reported by Chambers and Zweifach (1947) in support of the formation of an endocapillary layer due to the adsorption of a plasma protein.

Chambers and Copley (1947, 1953) developed a method for testing capillary fragility under biomicroscopic observation. The test agent was injected intradermally into the nictitating membrane of the rabbit's eye, and the corresponding membrane of the other eye was used as control. With this method, we studied many capillary hemorrhage producing or so-called capillorrhagic agents of chemical, bacterial, plant and animal origins (Copley and Chambers, 1953).

In later investigations using the Chambers-Copley method, the author produced numerous petechial hemorrhages in experiments with fibrinolysin (plasmin). What was striking in these experiments was a long latent period from 24 to 64 min, when the first petechiae appeared suddenly and rather explosively. The evaluation of these experimental findings led him to postulate the concept of the endoendothelial fibrin lining (EEFL), which was presented in 1953 at the XIXth International Physiological Congress in Montreal (Copley, 1953, 1954, 1983).

Most electron microscopists denied the existence of an endovascular layer, lining the luminal site of capillary or minute blood vessels. This changed in 1964, when Luft, 1965, 1966 (see also Copley, 1983), employing his new technique of ruthenium red staining, reported a thin, delicate layer. He thought that this endovascular layer, which he also found to extend to the interendothelial junction (Luft, 1966), consists solely of certain acid mucopolysaccharides. However, Copley and Scheinthal reported in 1970 (Copley, 1983) that both fibrinogen and fibrin are stained with ruthenium red, as well.

In using uranyl acetate staining, Palade and Bruns (1964) reported in 1964 diaphragms closing the fenestrae of the endothelium of visceral capillaries and the opening of endothelial vesicles in visceral and muscle capillaries (see also Palade, 1968). In 1964 Palade and Bruns postulated these diaphragms to be either part of a continuous, independent layer supposedly made up of proteins, covering the cell membranes of the endothelium on both the luminal and tissue sites, or layers of cell membrane itself, left behind by a process of cell membrane-vesicle fusion.

During the past few years, Michel (1979, 1980, 1981, 1984), Curry and Michel (1980) reported their findings of a porous endovascular lining on the endothelial cells extending to the interendothelial junctions, which were discussed in some detail in the author's recent publications (Copley, 1983a, b, 1984b). Michel described, in 1979, findings regarding measurements of filtration coefficients and osmotic reflection coefficients of single capillaries in the frog mesentery. His studies led him to postulate that the "selectivity of the capillary pore system lies in a three-dimensional net of extracellular material which covers the surface of the endothelial cells and fills the cracks between them (Michel, 1979)." This evaluation of his experimental findings supports strongly the concept of the EEFL, as well as its extension in surrounding the endothelial cells.

Other Findings and Phenomena Pertaining to the EEFL

As stated in the introductory remarks, it is not possible to deal in this presentation with all findings and phenomena regarding the EEFL. However, certain findings and their interpretations are highly significant in the physiology and pathophysiology of the vessel-blood organ.

Silberberg (1983) considered the EEFL on the basis of present knowledge on the adsorption of macromolecules to solid/liquid interfaces. He concluded that it is possible "to conceive of mechanisms by which an EEFL is not only built up but would also function as proposed by Copley."

The Copley-Scott Blair phenomenon, i.e., the lowering of apparent viscosity of blood and plasma in fibrin-lined capillary viscometers (Oka, 1981, 1983a, b, 1984, this book; Sigal, 1984) has been dealt with by Oka in his presentation (this book). It may be expected that this phenomenon aids the action of the heart in the microcirculation, because of the immense surface area of the EEFL in all capillary blood vessels (Copley, 1981).

The liberation of fibrinopeptides A and B during the conversion of fibrinogen to fibrin and that of plasminopeptides in the conversion of plasminogen to plasmin occur in close proximity to the endothelium. Since we found that these peptides augment capillary permeability, their occurrence at this site contributes directly to the physiological leakiness of the capillary blood vessels (Copley, 1964a; Copley et al., 1967). The quantitative determinations of capillary permeability were made with the Aschheim-Zweifach method (Aschheim et al., 1963), employing radioiodinated albumin, and with the Copley-Carol method, using horseradish peroxidase, which we introduced in 1964 as an indicator in the physiology of the microcirculation (Copley and Carol, 1964). Both methods gave similar results.

Pigman et al. (1961) found that in the presence of some proteins a slowly dissociable bond is formed between the protein and the gel structure of hyaluronic acid, which they considered important in the permeability of the intercellular ground substance in connective tissue. Based on these findings a dissociable bond may exist between hyaluronic acid and fibrin (Copley, 1963, 1964a). Furthermore, hyaluronic acid may be present in close proximity to the EEFL. It may act to liberate or dissociate fibrinolysin or plasmin, or an activator of plasminogen, and make it available for fibrino(geno)lysis. The

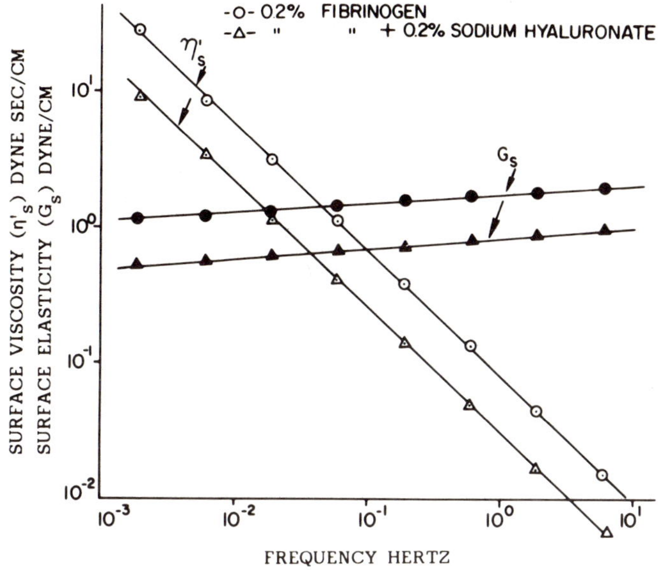

FIG. 2. Surface viscosity and surface elasticity versus frequency of 0.2% fibrinogen solution, as control, compared with 0.2% fibrinogen solution to which 0.2% sodium hyaluronate was added. See: Copley and King (1984).

marked inhibition of fibrinogenin formation by sodium hyaluronate, shown in Fig. 2, is of interest in this connection. The figure shows a decrease of about 50% in viscosity and elasticity of surface layers of solutions of 0.2% fibrinogen, to which 0.2% sodium hyaluronate was added (Copley and King, 1984). A relationship may exist between the release of plasmin and/or the plasminogen activator from the EEFL by hyaluronic acid and the latter's action in inhibiting fibrinogenin gelation. The release of plasmin may well have a regulatory action upon the integrity of the capillary wall, affecting both capillary permeability and capillary fragility, two physical phenomena which we discovered to behave antagonistically (Copley, 1964, 1980; Copley and Tsuluca, 1962).

By measuring contact angles of fibrin surfaces, we found that fibrin surface is wettable (Copley et al., 1964). We also established wettability of the inner lining of the blood vessel in the living animal (Copley, 1962).

The extremely high rigidity and, as shown in Fig. 3, very high viscoelasticity values, secured in measurements of surface layers of fibrinogen solutions demonstrate that the patency of the capillary blood vessel and the elasticity of its wall (Copley, 1974, 1976, 1981) are aided by the EEFL exposed to high shearing forces. They are particularly high at the walls of vessels of the microcirculation (Copley and King, 1976), as shown diagrammatically in Fig. 4.

An increased concentration of fibrinogen might occur, according to Fry (1973), in an interfacial region and this would exist at the interface between

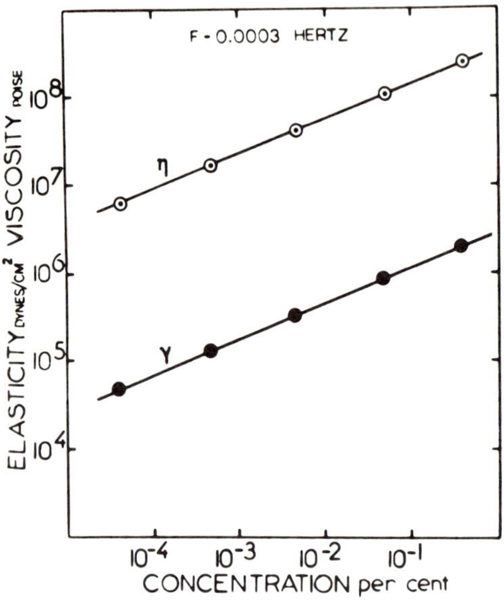

FIG. 3. Comparison of surface viscosity (η'_s) and surface elasticity (γ_s) plotted against different concentrations of human fibrinogen at frequency F=0.0003 Hertz. See: Copley (1984a).

the two portions of the vessel-blood organ, *viz.*, at the EEFL. Fry considers it possible that the maintenance of these chemical concentration gradients within certain limits is vital to the survival of the endothelial cells. His considerations appear to be in support of the existence of the EEFL.

The immigration of leukocytes across the capillary wall was recently proposed to occur according to a hypothesis by the author (Copley, 1983).

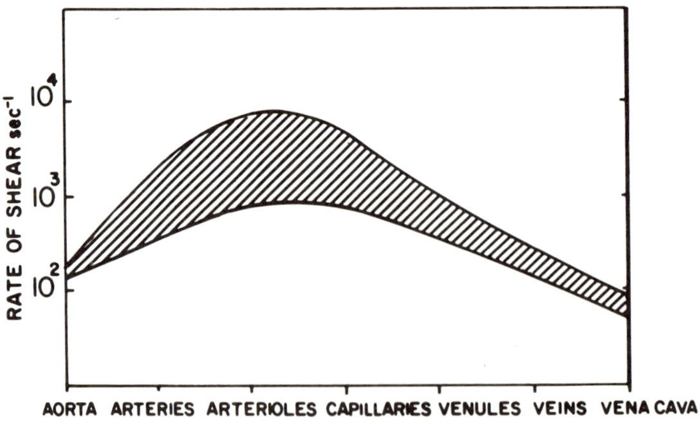

FIG. 4. Compilation of values of wall shear rates in different blood vessels from data by Whitmore (1968), Chien (1972) and Charm and Kurland (1974). See: Copley and King (1976).

It is based on fibrino(geno)lysis produced or initiated either *via* the plasmin system or *via* the alternative pathway of fibrinolytic proteases of the leukocytes. This concerns the EEFL, as well as other fibrin(ogenin) containing structures of the capillary blood vessel wall.

Palade, Simionescu and Simionescu reported findings pertaining to microdomains on the luminal site of the endothelium (Palade et al., 1979, 1981; Simionescu, M., 1981, 1982; Simionescu, N., 1981). These investigators expected that the structures corresponding to the differentiated domains would select, in addition to size, permeant molecules according to charge. They anticipate that fenestral diaphragms discriminate against anionic molecules. Stomatal diaphragms, plasmalemmal vesicles, and transendothelial channels are considered by them to favor the penetration of ionic molecules for diffusion, filtration, and vesicular transport. They pointed out that the majority of plasma proteins are anionic and that the size range remains to be established at which discrimination becomes effective.

The author emphasized that fibrinogen which is negatively charged appears to be selective regarding the adsorption of plasma proteins to its surface layers (Copley, 1971, 1983). Copley (1983) and Copley and King (1974) found that highly purified β-lipoprotein and highly purified γ-globulin nullified the extremely high viscosity and elasticity of the surface layers of the fibrinogen system.

It should be noted that the elastic modulus is a function of the cross-linking within the gel regardless of whether van der Waals forces or covalent bonds are involved. Data concerning the organization of the gel structure are provided by the magnitude of the elastic modulus (Copley, 1983).

Selectivity exists also concerning the adsorption of plasma proteins to the living endoendothelial lining as found by Witte (1981, 1983). Fluorescent labeled fibrinogen and fibronectin, injected intravenously into rats, were adsorbed at the luminal site in the microcirculation of the mesentery, i.e., on the EEFL.

In discussing the observations by Palade, Simionescu and Simionescu, the author stated that these microdomains may well be related to, intertwined with, or in close contact with the EEFL (Copley, 1983).

Of particular interest are Luft's findings (1966) regarding the contents of the vesicles stained with ruthenium red, "as if their contents might in some way be related to the fluffy layer" or endocapillary layer. Luft's observations suggest that the vesicles may contain — as we see it — cement fibrin. They also suggest that the endothelial cells may secrete or liberate into their vesicles substances which — again as we see it — may activate fibrin formation and fibrino(geno)lysis. Such possibilities about the roles of vesicles, which hitherto have not been considered, would offer, in addition to the transport function, other functions for the presence of vesicles and their contents in endothelial cells.

It should be noted that Chien et al. (1981, 1982) used ruthenium red as an extracellular marker in studies of endothelial vesicles *in situ*. They differentiated between vesicles which were free in the cytoplasm and vesicles with a stalk which were attached as temporary invaginations of the plasma membrane. The contents of the attached vesicles were stained with ruthenium red in contrast to those of the free vesicles. The findings of free vesicles by

Chien et al. (1982) are probably due to the procedure they employed of applying ruthenium red as an extracellular marker. Nevertheless, there possibly could be non-stained free vesicles following ruthenium red staining if the procedure which Luft originally used is followed. In such a case, certain open vesicles might not contain fibrinogen and plasminogen, but could contain factors, liberated from the endothelial cell, which would promote fibrin(ogenin) formation and fibrino(geno)lysis.

It appears from Luft's observations (1966) that the contents of both stalked and free vesicles are stained by ruthenium red. Since it is not a specific stain, as we found (Copley and Scheinthal, 1970), the electrodense stain, which filled the contents of the stalked and free vesicles and the interendothelial junctions, could not be interpreted to exclude fibrin and/or fibrinogenin.

Luft's findings regarding the contents of the vesicles appear to provide additional evidence that pinocytosis, traversing the endothelial cell, exists besides the transcapillary transport *via* the interendothelial junctions. In case fibrin(ogenin) is actually contained in the vesicles, the question becomes highly significant, whether fibrin and/or fibrinogenin are also important in vesicular transport.

The Structures of the Blood Capillary Wall and Transcapillary Transport

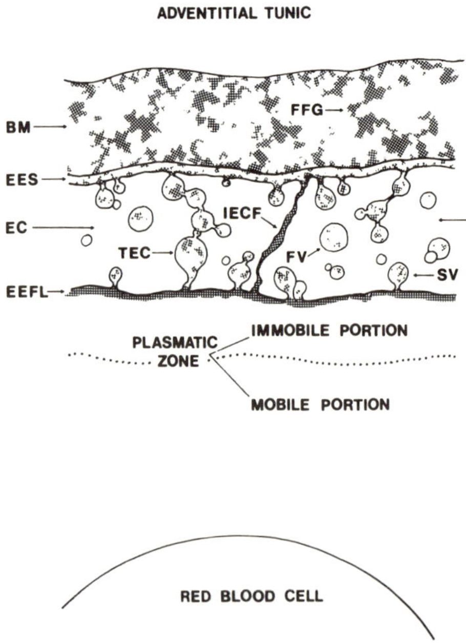

FIG. 5. Diagram illustrating the layers of the blood capillary wall and the location of the 'cement fibrin' in the basement membrane (BM) and surrounding the endothelial cell (EC) including the endo-endothelial fibrin lining (EEFL) in accordance with Copley's theory. Adventitial tunic (AT); focal fibrin(ogenin) gel (FFG); exoendothelial space (EES); free vesicle (FV); stalked vesicle (SV); transendothelial channel (TEC); interendothelial cement fibrin (IECF); plasmatic zone (PZ); immobile portion (IP); mobile portion (MP); red blood cell (RBC).

In Fig. 5, a diagrammatic picture of the microstructure of the blood capillary wall is given which illustrates its different layers. The diagram is meant to convey a general idea without suggesting scale and dimensions and without necessarily simulating the appearance of elements in the microstructure of the capillary wall.

The term "blood capillary" is used as a generic term for any capillary or minute blood vessel of the microcirculation (Copley, 1983a).

The layers and spaces, comprising the capillary wall are: (I) the immobile portion of the plasmatic zone, (II) the endoendothelial fibrin lining (EEFL), (III) the endothelium, consisting of (A) the endothelial cells and (B) the interendothelial cement filling the clefts or junctions, (IV) the exoendothelial space, (V) the basement membrane (BM), and (VI) the adventitial tunic.

The author considers the EEFL and its extension not merely between the endothelial cells, but also surrounding them, and the foci of fibrin and/or fibrinogenin structures in the BM as the principal filtration barriers in transcapillary transport. In these considerations the EEFL is the crucial barrier in all capillary blood vessels. Although this concept does not ascribe to the endothelial cells a role as the primary transcapillary barrier, he emphasized in recent publications (Copley, 1983, 1984b), that the endothelial cells are of great significance in the exchanges between the blood and the tissues.

Moreover, it is stressed that the endothelial cells may have a regulatory function for the formation and lysis of fibrin and fibrinogenin.

Since several speakers at this symposium deal with the endothelial cells and their functions, the author's remarks are limited to what is stated above. However, it is reemphasized that the endothelium consists of the endothelial cells and the interendothelial cement. This fact is contrary to the assumption, which equates the endothelium with the endothelial cells. This assumption also supports the belief that findings secured from cultured endothelial cells mirror fully processes in the entire endothelium. There can be no question that studies on endothelial cell cultures promise continued advancement of knowledge on the endothelium, but they cannot replace studies made *in situ* with adequate precautions, procedures and controls.

Later, in this presentation, the BM will be dealt with.

FIBRINOGENIN FORMATION *EXTRA VIVUM* AND *IN VIVO*

Initial fibrinogen aggregation and subsequent fibrinogen gelation comprise the two phases of fibrinogenin formation as shown in Fig. 6. Cohen and her associates (1983) claimed that their combined studies of electron microscopy and x-ray crystallography of preparations of aggregates and gels of modified fibrinogen account as well for the architecture of fibrin gels.

Gollwitzer et al. (1983a, b) studied aggregates and gels of non-altered or non-modified human and bovine fibrinogen without thrombin action *extra vivum* from segment-like precipitates to highly ordered paracrystals. Their studies proved that solutions of crude or highly purified fibrinogen will aggregate and form gels *extra vivum* without thrombin. Fibrinogen aggregates appeared identical to fibrin in electron microscopic studies by Weisel et al. (1983). They obtained fibrin-like arrays at high ionic strength, where the

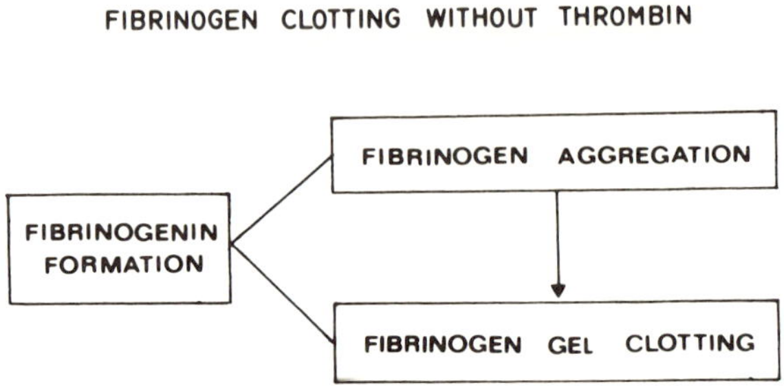

FIG. 6. The two phases of fibrinogenin formation. See: Copley (1983).

charges on fibrinogen are shielded, allowing otherwise not occurring interactions between fibrinogen molecules.

Witte (1980) observed biomicroscopically the formation of fibrinogenin gels in the microcirculation. *In vivo* fibrinogenin formation, which is significant in thrombogenesis and in the initiation of hemostasis, may well contribute to the integrity of the capillary wall and constitute one of its microstructures. Fibrinogen molecules, possibly adsorbed to the EEFL, would aggregate and form fibrinogenin gels.

Cement Fibrin and the Role of Calcium-Fibrin(ogenin) Complexes

There appear to be seven constitutents of cement fibrin, shown in Fig. 7. The concept of a cement substance, originating from a plasma protein and filling the clefts between the endothelial cells, is based on biomicroscopic findings by Chambers and Zweifach (1947). They considered this substance as a calcium-protein complex, which they named 'calcium proteinate' (Chambers and Zweifach, 1944).

The concept of 'cement fibrin' was first proposed by the author in 1962 (1964a), at which time the *in vivo* occurrence of fibrinogenin was not yet known. Cement fibrin was originally considered to consist of "at least three components: one, fibrin particles in initial stages of polymerization; two, a calcium containing fibrin or 'calcium fibrinate'; and three, fibrin breakdown particles due to fibrinolysis." Cement fibrin was thought to constitute the EEFL, and "to surround the endothelial cells" probably not in form of a continuous lining, but rather dispersed, as suggested above between the endothelial cells, in the exoendothelial space and in the BM itself (Copley, 1964b)".

'Atypical fibrin' in Fig. 7 refers to a fibrin formed by thrombin action on fibrinogen, partially altered by fibrinogenolysis. Fibrinogen-fibrin complexes have been described by Copley et al. (1964, 1968, 1970) and other authors (Stathakis et al., 1978). There are also fibrin fragments due to partial fibrinolysis.

Majno and Palade described the presence of fibrin in 1961 (Majno and Palade, 1961; see also Copley, 1964a, b) in their electron microscopic observations on the effect of histamine and serotonin at the 12 min stage as follows: "It was fairly common to observe filaments of fibrin, recognizable

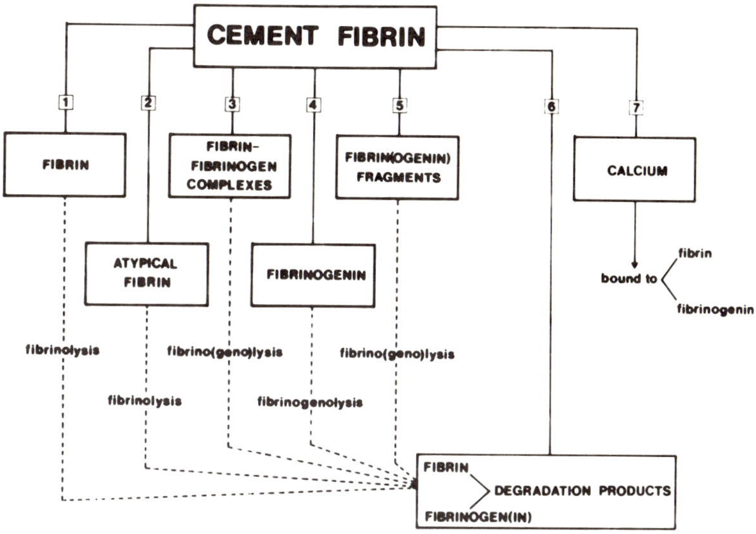

FIG. 7. Diagram illustrating the composition of 'cement fibrin'.

by the characteristic transverse striation with a period of 220Å." "Scattered among the filaments of fibrin were small masses or pools of granular material (Fig. 17, pp. 598–599); whether these represented, in part at least, fibrin at an early stage of polymerization could not be determined. No fibrin filaments were seen outside the basement membrane in the connective tissue." The granular masses might be interpreted, at least in part as fibrin(ogenin) fragments or breakdown particles of fibrin (and fibrinogenin) due to fibrino(geno)-lysis.

Certain proteins and other substances may be adsorbed to cement fibrin due to their affinity to fibrin surface.

It appears not yet to be generally known that the anticoagulant and antithrombotic actions of the endothelium can be due to the adsorption of proteins and other plasma constituents, such as thrombin or plasmin, to fibrin surface, as reported already nearly a quarter of a century ago (Copley, 1964b).

Calcium is considered to be bound to fibrin and possibly also to fibrinogenin. The latter possibility is supported by our recently published findings on the effect of calcium on the viscoelasticity of surface layers of fibrinogen. As shown in Fig. 8, the addition of 0.5 mM calcium chloride to the 0.2% solution of highly purified human fibrinogen caused an increase in the values of surface viscosity and surface elasticity of 30 and 40%, respectively (Copley and King, 1983). These findings are of particular significance with regard to the patency of the vascular lumen (Copley, 1974) and the elasticity of the vascular wall.

It is known that the addition of calcium ions to a plasma or a fibrinogen solution, to which thrombin is added, results in large increases in the rigidity and viscoelasticity of these gels (Copley, 1970; Shen et al., 1975).

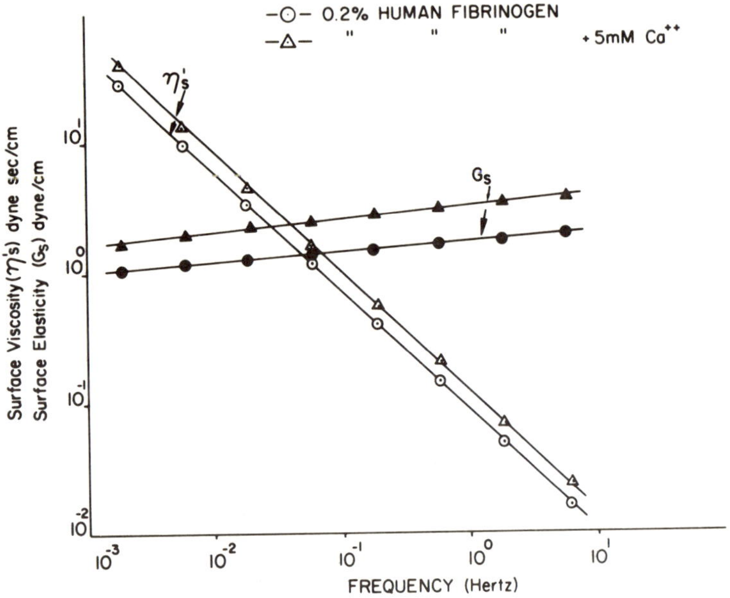

FIG. 8. Values of surface viscosity η'_s —○— and surface elasticity G'_s —●— of a 0.2% fibrinogen solution as control, compared with values of η'_s —△—, and G'_s —▲— upon the addition of 5mMCa^{2+}. See: Copley and King (1983).

Blombäck and Okada (1983) found that increasing calcium concentrations in fibrin formation favored more porous and plastic gels, whereas a decrease in calcium concentration resulted in tight and friable gels.

Henschen (1983) stated that, since the complete covalent structure of human fibrinogen is known, it is now possible to establish structure-function relationships. She pointed out that fibrinogen was found to contain several calcium-binding sites and that calcium ions are known to serve often in the stabilization of protein structure. She refers to the author's suggestion that the fibrin of the EEFL may exist as a calcium-fibrin complex (Copley, 1981). Since several calcium-binding sites exist in fibrinogen, calcium is probably also bound to fibrinogenin.

ENDOTHELIAL CELL SURFACE, INTERENDOTHELIAL JUNCTIONS, AND THE EEFL

The high resolution views of surface replication of the luminal surface of the endothelium, presented last year by Ryan and Ryan (1984a), showed an organized glycocalyx coating, which they consider to play a role in regulating capillary permeability. What, however, these authors did not take into account is the probability that their preparations for electron microscopy neglected taking proper precautions to secure the intactness of the EEFL and the interendothelial cement. Nevertheless, they appear to be aware of the presence of an endocapillary lining and the interendothelial cement. In this connection, they also referred to the EEFL.

In another communication, Ryan and Ryan (1984b) showed the endothelial surface to be "an ever changing one" and at times covered with fingerlike projections and carpeted with a polymeric coat of extracellular materials. They contended that the endothelial surface influences, among other activities, coagulation and fibrinolysis and, *via* carbonic anhydrase, controls the pH (Ryan and Ryan, 1984b).

In addition to surface enzymes, Ryan and Ryan considered endothelial receptors to provide direct cellular responses (Ryan and Ryan, 1984b). They claimed that "blood-borne signals received by surface receptors are translated into intracellular actions (including synthesis and release of active compounds, changes in cell shape, and alterations in vascular tone and permeability)" and that local differences in charge during agonist-receptor binding may be produced. They concluded that endothelial functions and structural correlates of these functions are "more complex than previously recognized."

The passive transport of water through the endothelial cell layer from the standpoint of hydrodynamic theories, based on ultrastructural information, was examined last year by Hsiung and Skalak (1984). They modeled the local geometry of tight junctions, based on molecular level forces and elastic membrane properties, which led to estimates of the hydraulic resistance of the clefts. They claimed that their model accounts for the large resistance measured experimentally. These authors contended that recent experimental data do not appear to support as a primary pathway the transport of large macromolecules *via* vesicles and considered fused vesicles forming an open channel to be rare. They claim that leaky junctions, such as around dying endothelial cells or produced within the cells by cytochemical changes to be important in endothelial permeability.

Hsiung and Skalak discussed the fiber matrix model of the endocapillary layer entending into the intercellular clefts as the other kind of model and considered the stress required to further widen the interendothelial junctions. On the basis of their computations, they suggested that the normal spacing of approximately $100-150$ Å is controlled by bridging molecules in the interendothelial cleft which are transparent under electron microscopy. As an example of this invisibility under the electron microscope, they referred to observations of the formation of rouleaux of red blood cells that the aggregating molecules, such as dextran, "control the width of the spacing between adjacent cell membranes." These authors stressed that "such molecular bridging would not necessarily need to provide a barrier to the passage of large molecular species, or increase the pressure drop, or the resistance to flow through the junctions greatly." These effects were considered to depend on the diameters of the fibers and their spacing (Hsiung and Skalak, 1984).

Hsiung and Skalak (1984) discussed the fibrin network as the principal structure in the endoendothelial lining. They suggested the making of detailed mathematical models, when the molecular structure of the EEFL becomes more fully known. Although *extra vivum* fibrin gel structures cannot be fully equated with the structure of the EEFL, the recent studies by Blombäck et al. (1984) may well give an approximation for such models.

THE BASEMENT MEMBRANE AND ITS FOCAL FIBRIN(OGENIN) GELS

The vascular basement membrane (BM), first recognized by Chrozonszczewski in 1866 (Copley, 1983), is an extracellular matrix composed of collagenous and non-collagenous glycoproteins (Copley, 1964a, 1965, 1969; Kuehn et al., 1982; Farquhar et al., 1983).

The BM consists of different zones which may vary rather widely in thickness. Among the components which constitute the BM are type IV collagen, laminin, heparan sulfate, proteoglycan and fibronectin (Farquhar, 1983). Its other component is fibrin and/or fibrinogenin. In 1957 and 1958 we reported the experimental production of (non-thrombocytopenic) vascular purpura in guinea-pigs and hamsters with fibrin antiserum of rabbits (Copley and Marēchal, 1957; Copley 1958). These findings provide direct evidence for the presence of fibrin in the BM. This component of the BM is essential for the integrity of the blood vessel wall, both pertaining to capillary permeability and capillary fragility.

The processes concerning the existence of fibrin(ogenin) gels in the BM were pictured by the author as follows: "Fibrinogen molecules enter the BM after their passage *via* the EEFL, the interendothelial junctions and the exoendothelial space. Such passage of fibrinogen molecules *via* the fibrin(ogenin) gels of these structures is expected to occur readily. Any further passage is halted in the matrix of the BM, where as continuous processes thrombin-induced fibrin gels and fibrinogenin gels are formed at numerous locations. These gels constitute, together with other components of the BM, the third filtration barrier of the blood capillary wall. Continuous fibrinolysis and fibrinogenolysis maintain homeostasis, preventing the clogging of the pores in the BM and thus keeping them open for transcapillary transport" (Copley, 1984b).

Gollwitzer et al. (1983a) emphasized that fibronectin possesses binding sites for fibrinogen and collagen and thus could act as the mediator of the two proteins. Mosher and Johnson (1983) reported that cross-linking of fibronectin to fibrin is known to occur. It may well take place in the BM. Fibronectin is rapidly incorporated into fibrin gels according to Blombäck and Okada (1983) despite the fact that γ- and α-chains were fully cross-linked. These authors contend that the binding of fibronectin to fibrin gel could serve as an anchor between fibrin gels and other structures.

On the basis of the above mentioned findings, the author contended that fibronectin has an affinity to fibrin surface to which it may be adsorbed (Copley, 1984b). Of particular interest is the location of focal fibrin gels in connection with the integrity of the capillary wall and the assessment of capillary fragility. These focal fibrin gels in the BM may occur with or without association to fibronectin and may be found at certain sites of the BM where fibronectin is present, regardless whether or not it is incorporated into the focal fibrin gels.

Fibrin Gels as Ordered Network Structures and the Porosity of the Capillary Wall

Blombäck and Okada (1983) pointed out that fibrinogen is a gel-forming protein which is not only of importance in hemostasis for the sealing of wounds or defects in the vasculature or, it should be added, in processes of thrombosis, but plays a role in compartmentalizing processes. They mentioned the well-known observation that infectious loci in tuberculosis are usually surrounded by masses of fibrin which are most likely gel structures. They stated that fibrinogen has to undergo activation in order to form a gel. Most commonly the activation is brought about enzymatically by thrombin, but that fibrinogenin formation, which we discussed in many publications (Copley, 1981, 1983a, 1983b, 1984a), is another type of fibrinogen activation, in which thrombin does not play a role. Polymers are formed as a result of activation and eventually gelation occurs.

Liquid and particle permeation experiments with fibrin gels, produced both with thrombin and Batroxobin, were performed by Blombäck and Okada (1983). While thrombin removes fibrinopeptides A and B. Batroxobin, an enzyme from the venom of the Brazilian snake *Bothrops atrox*, removes fibrinopeptide A only. From their experiments, they concluded that "the coagulant forces generated in blood and expressed as thrombin activity will determine the overall permeability and mechanical properties of any fibrin gel structure formed in blood, whether it be physiological hemostatic plugs, the EEFL or thrombin. They also found that changes in electrolyte or protein composition modify their gel formation.

Last year, Blombäck, Okada, Forslind and Larsson (1984) presented data which are of great significance in relation to the EEFL. They demonstrated that fibrin gels are ordered network structures and that their porosity is determined by the amount of thrombin present during the activation step preceding gelation. Fibrinopeptides are released during the action of thrombin on fibrinogen molecules with simultaneous formation of polymers, obeying apparent first order kinetics. These authors found the pore size of the network to be inversely related to the rate of polymer formation. They proposed that the polymers form an ordered lattice structure at the time of gelation and considered this structure to serve as a biological interface in the organism.

Blomback et al. (1984) presented evidence that fibrin gels formed under physiological conditions show considerable regularity. They gave a tentative explanation for the ordered structure which they found visualized by scanning electron micrographs (SEM) in fibrin gels. They considered conformational changes in fibrinogen as the driving force in this polymerization-gelation process. Such conformational changes may create in the solution phase density heterogeneity, which creates a chemical potential. This potential is the result "in flow of non-activated fibrinogen to the intiation points, as a first step in creation of order, out of an initially chaotic situation." They contended that the heterogeneity may also be based on differences in charge, created by the activation, but would have the same end results.

Blombäck et al. discussed the domain character, visualized by their SEM micrographs. Within each domain a lattice of fibrin strands is formed. With the growth of the lattice, its expansion will cause the lattice to come into close contact with similar lattices which originate in other domains. On the basis of their liquid and particle permeation studies, Blombäck et al. assumed that each domain has the same average pore size. From their findings, they raised the question regarding a primordial role of fibrinogen in the organism "for creation of dynamic interfaces for compartmentalization of cells and tissues." They referred to the theory of the EEFL and, after giving certain examples, concluded that "fibrin gels have the potentiality to serve both as

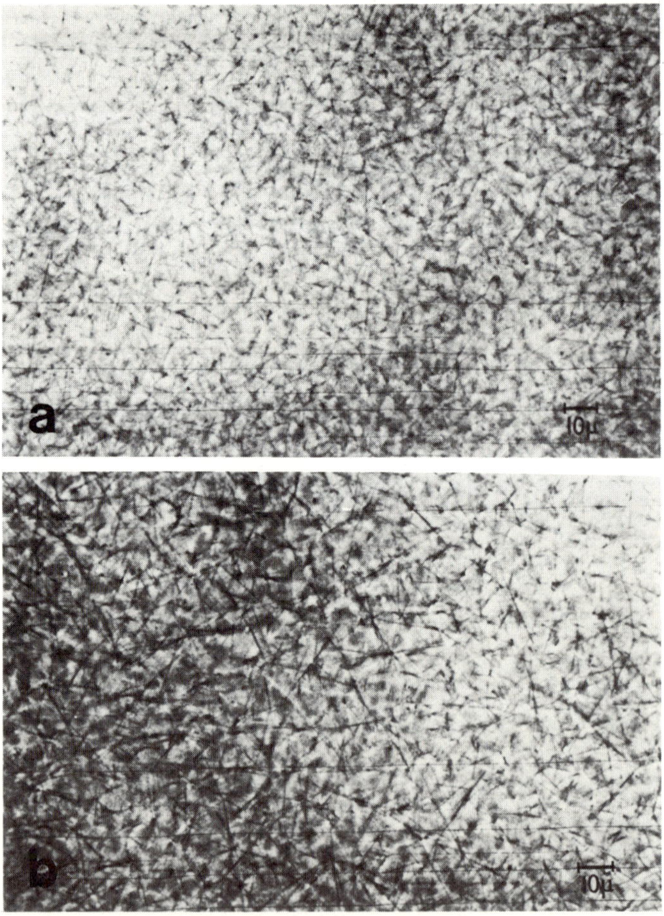

FIG. 9. Fibrin gel matrices observed by Blombäck et al. (1984) by phase contrast microscopy. Note: (a) length and thickness of fibrin strands, crossing at numerous points. (b) smaller pores due to increased enzyme concentration. For detailed description see: Blombäck et al. (1984).

filters and efficient interfaces for the exclusion of cells and particles while, at the same time, allowing for exchange of water, crystalloids and proteins."

Figs. 9 and 10 show fibrin gel matrices produced by Blombäck et al. (1984) and observed by phase contrast light microscopy and scanning electron microscopy. Figs. 9a and 9b revealed straight structures of fibrin strands of rather uniform thickness and length, shown by light microscopy. These strands cross at numerous points. The exact geometry of the network cannot be established in such studies. In Fig. 9b, the strands decrease in thickness and length and the pores become smaller by increasing the enzyme concentration. In Figs. 10a and 10b, the fibrin network structure is visualized by SEM. In Fig. 10a a "honeycomb"-like pore structure is shown. Since some shrinkage

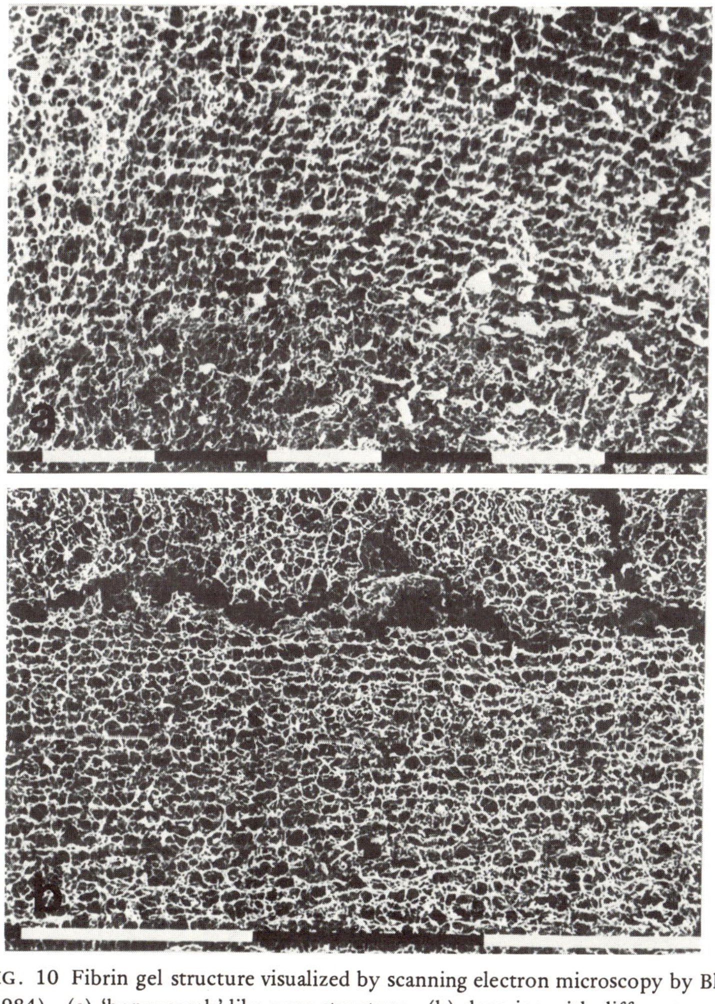

FIG. 10 Fibrin gel structure visualized by scanning electron microscopy by Blombäck et al. (1984). (a) 'honeycomb'-like pore structure; (b) domains with different pore orientation. For detailed description see: Blombäck et al. (1984).

of the matrix structure took place during drying, the exact geometry of the pores could not be defined, but hexagonal and/or rhomboid shaped surfaces are possible. The theoretical average pore size, calculated from liquid permeation data, was of similar magnitude as that estimated from the SEM pictures. Blombäck et al., who gave detailed descriptions of the procedures for securing these pictures, observed, as shown in Fig. 10b, "what appear to be domains with different pore orientation separated by rifts and 'grain boundaries' in the gel matrix (Blombäck et al., 1984)."

ULTRASTRUCTURAL CRITERIA OF GLOMERULAR CAPILLARIES AND LIVER SINUSOIDS WITH THE EEFL AS CRUCIAL FILTRATION BARRIER

In the author's view, the EEFL would be expected as the first filtration barrier in vessels in which the endothelium is discontinuous or where it is fenestrated. The glomerular capillaries have endothelial cells with large fenestrae. Certain blood vessels have no BM, such as the sinusoids of the liver in which the first filtration barrier would also be expected to be the EEFL. Thus, in all blood vessels, whether they have a discontinuous or fenestrated endothelium or where the BM does not exist, the crucial filtration barrier would be the EEFL, as in the author's theory it is expected to be in any blood vessel which contains both the endothelial cells and the BM.

The vessel-blood organ as it concerns the glomeruli of the kidney is indeed very special. According to Farquhar (1983), the glomerular capillaries differ from other capillaries in a number of different respects. Farquhar, Wissig and Palade (1961) studied the localization of the permeability barrier by the use of electron-dense ultrastructural tracers and found ferritin to be most satisfactory. They observed that there was an accumulation of ferritin against the BM in the exoendothelial space, i.e., between the endothelium and the BM, especially in the mesangial or axial regions. Farquhar concluded that these studies support "the concept that the BM acts as the main barrier to the passage of molecules in the same size range as plasma proteins" (Farquhar, 1975).

In physiological studies it has been demonstrated by Brenner et al. (1977, 1978) and Rennke et al. (1978) that the glomerular capillaries function as a size-and charge-selective barrier in the retention of plasma proteins in the circulation and in the production of the glomerular filtrates. Sialyl residues were detected in isolated glomerular BMs. Kanwar and Farquhar (1979a) showed the presence of a quasiregular network of anionic sites in the *laminae rarae* (internal and external) of the glomerular basement membrane (GBM). These authors found the occurrence of sulfated glycosaminoglycans rich in heparan sulfate, which are highly negatively charged components.

Kanwar, Linker and Farquhar (1980) demonstrated in a subsequent paper that "heparan sulfate plays a role in creating the normal restrictive permeability properties of the GBM to macromolecules." Anionic sites, similar to those in the GBM, are widely distributed in BMs, as shown in earlier findings by Farquhar (1975).

In histochemical and electron microscopic investigations of rat kidney and liver, Seno, Ono and Tsujii (1983) studied the role of charged groups of tissue components on the integrity of the blood capillary wall. Their findings indicate that anionic groups of proteins are "very important for the protection of plasma protein leakage through capillary walls." Such protein leakage was prevented by newly formed fibrin-fibrinogen layers lining the endothelial walls. In scanning electron microscopy (SEM) of the luminal surface of glomerular capillaries, perfused with cationic iron colloid (CI), they found increased endothelial desquamations and deformation adsorbing amorphous gross depositions. In transmission electron microscopy of the glomerular capillaries perfused with CI, they observed swollen and desquamating endothelial cells with the colloid particles on the luminal surface as well as in the BM, particularly in the *lamina rara interna*.

In the sinusoids of the liver, Seno et al. found, following immuno-histochemical staining of fibrinogen, the occurrence of "thick fibrin-fibrinogen lining of the walls of sinusoids which had heavy CI deposition. Similar morphologic changes of the liver as in CI perfusion were found with protamine sulfate perfusion. They observed a thick fibrin-fibrinogen lining surrounding the sinusoidal walls with fibrin-fibrinogen deposition on the luminal site of the endothelial cells. No diffuse fibrinogen staining was found in neighboring tissues (Seno et al., 1983).

The findings by Seno et al. appear to support the concept that in the case of glomerular capillaries the EEFL is the main filtration barrier. This seems to be also the case in the liver sinusoids, where the endothelial cells appear to be surrounded by layers of fibrin and possibly containing also fibrinogenin. The amorphous gross depositions may be partially lysed fibrin and/or fibrinogenin similar to the granular deposits observed by Majno and Palade (1961), referred to earlier in this presentation.

For the documentation of the presence of proteoglycans in the BM, Kanwar and Farquhar (1979b, 1980) used ruthenium red. Earlier in this presentation the findings by Copley and Scheinthal were cited, which demonstrated that ruthenium red is not a specific stain for proteoglycans as it also stains fibrinogen and fibrin (Copley and Scheinthal, 1970). The glycosaminoglycans, as identified by ruthenium red staining in the BM by Kanwar and Farquhar (1979a, 1979b), may well be associated with fibrin(ogenin), located at these particular sites, since on the basis of their findings they cannot be excluded as constituent(s) of the BM. Moreover, Kanwar and Farquhar may possibly have provided the first electron microscopic evidence for the presence of fibrin(ogenin) in the BM.

On the Action of Fibrin(ogenin) as Main Constitutent for Filtration in All Capillary Blood Vessels

It is realized that the assignment of gels of fibrin and/or fibrinogenin as main constituent of capillary blood vessels is an extraordinary claim which can no longer be ignored in considerations of the physiology and pathophysiology of transcapillary transport.

The author can only reiterate what he stated recently (Copley, 1984b). "The question must be raised: Why were these fibrin or fibrin related substances never been observed, for instance in electron microscopic studies? This question can be readily answered. In securing tissue samples for such studies, blood vessels will have to be severed in the living animal. This will result instantaneously in the generation of fibrinolytic enzymes. These enzymes, which do not necessarily need to be plasmin or plasmin-like substances, will rapidly destroy any fibrin or fibrinogenin structures. To the author's knowledge, no attempts have been made by electron microscopists to counteract any fibrinolytic action by the use of inhibitors not only directed against plasmin or plasmin-like enzymes, e.g., by Trasylol. Other enzymes, such as cathepsins, elastase, etc. have also not been considered to be counteracted in their fibrinolytic or fibrinogenolytic actions. However, such precautions are not enough.

One also needs to prevent the collapse of a fibrin(ogenin) gel during the preparation procedure prior to electron microscopy. With the techniques hitherto used, such precautions were not possible. The specimen was dehydrated and the prior fixation with glutaraldehyde may not be necessarily sufficient, since the collapse of the gel structures may already have taken place. In this context, it should be emphasized that the fractional volume of the gel matrix is exceedingly minute and even for high fibrinogen concentrations it is usually less than 1% (Blombäck, 1983). This means that the gel matrix can easily be overlooked, especially if the gel is collapsed and what remains may be merely a strand even though precautions against fibrin(ogen)olysis were made.

It is quite possible that better information could be obtained by the use of other electron microscopic techniques, such as freeze-etching. In this connection, the approach recently developed by Blombäck et al. (1984) is of great interest. They showed that sectioning fibrin gels, produced *extra vivum*, resulted in collapse of the gels. On the other hand, observations by scanning electron microscopy of crack surfaces, which appeared naturally during the freeze-drying process, revealed the ordered nature of the fibrin network (Figs. 10a, 10b).

The approach by Blombäck et al. has certain similarities with the freeze-etching technique and, anyway, shows that entirely new approaches may yield rewarding results. It is now up to the morphologists to find or invent new approaches to make, in the microstructure of the blood capillary wall, the hitherto unseen *in vivo* fibrin and fibrinogenin visible" (Copley, 1984b).

Abstract

The endoendothelial fibrin(ogenin) lining (EEFL) is considered by the author to be *the* interface between the two portions of the 'vessel-blood organ', *viz.*, the vessel wall and the circulating blood. The view is no longer tenable that the endothelium, consisting of the endothelial cells and the interendothelial cement, is the primary filtration barrier in transcapillary transport. Considerable experimental evidence exists that the primary barrier is the EEFL, which is formed in close proximity to the vessel wall in the more or less immobile portion of the plasmatic zone. There, homeostatic processes of fibrin(ogenin) formation and fibrino(geno)lysis can occur, undisturbed by the flow of blood. The EEFL may contain calcium as calcium fibrinate, and fibrinogenin, i.e. aggregates or gels of fibrinogen formed without thrombin, and fibrinogen-fibrin complexes. These and other substances constitute the 'cement fibrin', contained in the interendothelial junctions, the basement membrane (BM), and possibly also in the stalked and free pinocytic vesicles. The EEFL is also considered to be the crucial barrier in capillaries where the endothelium is discontinuous or, as in the glomerular capillaries, is fenestrated, as well as in vessels which have no BM, as the sinusoids of the liver. Proteins and other substances in plasma may have affinity to fibrin and fibrinogenin surface and thus be adsorbed to the EEFL. A dissociable bond may exist between hyaluronic acid and the EEFL. It may dissociate plasmin or an activator of plasminogen and make it available for fibrino(geno)lysis. Fibrin(ogenin) gels are considered among the main constituents in each of the three structures in the architecture of the blood capillary wall, *viz.*, as EEFL, interendothelial cement, and foci in the BM. The apparently selective properties of gels of fibrin and fibrinogenin, their porosity and the possibly adjustable pore size, serve in transcapillary transport. The EEFL interface is significant in different physiological processes. They concern the Copley-Scott Blair phenomenon which affects the circulating blood in aiding the action of the heart in the microcirculation. The EEFL is likewise significant in its anticlotting and antithrombotic functions, in maintaining vascular patency among other vital functions. Certain precautions must be made and *in situ* techniques will need to be developed and invented pertaining to light and electron microscopy to make the hitherto unseen *in vivo* fibrin and fibrinogenin visible as cement fibrin.

Acknowledgement

The author thanks Birger Blombäck of the Karolinska Institute, Stockholm, Sweden and the New York Blood Center, New York, NY, USA for providing the photomicrographs of Figs. 9a and 9b and the electron micrographs of Figs. 10a and 10b for publication in this presentation.

References

Aschheim, E., Tsuluca, V., and Copley, A.L. (1963). Quantitative relation between certain fibrinolysis factors and inflammation. *Proc. Soc. Exp. Biol. Med.* **112**, 434–436.

Blombäck, B. (1983). Personal communication, 6. June.

Blombäck, B., Okada, M., Forslind, B., and Larsson, U. (1984). Fibrin gels as biological filters and interfaces. *Biorheology* **21**, 93–104.

Blombäck, B., and Okada, M. (1983). Fibrin gels and their possible implication for surface hemorheology in health and disease. *Ann. N.Y. Acad. Sci.* **416**, 397–409.

Brenner, B.M., Bohrer, M.P., Baylis, C., and Deen, W.M. (1977). Determinants of glomerular permselectivity. Insights derived from observations *in vivo*. *Kidney Int.* **12**, 229–237.

Brenner, B.M., Hostetter, T.H., and Humes, H.D. (1978). Molecular basis of proteinuria of glomerular origin. *N. Engl. J. Med.* **298**, 826–833.

Chambers, R., and Zweifach, B.W. (1940). Capillary endothelial cement in relation to permeability. *J. Cellular Comp. Physiol.* **15**, 255–273.

Chambers, R., and Zweifach, B.W. (1944). Topography and function of mesenteric capillary circulation. *Am. J. Anat.* **75**, 173–205.

Chambers, R., and Zweifach, B.W. (1947). Intercellular cement and capillary permeability. *Physiol. Rev.* **27**, 436–463.

Chambers, R., and Copley, A.L. (1947). A method and observations on capillary fragility in rabbits. *Fed. Proc., Fed. Am. Soc. Exp. Biol.* **6**, 88.

Chien, S., Lee, M.M.L., Laufer, L.S., Handley, D.A., Weinbaum, S., Caro, C.G., and Usami, S. (1981). Effects of oscillatory mechanical disturbance on macromolecular uptake by arterial wall. *Arteriosclerosis* **1**, 326–336.

Chien, S., Laufer, L., and Handley, D.A. (1982). Vesicle distribution in the arterial endothelium determined with ruthenium red as an extracellular marker. *J. Ultrastruct. Res.* **79**, 198–206.

Cohen, C., Weisel, J.W., Phillips, Jr., G.N., Stauffacher, C.U., Fillers, J.P., and Daub, E. (1983). The structure of fibrinogen and fibrin. I. Electron microscopy and X-ray crystallography of fibrinogen. *Ann. N.Y. Acad. Sci.* **408**, 194–213.

Cohnheim, J. (1873). Neue Untersuchungen ueber die Entzuendung. Berlin, A. Hirschwald.

Copley, A.L., and Chambers, R. (1953). Experimentally induced petechial hemorrhage and white embolization in the rabbit's nictitating membrane. *Am. Heart J.* **45**, 237–251.

Copley, A.L. (1953). On a new physiologic role of fibrin and the capillorrhagic effect of fibrinolysis in normal and x-irradiated rabbits. *In* "Abstracts of Communic. XIXth Internat. Physiol. Congr. Montreal, Canada" pp. 280–281.

Copley, A.L. (1954). Effet capillorrhagique de la fibrinolysine et de l'antifibrinolysine sur la membrane nictitante du lapin normal et exposé aux rayons X. *Arch. Int. Pharmacodyn. Tér.* **99**, 426–434.

Copley, A.L., and Maréchal, J. (1957). Le taux de fibrinogène et la numeration des plaquettes dans le purpura vasculaire produit chez le cobaye par du sérum de lapin anti-fibrine de cobaye. *J. de Physiol.* **49**, 987–991.

Copley, A.L. (1958). Vascular purpura in guinea-pigs and hamsters produced by guinea-pig antifibrin rabbit serum. *In* "Transact. 6th Congr. Europ. Soc. Haemat., Copenhagen 1957" pp. 518–522. S. Karger, Basel, New York.

Copley, A.L., and Staple, P.H. (1962). Haemorheological studies on the plasmatic zone in the microcirculation of the cheek pouch of Chinese and Syrian hamsters. *Biorheology* **1**, 3–14.

Copley, A.L. (1962). The endoendothelial fibrin film and fibrinolysis. *In* "Proc. VIIIth Internat. Congr. Hematol. Tokyo, 1960" Vol. 3, pp. 1648–1666. Pan-Pacific Press, Tokyo.

Copley, A.L., and Tsuluca, V. (1962). The antibradykinin action of fibrinolysin and other studies on capillary permeability employing different mediators and synthetic bradykinin. *In* "Proc. 1st Internat. Pharmacological Meeting Stockholm 1961" (M. Rocha e Silva and U.S. von Euler, eds.), pp. 67–85. Pergamon Press, Oxford; *Biochem. Pharmacol.* **10**, 67–85.

Copley, A.L. (1963). On a dissociable bond between fibrinogen and surfaces of native fibrin and pseudo-cement fibrins. *Fed. Proc., Fed. Am. Soc. Exp. Biol.* 22, 619.

Copley, A.L. (1964a). Capillary permeability versus fragility and the significance of fibrin as a physiologic cement of the blood vessel wall. *In* "2nd Europ. Conf. on Microcirculation, Pavia, 1962" (H. Harders, ed.), S. Karger, Basel, New York, *Bibl. Anat.* 4, 3–19.

Copley, A.L. (1964b). On the anticoagulant action of fibrin in the prevention of thrombosis. *In* "Proc. IXth Congr. Internat. Soc. Hematol. Mexico City 1962" Vol. II, pp. 367–378. Universidad Nacional Autonoma de Mexico, Mexico City.

Copley, A.L., and Carol, B. (1964). Inhibiting action of epsilon aminocaproic acid on capillary permeability in guinea-pigs tested with new quantitative method based on Straus' peroxidase procedure. Variance and covariance analyses. *Life Sci.* 3, 65–76.

Copley, A.L., Glover, F.A., and Scott Blair, G.W. (1964). The wettability of fibrinized surfaces and of living vascular endothelium by blood. *Biorheology* 2, 29–35.

Copley, A.L., and Luchini, B.W. (1964). The binding of human fibrinogen to native fraction fibrins and the inhibition of polymerization of a new human fibrin monomer by fibrinogen. *Life Sci.* 3, 1293–1305.

Copley, A.L. (1965). Capillary permeability, capillary incontinence, compaction stasis and basement membrane breakdown. *Bibl. Anat.* 7, 148–155.

Copley, A.L., Hanig, J.P., Luchini, B.W., and Allen, Jr., R.L. (1967). On the capillary permeability enhancing activity of isolated fibrinopeptides and their role in the physiology of the blood capillary wall. *In* "Proc. IVth Europ. Conf. Microcirculation. Cambridge, England, 1966" (H. Harders, ed.), pp. 475–481. S. Karger, Basel, New York; *Bibl. Anat.* 9, 475–481.

Copley, A.L., Luchini, B.W., and Whelan, E.W. (1968). On the role of fibrinogen-fibrin complexes in flow properties and suspension stability of blood systems. *In* "Hemorheology. Proc. 1st Internat. Conf. Univ. of Iceland, Reykjavik 1966" (A.L. Copley, ed.), pp. 375–388. Pergamon Press, Oxford, New York.

Copley, A.L. (1969). On cement fibrin, a proposed constituent of the capillary basement membrane, and on lesions in the capillary wall in diabetes mellitus. *In* "Diabetes. Proc. 6th Congr. Internat. Diabetes Fed., Stockholm, Sweden, 1967" (J. Östman and R.D.G. Milner, eds.), pp. 606–609. Excerpta Medica Foundation, Amsterdam.

Copley, A.L., and Scheinthal, B.M. (1970). Nature of the endoendothelial layer as demonstrated by ruthenium red. *Exp. Cell Res.* 59, 491–492.

Copley, A.L. (1970). Some problems in hemorheology. *In* "Proc. 5th Internat. Congr. Rheology" (S. Onogi, ed.), Vol. 2, pp. 3–25. Univ. of Tokyo Press and Univ. Park Press, Tokyo, Baltimore, Manchester.

Copley, A.L. (1971). Non-Newtonian behavior of surface layers of human plasma protein systems and a new concept of the initiation of thrombosis. *Biorheology* 8, 79–84.

Copley, A.L. (1974). Hemorheological aspects of the endothelium-plasma interface. *Microvasc. Res.* **8**, 192–212.

Copley, A.L., and King, R.G. (1972). Viscous resistance of thromboid (thrombus-like) surface layers in systems of plasma proteins including fibrinogen. *Thromb. Res.* **1**, 5–17.

Copley, A.L., and King, R.G. (1974). The reducing action of highly purified γ globulin and β lipoprotein on the viscous resistance of surface layers of fibrinogen. *Thromb. Res.* **4**, 193–198.

Copley, A.L., and King, R.G. (1976). Polymolecular layer of fibrinogen systems and the genesis of thrombosis. *In* "Hemorheology and Thrombosis" (A.L. Copley and S. Okamoto, eds.), pp. 393–409. Pergamon Press, Oxford, New York; *Thromb. Res. Suppl.* **II**, 393–409.

Copley, A.L. (1980). Pathophysiological significance of hemorheological aspects of the endoendothelial fibrin and of fibrinogen gel clotting. *In* "Hemorheology and Diseases" (J.F. Stoltz and P. Drouin, eds.), pp. 293–325. Doin Editeurs, Paris.

Copley, A.L. (1981). Hemorheological aspects of the endoendothelial fibrin lining and of fibrinogen gel clotting. Their importance in physiology and pathological conditions. *Clin. Hemorheology*, 9–72.

Copley, A.L. (1982). Plenary lecture. The future of the science of biorheology. *Biorheology* **19**, 47–69.

Copley, A.L. (Ed.) (1983a). "The Endoendothelial Fibrin Lining, Symposium of the XIIth Europ. Conf. on Microcirculation, Jerusalem, Israel, 7 September 1982" p. 160. Pergamon Press, New York, Oxford; *Thromb. Res. Suppl.* **V**.

Copley, A.L. (1983b). The endoendothelial fibrin lining. A historical account. *In* "The Endoendothelial Fibrin Lining, Symposium of the XIIth Europ. Conf. on Microcirculation, Jerusalem, Israel, 7 September 1982" (A.L. Copley, ed.), pp. 1–26. Pergamon Press New York, Oxford.

Copley, A.L. (1983c). The physiological significance of the endoendothelial fibrin lining (EEFL) as the critical interface in the 'vessel-blood organ' and the importance of *in vivo* 'fibrinogenin formation' in health and disease. *In* 1983a, pp. 105–145.

Copley, A.L. (1983d). The endoendothelial fibrin lining, fibrinogenin gel clotting, and the endothelium-blood interface. *Ann. N.Y. Acad. Sci.* **416**, 377–396.

Copley, A.L., and Seaman, G.V.F. (Eds.) (1983). Surface phenomena in hemorheology: Their theoretical, experimental and clinical aspects. *Ann. N.Y. Acad. Sci.* **416**, p. 761.

Copley, A.L., and King, R.G. (1983). A note on the effect of Ca^{2+} on the viscous and elastic moduli of surface layers of fibrinogen. *Progr. Colloid and Polymer Sci.* **68**, 131–132.

Copley, A.L. (1984a). The importance of hemorheology in the pathophysiology of the vessel-blood organ. *In* "Techniques Avancées en Hémorhéologie. Nancy, France 16–18 Novembre 1983" (M.L. Viriot, J.C. André, M. Lucius and J.F. Stoltz, eds.), pp. 15–62. DPIC-Institut National Polytechnique de Lorraine, Nancy.

Copley, A.L. (1984b). The endoendothelial fibrin lining as the crucial barrier and the role of fibrin(ogenin) gels in controlling transcapillary transport. *Biorheology* **21**, 135–153.

Copley, A.L., and King, R.G. (1984). A survey of surface rheological experiments on the inhibition of fibrinogenin formation employing surface layers of fibrinogen systems with heparins and other substances. A contribution on antithrombogenic action. *Thromb. Res.* **35**, 237–256.

Curry, F.E., and Michel, C.C. (1980). A fibre matrix model of capillary permeability. *Microvasc. Res.* **20**, 96–99.

Danielli, J.F. (1940). Capillary permeability and oedema in the perfused frog. *J. Physiol.* **98**, 109–129.

Farquhar, M.G., Wissig, S.L., and Palade, G.E. (1961). Glomerular permeability. I. Ferritin transfer across the normal capillary wall. *J. Exp. Med.* **113**, 47–66.

Farquhar, M.G. (1975). The primary glomerular filtration barrier — basement membrane or epithelial slits? *Kidney Int.* **8**, 197–211.

Farquhar, M.G. (1983). The glomerular basement membrane. A selective macromolecular filter. *In* "Cell Biology of Extracellular Matrix" (E.D. Hay, ed.), pp. 335–378. Plenum, New York.

Farquhar, M.G., Courtoy, P.J., Lemkin, M.C., and Kanwar, Y.S. (1982). Current knowledge of the functional architecture of the glomerular basement membrane. *In* "New Trends in Basement Membrane Research" (K. Kuehn, H. Schoene and R. Timpl, eds.), pp. 9–29. Raven Press, New York.

Fry, D.L. (1973). Responses of the arterial wall to certain physical factors. *In* "Atherogenesis: Initiating Factors. A Ciba Foundation Symposium 1972" (R. Porter and J. Knight, eds.), pp. 93–125. Elsevier-North Holland, Amsterdam.

Gollwitzer, R., Bode, W., and Karges, H.E. (1983a). On the aggregation of fibrinogen molecules. *In* "The Endoendothelial Fibrin Lining, Symposium of the XIIth Europ. Conf. on Microcirculation, Jerusalem, Israel, 7 September, 1982" (A.L. Copley, ed.), pp. 41–53. Pergamon Press, New York, Oxford.

Gollwitzer, R., Bode, W., Schramm, H.J., Typke, D., and Gucken-Berger, R. (1983b). Laser diffraction of oriented fibrinogen molecules. *Ann. N.Y. Acad. Sci.* **408**, 214–225.

Henschen, A. (1983). On the structure of functional sites in fibrinogen. *In* "The Endoendothelial Fibrin Lining, Symposium of the XIIth Europ. Conf. on Microcirculation, Jerusalem, Israel, 7 September 1982" (A.L. Copley, ed.), pp. 27–39. Pergamon Press, New York, Oxford.

Herbst, C. (1900). Über das Auseinandergehen von Furchungs-und Gewebszellen in Kalk freien Medium. *Arch. f. Entw. Mech.* **9**, 424–463.

Hsiung, C.C., and Skalak, R. (1984). Hydrodynamic and mechanical aspects of endothelial permeability. *Biorheology* **21**, 207–221.

Kanwar, Y.S., and Farquhar, M.G. (1979a). Presence of heparan sulfate in the glomerular basement membrane. *Proc. Natl. Acad. Sci. U.S.A.* **76**, 1303–1307.

Kanwar, Y.S., and Farquhar, M.G. (1979b). Anionic sites in the glomerular basement membrane. *In vivo* and *in vitro* localization to the laminae rarae by cationic probes. *J. Cell Biol.* **81**, 137–153.

Kanwar, Y.S., Linker, A., and Farquhar, M.G. (1980). Increased permeability of the glomerular basement membrane to ferritin after removal of glycosaminoglycans (heparan sulfate) by enzyme digestion. *J. Cell Biol.* **86**, 688–693.

Kuehn, K., Schoene, H.-H., and Timpl, R. (Eds.) (1982). "New Trends in Basement Membrane Research, 10th Workshop Conference Hoechst, Eibsee, F.R.G., 11–14 May 1981" p. 293. Raven Press, New York.

Luft, J.H. (1965). *J. Cell Biol.* **23**, 54A, 1964. Cited by Luft J.H. The ultrastructural basis of capillary permeability. *In* "The Inflammatory Process" (B.W. Zweifach, L. Grant and R.T. McCluskey eds.), pp. 121–159. Academic Press, New York, London.

Luft, J.H. (1966). Fine structure of capillary and endocapillary layer as revealed by ruthenium red. *Fed. Proc. Fed. Am. Soc. Exp. Biol.* **25**, 1173–1183.

Michel, C. (1979). The investigation of capillary permeability in single vessels. *Acta Physiol. Scand. Suppl.* **463**, 67–74.

Michel, C.C. (1980). Filtration coefficients and osmotic reflexion coefficients of the walls of single frog mesenteric capillaries. *J. Physiol. (London)* **309**, 341–355.

Michel, C.C. (1981). The flow of water through the capillary wall. *In* "Water Transport Across Epithelia" (H.H. Ussing, N. Bindslev, N.A. Lassen and O. Sten-Knudsen, eds.), pp. 268–279. Munksgaard, Copenhagen.

Michel, C.C. (1983). The effects of certain proteins on capillary permeability to fluid and macromolecules. *In* "The Pathogenicity of Cationic Proteins" (P.P. Lambert, P. Bergmann and R. Beauwens, eds.), pp. 125–143, Raven Press, New York.

Majno, C., and Palade, G.E. (1961). The effect of histamine and serotonin on vascular permeability: An electron microscopic study. *J. Biophys. Biochem. Cytol.* **11**, 571–605.

Mosher, D.F., and Johnson, R.B. (1983). Specificity of fibronectin-fibrin crosslinking. *Ann. N.Y. Acad. Sci.* **408**, 583–594.

Nolf, P. (1908). Contribution à l'étude de la coagulation du sang. 5ème mémoire. La fibrinolyse. *Archives Internationales de Physiologie* **6**, 306–359.

Oka, S. (1981). Cardiovascular Hemorheology. pp. 57–60. Cambridge University Press, Cambridge.

Oka, S. (1983a). Physical theory of some interface phenomena in hemorheology. *Ann. N.Y. Acad. Sci.* **416**, 115–127.

Oka, S. (1983b). Biorheological aspect in relation to endoendothelial fibrin lining. *Thromb. Res.* **32**, 649–653.

Oka, S. (1984). Copley-Scott Blair phenomenon and electric double layer. *Biorheology* **21**, 417.

Oka, S. (1985). Electric aspect of interface between blood and endoendothelium. *In* "Biopathology of Vascular Wall and Glomerular Dysfunction" (S. Seno, A.L. Copley, M.A. Venkatachalam and Y. Hamashima, eds.), pp. 53–58. Academic Press, Tokyo.

Okada, M., and Blombäck, B. (1983). Factors influencing gel structure studied by flow measurement. *Ann. N.Y. Acad. Sci.* **408**, 233–253.

Okada, M., Chang, M.Y., Horowitz, B., and Blombäck, B. (1983). Effect of fibronectin on fibrin gel structure. *Thromb. Haemost.* **50**, 185.

Overton, E. (1904). Beiträge zur allgemeinen Muskel- und Nervenphysiologie.

III. Studien über die Wirkung der Alkali-und Erdalkalisalze auf Skelettmuskeln und Nerven. *Pflügers Archiv.* **105**, 179–290. (see pp. 279–281).

Palade, G.E., and Bruns, R.R. (1964). Structure and function in normal muscle capillaries. *In* "Small Blood Vessel Involvement in Diabetes Mellitus" (M.D. Silverstein, A.R. Colwell, Sr. and K. Meyer, eds.) pp. 39–55. American Institute of Biological Sciences, Washington, D.C.

Palade, G.E. (1968). Small pore and large pore systems in capillary permeability. *In* "Hemorheology" (A.L. Copley, ed.), pp. 703–718. Pergamon Press, New York, Oxford.

Palade, G.E., Simionescu, M., and Simionescu, N. (1979). Structural aspects of the permeability of the microvascular endothelium. *Acta Physiol. Scand. Suppl.* **463**, 11–32.

Palade, G.E., Simionescu, M., and Simionescu, N. (1981). Differentiated microdomains on the luminal surface of the capillary endothelium. *In* "Perspectives in Biorheology. Festschrift for A.L. Copley" (A. Silberberg, ed.), pp. 563–568. Pergamon Press, New York, Oxford; *Biorheology* **17**, 563–568.

Pigman, W., Gramling, E., and Holley, H.L. (1961). Interactions of hyaluronic acid with serum albumin. *Biochim. Biophys. Acta* **46**, 100–107.

Poiseuille, J.L.M. (1839). Recherches sur les causes du mouvement du sang dans les vaisseaux capillaires. Acad. Sciences. Séance publique du 28 décembre 1835, Tome VII des Savants étrangers. Impr. Royale, Paris.

Rennke, H.C., Patel, Y., and Venkatachalam, M.A. (1978). Glomerular filtration of proteins: Clearance of anionic, neutral, and cationic horseradish peroxidase in the rat. *Kidney Int.* **13**, 324–328.

Ryan, U.S., and Ryan, J.W. (1984). The ultrastructural basis of endothelial cell surface functions. *Biorheology* **21**, 155–170.

Ryan, U.S., and Ryan, J.W. (1984). The endothelial cell surface. *Biorheology* **21**, 39–56.

Seno, S., Ono, T., and Tsujii, T. (1983). Macromolecular charge and cellular surface charge in adhesion, ingestion, and blood vessel leakage. *Ann. N.Y. Acad. Sci.* **416**, 410–425.

Shen, L.L., Hermans, J., McDonagh, J., McDonagh, R.P., and Carr, M. (1975). Effects of calcium ion and covalent cross-linking on formation and elasticity of fibrin gels. *Thromb. Res.* **6**, 255–265.

Sigal, V.L. (1984). The Copley-Scott Blair phenomenon. Will it be explained by the effect of an electric double layer? *Biorheology* **21**, 297–302.

Silberberg, A. (Ed.) (1984). 5th Internat. Congr. of Biorheology, Baden-Baden, FRG, 20–24 August 1983. Symposium on Permeability and the Blood Vessel Wall. *Biorheology* **21**, 105–223.

Silberberg, A. (1983). Macromolecular surface films at a solid/liquid interface. *In* "The Endoendothelial Fibrin Lining, Symposium of the XIIth Europ. Conf. on Microcirculation, Jerusalem, Israel, 7 September 1982" (A.L. Copley, ed.), pp. 55–59. Pergamon Press, New York, Oxford.

Simionescu, N., Simionescu, M., and Palade, G.E. (1981). Differentiated microdomains on the luminal surface of the capillary endothelium. I. Preferential distribution of anionic sites. *J. Cell Biol.* **90**, 605–613.

Simionescu, M., Simionescu, N., and Palade, G.E. (1981). Differential microdomains on the luminal surface of the capillary endothelium. II. Partial characterization of their anionic sites. *J. Cell Biol.* **90**, 614–621.

Simionescu, M., Simionescu, N., and Palade, G.E. (1982). Biochemically differentiated microdomains of the cell surface of capillary endothelium. *Ann. N.Y. Acad. Sci.* **401**, 9–24.

Stathakis, N.E., Mosesson, M.W., Chen, A.B., and Galanakis, D.K. (1978). Cryoprecipitation of fibrin-fibrinogen complexes induced by the cold-insoluble globulin of plasma. *Blood* **51**, 1211–1222.

Weisel, J.W., Phillips, Jr., G.N., and Cohen, C. (1983). The structure of fibrinogen and fibrin: II. Architecture of the fibrin clot. *Ann. N.Y. Acad. Sci.* **408**, 367–379.

Witte, S. (1980). Vitalmikroskopische Untersuchungen über das Verhalten von Fibrinogen in der Mikrozirkulation. *In* "Fibrinogen, Fibrin and Fibrin Glue. Side Effects of Therapy with Clotting Factor Concentrates" (K. Schimpf, ed.), pp. 85–89. F.K. Schattauer Verlag, Stuttgart, New York.

Witte, S. (1981). The affinity of fluorescent labeled fibrinogen to the vessel wall as seen by vital microscopy. *In* "Perspectives in Biorheology. Festschrift for A.L. Copley" (A. Silberberg, ed.), pp. 579–588. Pergamon Press, New York, Oxford; *Biorheology* **17**, 579–588.

Witte, S. (1983). The endoendothelial lining as studied by a fluorescent labeling technique *in situ*. *In* "Endoendothelial Fibrin Lining, Symposium of the XIIth Europ. Conf. on Microcirculation, Jerusalem, Israel, 7 September 1982" (A.L. Copley, ed.), pp. 93–104. Pergamon Press, New York, Oxford.

TRANSCYTOSIS OF LOW DENSITY LIPOPROTEIN THROUGH VASCULAR ENDOTHELIUM

Eliza Vasile and Nicolae Simionescu[1]

Institute of Cellular Biology and Pathology, Bucharest

There is a strong evidence that cells have a specific mechanism for extracting from circulating lipoproteins the cholesterol needed for their membrane biogenesis (Anderson et al., 1976; Goldstein et al., 1979). In humans and some animal species, the main cholesterol carrier is the low density lipoprotein (LDL) (Chapman, 1980).

It is obvious that, in order to reach different tissues, LDL has first to pass through vascular endothelium. In relation to this process, two major questions arise: (a) how LDL cross the endothelial cell; (b) to what extent LDL molecule is modified during this passage. At present, there are two important lines of information. One is the identification of the "LDL receptor pathway" extensively documented *in vitro* on fibroblasts, macrophages, and smooth muscle cells (Anderson et al., 1976; Drevon et al., 1981; Goldstein et al., 1979). The other comes mostly from work in Steinberg's laboratory indicating that upon incubation with endothelial cells in culture, LDL is significantly modified ("endothelial-modified LDL") (Henriksen et al., 1982).

Since the accumulation of LDL is a hallmark of the atheromatous plaque (Hollander, 1977), the understanding of LDL transport through vascular endothelium is a prerequisite for getting insights into the cellular and molecular basis of atherogenesis.

The findings reported hereafter referring mainly to LDL transcytosis through endothelium, are derived from the following lines of investigation:

(1) observations on the transport of endogenous rat LDL *in vivo*;
(2) observations on transport of exogenous LDL perfused *in situ*;
(3) transport of native or methylated Apo B-gold complexes perfused *in situ* or incubated with endothelial cells in culture;
(4) uptake of radiolabeled native or methylated LDL perfused *in situ*.

A more detailed account of the experimental approaches used is given in Table 1.

We have chosen to work mostly with rat LDL on rat endothelium, because of the great advantage of using homologous LDL as required by species specificity. We have been however aware of two major limitations: *a*) in rat, the main cholesterol carrier is HDL; however rat cells handle very well LDL; *b*) since rat LDL contains ~15% Apo E, the binding sites and routes detected with rat LDL reflect to some degree also sites and pathways for the uptake of HDL_1.

[1]Supported by the Ministry of Education, Romania and NIH, USA, Grant HL-26343.

TABLE 1

EXPERIMENTAL APPROACHES USED FOR STUDYING THE LDL TRANSCYTOSIS THROUGH VASCULAR ENDOTHELIUM

	Experimental conditions	Type of investigation
1. Endogenous rat LDL	*In vivo* observations in rats	Direct electron microscopic visualization of lipoprotein particles in endothelium
2. Exogenous rat LDL or human rat LDL	*In situ* perfusion in rats	Immunocytochemical detection of LDL and its pathways in and through the arterial endothelium
3. $[^{125}I]$-Apo B-gold	Incubation of bovine aortic endothelial cells in culture	Electron microscopic localization of Apo B-gold particles in endothelial cells in culture
4. Apo B-gold, and methylated Apo B-gold	*In situ* perfusion of coronary arteries and aorta in guinea pig	Electron microscopic visualization of native and methylated Apo B pathways through endothelium
5. $[^{125}I]$-native rat LDL and $[^{125}I]$-methylated rat LDL	*In situ* perfusion in rats	Spectrometric measurements of uptake of $[^{125}I]$ LDL by rat aorta
6. $[^{125}I]$-native human LDL, and $[^{125}I]$-methylated LDL	*In situ* perfusion in guinea pigs	Spectrometric measurements of uptake of LDL by guinea pig aorta

TRANSCYTOSIS OF ENDOGENOUS LIPOPROTEINS *IN VIVO*

Working on some old Sprague-Dawley rats, by chance we found that their vessels were filled with lipoproteins (LP). The electron opacity of these particles was much enhanced because the specimens were treated in bloc with tannic acid as mordant (Simionescu, N., and Simionescu, M., 1976). The particles covered the whole dimensional spectrum of plasma lipoproteins, most of them being in the range of 20 to 25 nm (probably LDL and HDL_1) and 30 to 70 nm (probably VLDL). Observations were made both on large vessels as well as capillaries. The illustrations in Fig. 1 are from diaphragm capillaries provided with a continuous endothelium, the most commonly encountered type of endothelium.

FIG. 1. Interaction of plasma lipoproteins (LP) with vascular endothelium *in vivo* (diaphragm capillaries in spontaneously hyperlipidemic rats). (*a*) Particles of the size of LDL (~ 20–25 nm in diameter) can be seen in the vessel lumen (*arrow*) and in plasmalemmal vesicle open on the luminal front (*arrowhead*). x 82,000; (*b*) In other locations LP particles occur in high density in plasma (*arrows*), and some particles are found in cytoplasmic plasmalemmal vesicles (*arrowhead*). *rb*, red blood cell. x 82,000; (*c*) Other particles could be observed in vesicles open on the abluminal front (*arrowhead*). x 82,000.

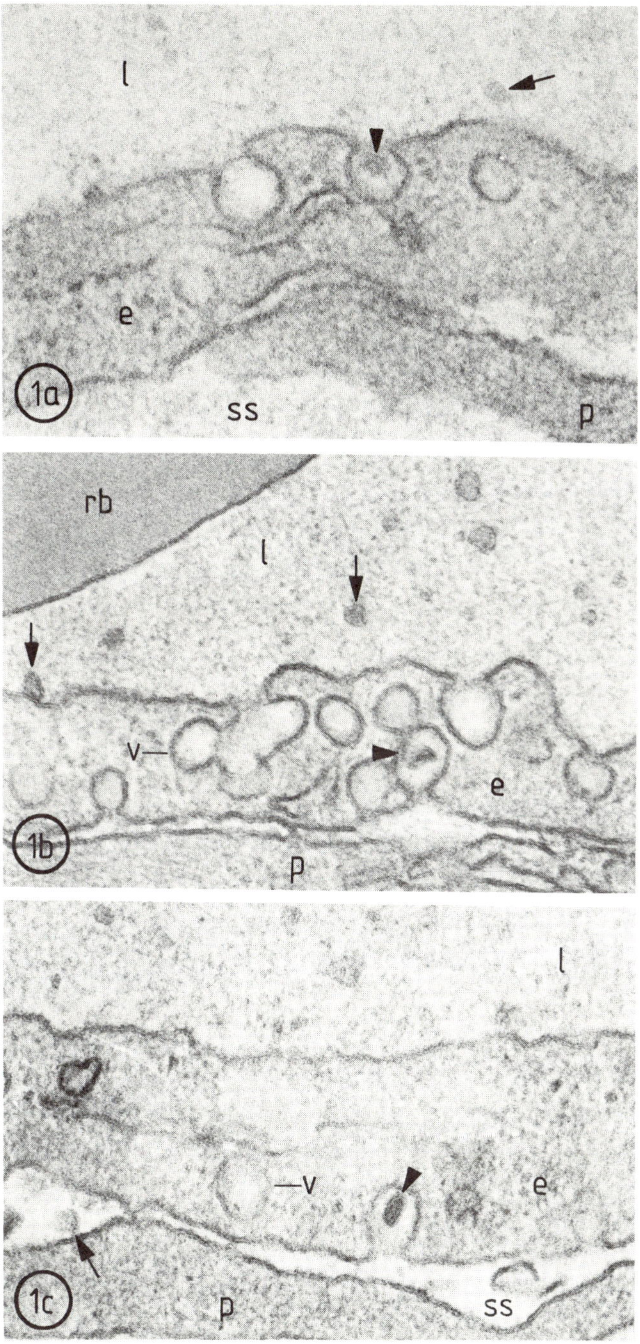

ABBREVIATIONS: *e*, endothelium; *l*, lumen; *p*, pericytes; *ss*, subendothelial space; *v*, plasmalemmal vesicle.

LP could be seen not only in the vascular lumen, but also in the endothelial structures known to be involved in the transport of water-soluble macromolecules to be delivered to the endothelial cell itself (endocytosis) or to the subendothelial components of a given tissue (transcytosis) (Simionescu, N., 1980, and 1983).

As indicated by the morphometric analysis, in the diaphragm capillaries, at a steady state, about 19% of LP particles ~20 to 25 nm large were detected in endothelial features potentially involved in receptor-mediated endocytosis (Table 2). The great majority of such LP particles were localized either attached to luminal plasma membrane (~40%), within plasmalemmal vesicles in different locations (~20%) or in the subendothelial space (~20%) (Simionescu, N., and Simionescu, M., 1985) (Table 2 and Fig. 1). Occasionally, LP particles of the size of LDL were detected in chains of fused vesicles (Fig. 2a) or in patent transendothelial channels (Fig. 2b). LP appeared also to be taken up by other cells of the vessel wall such as pericytes and smooth muscle cells.

In all specimens examined, no lipoproteins of any size could be detected in the intercellular spaces or intercellular junctions.

The possibility of a reverse pathway — from the subendothelial space to the vascular lumen — is highly unlikely because of the steep concentration gradient of LP existent between lumen and the pericapillary space (about 10 : 1).

The morphometric analysis carried out on a relatively large sampling indicates that *in vivo* (at least in hyperlipidemic conditions), as compared to endocytosis, transcytosis may be a prevalent process.

On our knowledge, these findings represent the first direct visualization

TABLE 2

RELATIVE OCCURRENCE OF THE ENDOGENOUS LDL* IN THE CAPILLARY ENDOTHELIUM IN THE DIAPHRAGM OF SPONTANEOUSLY HYPERLIPIDEMIC RATS (Percentage of detected particles)

Structures involved in endocytosis†	Plasma membrane	Luminal vesicles	Cytoplasmic vesicles	Abluminal vesicles	Subendothelial space
19 ± 2.3	40 ± 6.9	8 ± 2.4	7 ± 1.4	5 ± 1.2	20 ± 4.5

*Lipoprotein particles 20 to 25 nm in diameter, presumably representing LDL and HDL_1 (Simionescu, N., and Simionescu, M., 1985)

†Include coated pits, coated vesicles, endosomes, multivesicular bodies and secondary lysosomes

±, $\overline{SD}$ of the mean, determined by using the large sample theory. Sampling: 262 microvascular profiles randomly collected from thin sections obtained from 41 tissue specimens. Total endothelial length examined was 984 μm with an aggregate area of endothelial sections of 342 μm^2 : the number of lipoprotein particles in the size range of 20 to 25 nm was 1924.

of endogenous LDL at the level of the endothelial cell. Concomitantly, they constitute the first detection of an untagged physiologic constituent of blood plasma interacting with vascular endothelium.

The occurrence, *in vivo*, of LP particles in plasmalemmal vesicles in all locations, in transendothelial channels and in the subendothelial compartment, indicates that endothelial vesicles are active, dynamic carriers of plasma macromolecules and not just immobile invaginations of plasma membrane as claimed by some investigators based on serial morphologic reconstructions (Bundgaard et al., 1979; Frøkjaer-Jansen, 1980). The total absence of LP from intercellular spaces and junctions also indicates that the paracellular route excludes in normal conditions the transendothelial passage of plasma proteins (Simionescu N., 1983).

When spontaneously hyperlipidemic rats were injected intravenously with cationized ferritin (CF) pI 8.4, this tracer bound firmly to some LP forming CF-LP complexes. Examined at 5, 20, and 60 min after CF administration, CF-LP complexes were found to be taken up by endothelium only by endocytosis (adsorptive uptake *via* coated pits and vesicles, and probably also by fluid phase uptake through a fraction of plasmalemmal vesicles). CF-LP complexes were progressively accumulated within multivesicular bodies and lysosomes (Fig. 2c). These results revealed the importance of the net surface charge of macromolecular complexes for their intracellular sorting and fate (Simionescu N., and Simionescu M., 1985).

Transcytosis of Exogenous Rat LDL Perfused *In Situ*

In order to establish the kinetics of the LDL transport through arterial endothelium, native untagged rat LDL (at concentrations varying from 10 to 80 mg cholesterol/100 ml) was perfused *in situ* for time intervals of 2, 5, and 10 min, and then detected immunocytochemically using anti rat LDL IgG coupled to horseradish peroxidase (anti LDL-HRP) (Vasile et al., 1983). Similar experiments were carried out with human LDL. The results indicated that the exogenous LDL is taken up by the arterial endothelium through two parallel compartmented routes.

(a) A relatively small amout is taken up by endocytosis involving (i) a high affinity receptor-mediated process *via* coated pits, coated vesicles, and endosomes, and (ii) probably a receptor-independent uptake by fluid phase carried out by a fraction of plasmalemmal vesicles. By both mechanisms, LDL is brought to lysosomes to supply cholesterol for the metabolic needs of the endothelial cell.

(b) Most circulating LDL is transported through endothelial cell by transcytosis *via* plasmalemmal vesicles, thus delivering cholesterol to other cells. As demonstrated by Fig. 3a to c and Table 3, LDL transcytosis is a stepwise process. At any time, there was no intercellular passage of such molecules. Endocytosis was diminished at low temperature, but was not augmented by increasing LDL concentration. Conversely, transcytosis was less modified by lowering the temperature of the perfusates, but was markedly enhanced at high concentrations of LDL. Heparin was effective in removing LDL from coated pits.

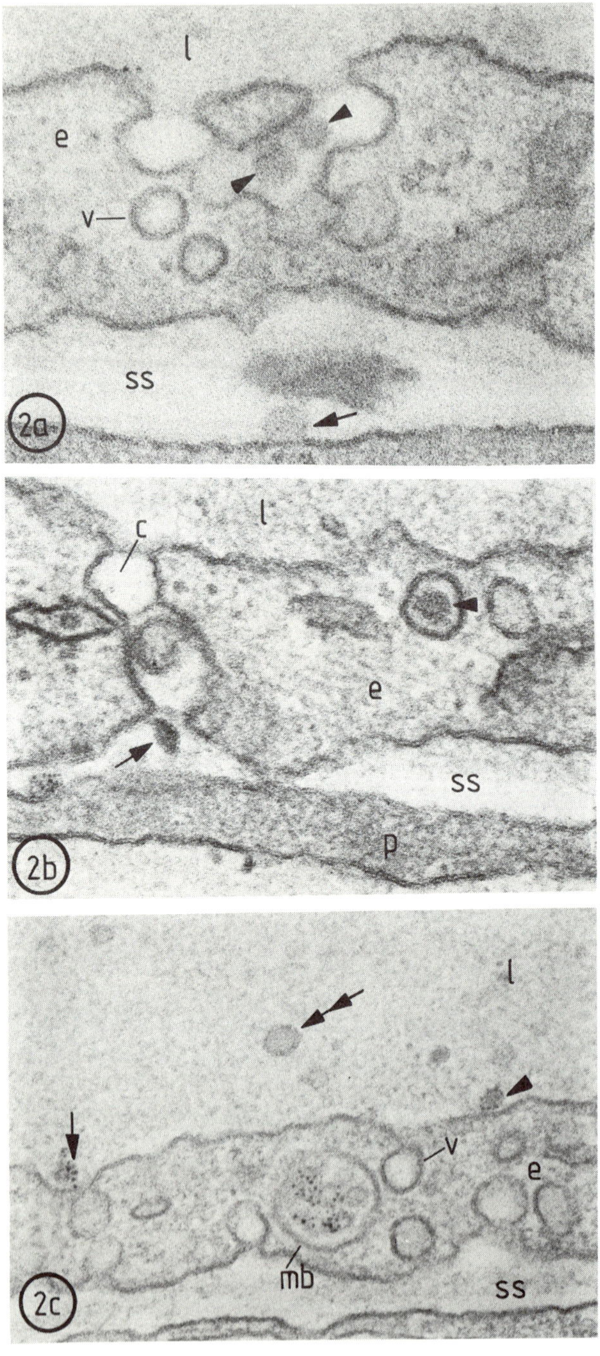
l
e
v
ss
2a
l
c
e
ss
p
2b
l
v
e
mb
ss
2c

TABLE 3

KINETICS OF TRANSCYTOSIS OF EXOGENOUS RAT LDL THROUGH RAT ARTERIAL ENDOTHELIUM
(percentage of detected particles)

Time interval**	Location of LDL particles†					
	Plasma membrane	Luminal vesicles	Cytoplasmic vesicles	Abluminal vesicles	Subendothelial space	Structure involved in endocytosis*
min						
2	55 ± 16.2	0	0	0	5 ± 2.1	40 ± 19.4
5	34 ± 12.4	10 ± 2.4	5 ± 1.4	3 ± 1.2	6 ± 2.3	42 ± 16.5
10	26 ± 11.2	0	0	0	13 ± 3.4	61 ± 21.3

±, $\overline{\text{SD}}$ of the mean determined by using large sample theory

* Include coated pits, coated vesicles, endosomes, multivesicular bodies and secondary lysosomes

† In these pulse-chasing experiments, the LDL concentration used was 10 – 30 mg cholesterol/100 ml

**Sampling: 10 – 13 rats for each time point, and 4 – 6 arterial specimens from each animal were collected and processed for electron microscopy. From each specimen 60 – 80 sections. Total length of endothelial profiles examined: 410 μm (2 min), 422 μm (5 min), and 478 μm (10 min). On randomly collected specimens, the number of LDL particles examined were 707 (2 min), 682 (5 min), and 728 (10 min). The endothelial surface was calculated by considering a section thickness of ~60 nm.

FIG. 2. Same type of capillaries as in Fig. 1, showing LP particles in a chain of fused vesicles (*a*) and at the level of a transendothelial channel (*c*) (*b*). In *c*, when animals were injected intravenously with cationized ferritin (CF), numerous LP-CF complexes (*arrow*) were formed. The latter were virtually taken up only by endocytosis and accumulated within multivesicular bodies (*mb*). *a* and *b*, x 86,000; *c*, x 58,000.

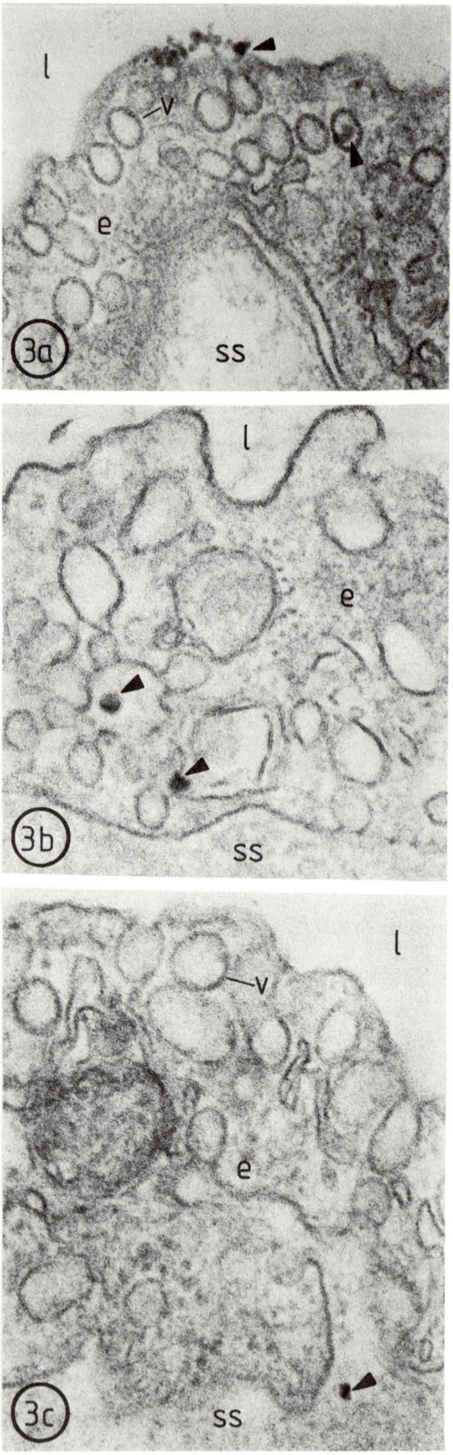
l
v
e
3a
ss
l
e
3b
ss
l
v
e
3c
ss

TRANSPORT OF NATIVE AND METHYLATED APO B-GOLD COMPLEX

To find out whether the endothelial handling of apoprotein B is the same as that revealed by the immunocytochemically-detected LDL, we used as electron dense probe an Apo B-gold conjugate. To check the involvement of a specific receptor, in parallel experiments we perfused methyl-Apo B, since it has been shown that reductive methylation renders the Apo B unable to interact with its receptor (Mahley et al., 1979, 1980). Soluble immunoreactive form of apoprotein B (Apo B), was prepared from human LDL by delipidation in the presence of Triton X-100 according to the method of Soccoro and Camejo (1979). Human and rat methylated LDL were obtained by the method of Weisgraber et al. (1978). Methylated Apo B was prepared from previously methylated LDL; the degree of methylation was assayed by the trinitrobenzensulfonic acid technique (Habeeb, 1966). Gold complexes with either native Apo B or methylated Apo B were obtained by adsorbing one of these protein species on ~15 nm diameter colloidal gold (Frens, 1973).

The biological activity of Apo B-gold particles was tested on bovine aortic endothelial cells in culture. Confluent endothelial cells in culture were maintained in a medium deficient of fetal calf serum, in presence of 5% lipoprotein-deficient serum, 24 hr before the experiment. The cells were incubated with [^{125}I]-Apo B-gold (10 cpm/ng protein) at different concentration (10 – 70 μg/ml, at 37 °C, for 2 hr. Surface binding and cellular uptake of [^{125}I]-Apo B-gold were also measured (Goldstein et al., 1976). The curves depicting the binding and the cellular uptake were similar with those for receptor-mediated processes. No degradation could be measured: probably the degradation products (polypeptides) remained bound to the gold core. The binding and the uptake of [^{125}I]-Apo B-gold was effectively competed by excess of cold LDL. Apo B-gold and methylated Apo B-gold (E_{520} = 1.4) at 37 °C were perfused *in situ* in guinea pigs, for 5 to 15 min. After washing and fixation *in situ*, specimens of thoracic aorta and coronary arteries were processed for electron microscopy. In controls, a polyethyleneglycol-gold complex (E_{520} = 2.8) was perfused for 15 min instead of Apo B-gold. In addition, endothelial cells (bovine aorta) in culture were incubated for 2 hr with [^{125}I]-Apo B-gold complex (50 μg/ml protein content), then cooled at 4 °C for 30 min, fixed with aldehydes and processed for electron microscopy.

Apo B-gold complex perfused *in situ* was found in features involved in endocytosis (coated pits/vesicles, endosomes, multivesicular bodies and lyso-

FIG. 3. Transcytosis of rat exogenous LDL through arterial endothelium in rat. LDL was detected immunocytochemically. (*a*) At 2 min of perfusion, LDL particles were detected bound on plasma membrane or in plasmalemmal vesicles (*arrowheads*). x 56,000; (*b*) At 5 min some LDL particles could be seen in vesicles approaching the abluminal front; x 68,000; and (*c*) at 10 min LDL particles (usually smaller than those occurring within vesicles) appeared in the subendothelial space (*arrowhead*). x 68,000.

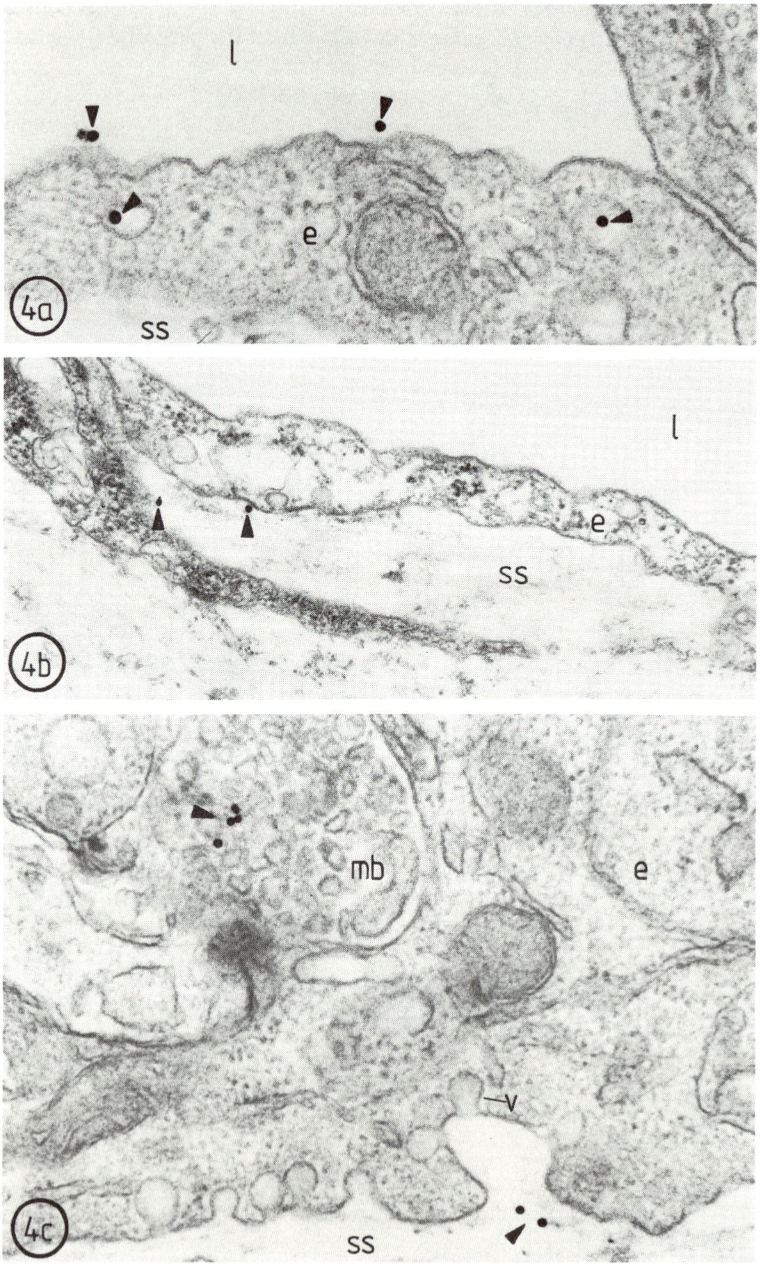
l
e
ss
4a
l
e
ss
4b
mb
e
v
ss
4c

TABLE 4

UPTAKE OF RAT NATIVE LDL AND METHYLATED LDL BY RAT AORTA
(double labeling: [^{125}I]-, and cholesteryl[^{14}C] oleate-LDL)

LDL concentration	ng LDL cholesterol/ mg aortic wet tissue/1 h		ratio methylated LDL / native LDL
	native LDL	methylated LDL	
10 mg LDL cholesterol/100 ml	6.02±1.37	5.69±2.76	0.94±0.16
20 mg LDL cholesterol/100 ml	15.74±7.90	14.7 ±10.3	0.94±0.16

Results are means ± $\overline{SD}$

TABLE 5

UPTAKE OF HUMAN NATIVE LDL AND METHYLATED LDL
BY GUINEA PIG AORTA (labeling: [^{125}I]-LDL)

LDL concentration	ng LDL cholesterol/ mg aortic wet tissue/1 h		ratio methylated LDL / native LDL
	native LDL	methylated LDL	
10 mg cholesterol/100 ml	4.21±2.5	3.63±1.71	0.87±0.13

Results are means ± $\overline{SD}$

somes) as well as in plasmalemmal vesicles in sequencial stages from the luminal (5 min) till the abluminal front of endothelial cell (10 and 15 min) (Figs. 4a and b). The uptake and accumulation within the aortic wall was almost similar for native and methylated LDL (Table 4), but methylated Apo B-gold particles, perfused in the same conditions as native Apo B-gold, were found located mostly in endothelial features involved in transcytosis: the labeling of the latter was 5 fold more frequent than the labeling of features participating in endocytosis.

In cultured bovine aortic endothelial cells, Apo B-gold particles were encountered mainly in coated pits/vesicles and multivesicular bodies, and less frequent in plasmalemmal vesicles and the subendothelial space (Fig. 4c).

FIG. 4. *In situ* perfusion of methylated Apo B-gold complexes in rat: (*a*) in the endothelium of coronary arteries the complexes occurred on the plasma membrane and in apparently internalized plasmalemmal vesicles; x 78,000; (*b*) At later time points, such complexes appeared in the subendothelial space (*arrowheads*). x 36,000. (*c*) In cultured endothelial cells (bovine aorta) the Apo B-gold complexes are mostly endocytosed and accumulated in multivesicular bodies (*mb*), and only occasionally such complexes reached the subendothelial space (*arrowhead*). x 78,000.

In controls, very rare polyethyleneglycol-gold particles were detected at the level of the endothelial cells.

These observations indicate that the transport pathways taken by Apo B are similar to those followed by LDL. *In situ*, transcytosis is the most pronounced process, whereas *in vitro* endocytosis prevails. Transcytosis *in situ* is particularly marked in the case of methylated LDL.

To obtain quantitative data about the influx of methyl-LDL through the rat arterial wall (reflecting a low-affinity or receptor-independent transcytosis), we perfused *in situ* [^{125}I]-, [^{14}C]-oleat cholesteryl LDL or its methylated form (10 mg or 20 mg LDL cholesterol/100 ml), at 37 ℃ for 1 hr. The LDL double labeling was performed by successive labeling with [^{14}C]-oleat cholesteryl (Krieger et al., 1977), and iodination with ^{125}INa by the ICl method (Billheimer et al., 1972). At the end of experiments, aortae were stripped of their intima, and spectrometry was carried out separately for the latter and the rest of the arterial wall. The comparative values of the uptake are given in Table 4. After 1 hr of LDL perfusion, 50 – 60% of radioactivity was confined to the intima. The total amount of native LDL accumulated within the arterial wall was comparable to that of methylated LDL. But in the case of the latter the fractional contribution of transcytosis is relatively much higher than that of the transcytosis. This assumption is based on the evidence obtained with the methylated Apo B-gold conjugate. Since by reductive methylation of its lysine residues, LDL loses the ability to bind to the LDL receptors, the values recorded largely represent the magnitude of the methylated LDL transcytosed and transiently found within the aortic wall, especially within the intima.

Uptake of Iodinated LDL by Guinea Pig Aorta

Human LDL largely interacts with guinea pig LDL receptor (Wriston, 1984). The [^{125}I]-human LDL or its methylated form was perfused *in situ* and measurements of radioactivity trapped in the aortic wall were made as in the above experiments. The values recorded are listed in Table 5. As in the rat, after 1 hr perfusion, about 50 to 60% of radioactivity was associated with the aortic intima. The comparative uptake of native *vs.* methyl-LDL was quite similar to that detected in the previously reported experiments in the rat.

Abstract

Vascular endothelium possesses a dual mechanism for handling the circulating LDL: *a*) receptor-mediated endocytosis supplies cholesterol for the endothelial cell needs, and *b*) transcytosis, a low affinity nonsaturable uptake which involves plasmalemmal (transcytotic) vesicles; the latter process increases with LDL concentration. LDL vectorial transport by transcytotic vesicles both *in vivo* and *in situ*, demonstrates that these features are mobile shuttling carriers. In none of the experimental conditions used, lipoprotein particles were detected in the intercellular spaces of junctions of capillary or arterial endothelium.

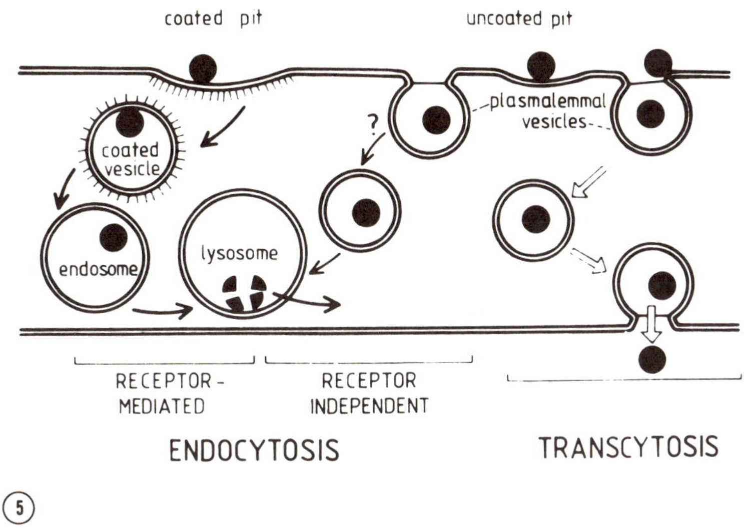

FIG. 5. Diagramatic representation of the dual pathway of endothelial transport of LDL.

Transcytotic pathways for LDL and Apo B are the same.

Transcytosis is the major endothelial transport process for both native and methylated LDL. Due to its very low endocytotic rate, the amount of methylated LDL transcytosed *in situ* appears particularly pronounced, although its total amount accumulated within the aortic wall is comparable to that of the native LDL.

Transcytosis of LDL supplies cholesterol to the other cells of the vessel wall and surrounding tissues and can monitor an excessive accumulation of plasma LDL.

ACKNOWLEDGEMENTS

The excellent editing and typing of this manuscript by Mihaela Mazilu is gratefully acknowledged.

REFERENCES

Anderson, R.G.W., Goldstein, J.L., and Brown M.S. (1976). Localization of low density lipoprotein receptors on plasma membrane of normal human fibroblasts and their absence in cells from a familiar hypercholesterolemia homozygote. *Proc. Natl. Acad. Sci. U.S.A.* **73**, 2434–2438.

Bilheimer, D., Eisenberg, S., and Levy, R.L. (1972). The metabolism of very low density lipoproteins. *Biochim. Biophys. Acta* **260**, 212–221.

Bundgaard, M., Frøkjaer-Jansen, J., and Crone, C. (1979). Endothelial plasmalemmal vesicles as elements in a system of branching invaginations from the cell surface. *Proc. Natl. Acad. Sci. U.S.A.* **76**, 6439–6442.

Chapman, M.J. (1980). Animal lipoproteins: chemistry, structure and comparative aspects. *J. Lipid Res.* **21**, 789–853.

Drevon, C.A., Attie, A.D., Pangburn, S.H., and Steinberg, D. (1981). Metabolism of homologous and heterologous lipoproteins by cultured rat and human skin fibroblasts. *J. Lipid Res.* **22**, 37–46.

Frens, G. (1973). Controlled nucleation for the regulation of the particle size in nondisperse suspensions. *Nature Physical Science* **241**, 20–22.

Frøkjaer-Jansen, J. (1980). Three-dimensional organization of plasmalemmal vesicles in endothelial cells. An analysis by serial sectioning of frog mesenteric capillaries. *J. Ultrastruct. Res.* **73**, 9–20.

Goldstein, J.L., Basu, S.K., Brunschede, V.Y., and Brown, M.S. (1976). Release of low density lipoprotein from its cell surface receptor by sulphated glycosaminoglycans. *Cell* **7**, 85–95.

Goldstein, J.L., Anderson, R.G.W., and Brown, M.S. (1979). Coated pits, coated vesicles, and receptor-mediated endocytosis. *Nature* **279**, 679–685.

Habeeb, A.F.S.A. (1966). Determination of free amino groups in proteins by trinitrobenzen sulfonic acid. *Anal. Biochem.* **14**, 328–336.

Henriksen, T., Mahoney, E.M., and Steinberg, D. (1982). Interactions of plasma lipoproteins with endothelial cells. *Ann. N.Y. Acad. Sci.* **401**, 102–116.

Hollander, W. (1977). Role of arterial lipoproteins in the formation of the fibrous plaque. *In* "Atherosclerosis: Metabolic, Morphologic, and Clinical Aspects" (G.W. Manning and M.D. Haust, eds.), pp. 793–799. Plenum Press, New York.

Krieger, M., Brown, M.S., Faust, J.R., and Goldstein, J.L. (1977). Replacement of endogenous cholesteryl esters of low density lipoprotein with exogenous cholesteryl linoleate. *J. Biol. Chem.* **252**, 4861–4871.

Mahley, R.W., Innerarity, T.L., Weisgraber, K.H., and Oh, S.Y. (1979). Altered metabolism (*in vivo* and *in vitro*) of plasma lipoproteins after selective chemical modification of lysine residues of the apoproteins. *J. Clin. Invest.* **64**, 743–750.

Mahley, R.W., Weisgraber, K.H., Melchior, G.W., Innerarity, T.L., and Holcombe, K.S. (1980). Inhibition of receptor-mediated clearance of lysine and arginine-modified lipoproteins from the plasma of rats and monkeys. *Proc. Natl. Acad. Sci. U.S.A.* **77**, 225–229.

Simionescu, N., and Simionescu, M. (1976). Galloylglucoses of low molecular weight as mordant in electron microscopy. I. Procedure and evidence for the mordanting effect. *J. Cell Biol.* **70**, 608–621.

Simionescu, N. (1981). Transcytosis and traffic of membranes in the endothelial cell. *In* "International Cell Biology 1980–1981" (H.G.

Schweiger, ed.), pp. 657–672, Springer Verlag, Berlin.
Simionescu, N. (1983). Cellular aspects of transcapillary exchange. *Physiol. Rev.* **63**, 1536–1579.
Simionescu, N., and Simionescu, M. (1985). Interactions of endogenous lipoproteins with capillary endothelium in spontaneously hyperlipoproteinemic rats. *Microvasc. Res.* (in press)
Socorro, L., and Camejo, G. (1979). Preparation and properties of soluble immunoreactive apo LDL. *J. Lipid Res.* **20**, 631–639.
Vasile, E., Simionescu, M., and Simionescu, N. (1983). Visualization of the binding, endocytosis and transcytosis of low density lipoprotein in the arterial endothelium *in situ*. *J. Cell Biol.* **96**, 1677–1689.
Weisgraber, K.H., Innerarity, T.L., and Mahley, R.W. (1978). Role of the lysine residues of plasma lipoproteins in high affinity binding to cell surface receptors on human fibroblasts. *J. Biol. Chem.* **253**, 9053–9062.
Wriston, Jr., J.C. (1984). Comparative biochemistry of the guinea-pig, a partial checklist. *Comp. Biochem. Physiol.* **77B**, 253–278.

MINUTE STRUCTURE OF HUMAN KIDNEY GLOMERULUS, ITS EMBRYONIC DEVELOPMENT AND AGE-RELATED CHANGES: A SCANNING ELECTRON MICROSCOPE STUDY OF VASCULAR CASTS

Takuro Murakami and Akio Kikuta

Department of Anatomy, Okayama University Medical School, Okayama

Tetsuji Kaneshige

Kidney Research Laboratory, Okayama Chuo Hospital, Okayama

Ichiro Naito

Division of Ultrastructure Research, Shigei Medical Research Institute, Okayama

The architecture of the kidney glomerular capillaries has been intensively studied in man and various animals by light microscopy of sectioned tissues with or without dye-injection, or cast samples (Bowman, 1842; Johnston, 1899; Vimtrup, 1928; Wilmer, 1941; Trabucco and Marquez, 1952; Hall, 1955; Boyer, 1956; Elias, 1957; Lewis, 1958). However, these conventional light microscope studies were insufficient to the clear three-dimensional analysis of such conglomerated capillaries as those of the kidney glomerulus, because of limited resolution and shallow focus of the light microscope (Murakami, 1971). Thus, the observations led to the erroneous models of the glomerular capillary tuft, *viz.* the non-anastomosing capillary model proposed by Bowman (1842) and supported by Vimtrup (1928), Wilmer (1941) and Elias (1957) and the sacculated capillary model by Trabucco and Marquez (1952). Among these, the plexus or anastomosing capillary model proposed by Johnston (1899) and supported by Hall (1955), Boyer (1956) and Lewis (1958) should be noted.

Recently developed scanning electron microscopy (SEM) of vascular casts has overcome the shortcoming of light microscopy and allowed a clear three-dimensional visualization of blood vascular beds, including those of the kidney glomerulus (Murakami, 1971). Thus, this microscopy has provided in man, monkey, rat and other animals a conclusive evidence to support the plexus model of Johnston (1899) in the glomerular capillary arrangement (Murakami, 1971, 1972, 1978; Murakami et al., 1971, 1985a; Lee et al., 1972; Spinelli, 1974; Anderson and Anderson, 1976; Morris and Campbell, 1978; Ohtani and Naito, 1980; Casellas and Mimran, 1981; Unehira, 1981). SEM combined with microdissections has further clarified that the glomerular capillary plexus is lobulated (Murakami et al., 1971, 1985a; Murakami, 1972, 1978; Unehira, 1981). In this paper the details of the human glomerular

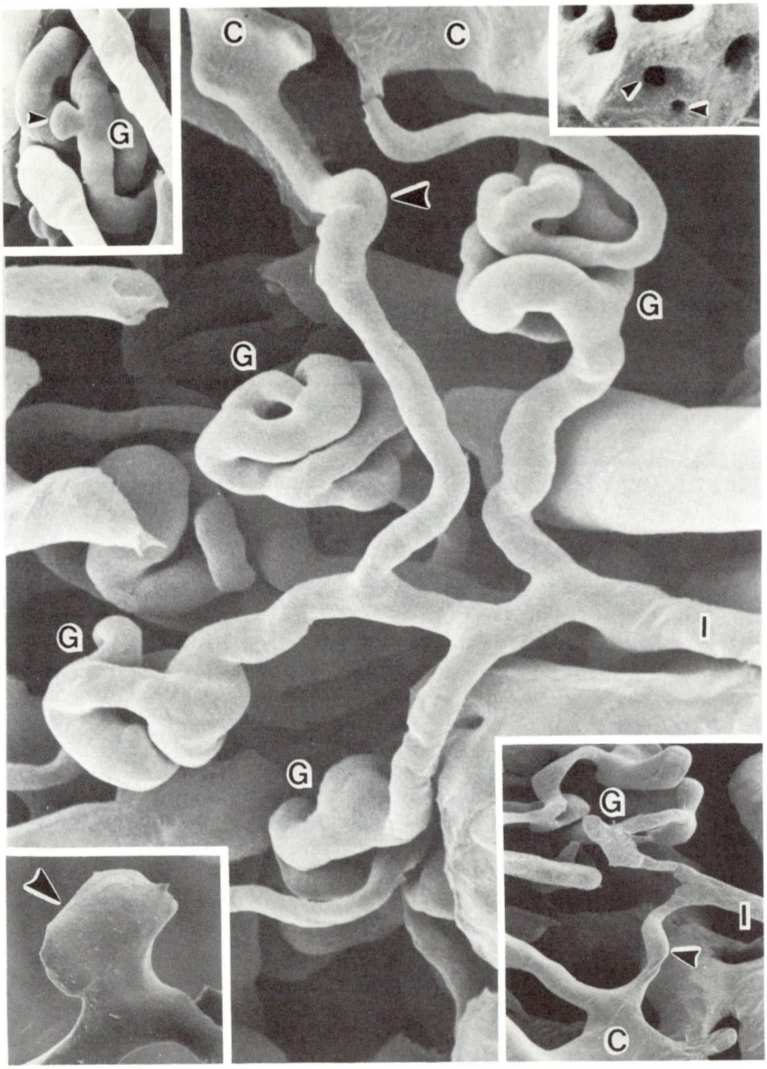

FIG. 1. SEM picture of the casts of subcapsular glomeruli and their connecting vessels in the kidney of a 6-month-old male fetus stillborn due to the umbilical cord coiling. Note the immature glomerular capillary tufts (G) and an U-shape winding (arrowhead). C, parenchymal capillaries; I, terminal branch of the interlobular artery. x 490. A simply widened form shown in *Lower right inset* (arrowhead) is probably the first stage of glomerulus formation. x 200. A marked protrusion shown in *Lower left inset* (arrowhead) will be of second-stage, the transient form from the straight to U-shaped vessel or a capillary island in the renal vesicle. x 600. A small round capillary protrusion appearing in *Upper left inset* (arrowhead) may be of new capillary formation by budding (see text) x 300. Two small pits penetrating the glomerular capillary loop are shown in *Upper right inset* (arrowhead) x 800. Method; see text.

vascular architecture at developing and aging stages revealed by SEM are demonstrated.

MATERIALS AND METHODS

The human healthy kidneys obtained at autopsy from 3 individuals, a male fetus (6 months old) and two adult men (45 and 76 years old), were perfused with physiological saline first and then with laboratory-prepared low viscosity methyl methacrylate media through the renal arteries (Murakami,

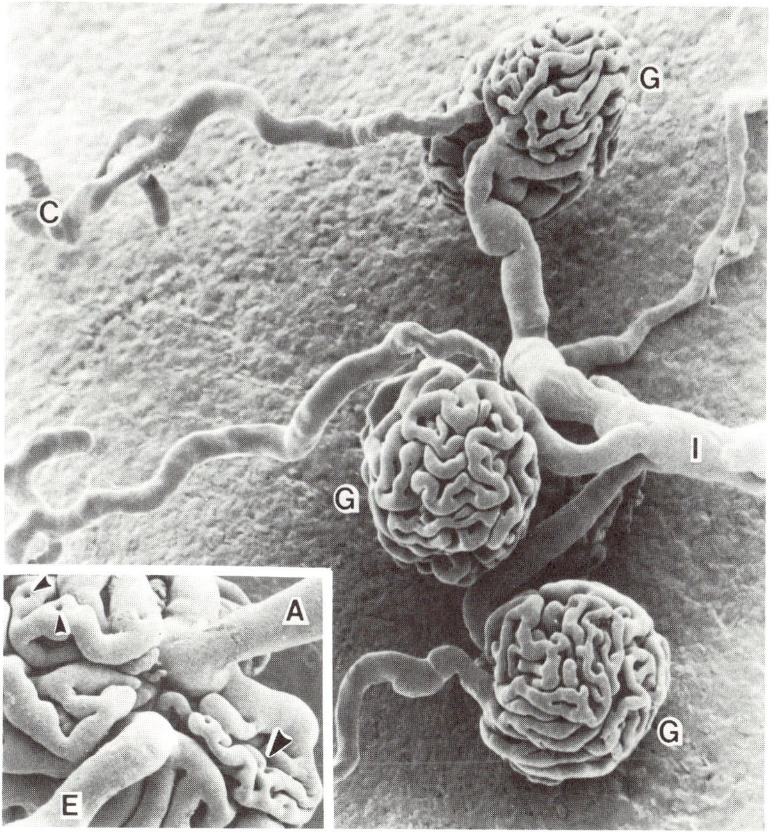

FIG. 2. SEM picture of the casts of subcapsular glomeruli with their connecting vessels. A sample from the kidney of a 45-year-old man dying of gastric cancer. Note that the adult glomerular tufts (G) contain numerous capillaries, compared with the fetal or immature ones (Fig. 1). C, parenchymal capillary; I, the interlobular artery. x 200. *Inset* shows a closer view of the vascular pole of a subcapsular glomerulus having small pits (smaller arrowhead) and very thin capillaries (bigger arrowhead). A and E, afferent and efferent arterioles. x 250.

1971; Murakami, et al., 1973). The infused kidneys were corroded in a hot NaOH solution (10%, 60 ℃), washed in running tap water, and dried in air

3

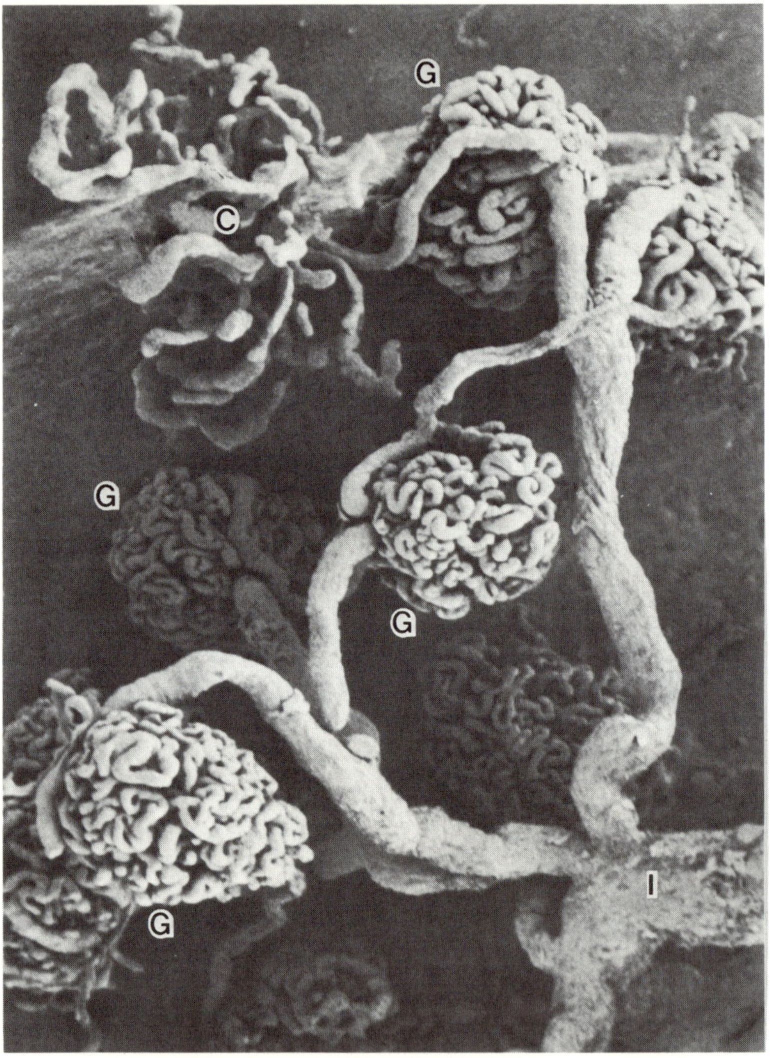

FIG. 3. SEM picture of the subcapsular glomeruli and their connecting vessels of a kidney from a 76-year-old man dying of gastric cancer. Note that the glomerular capillaries are extremely tortuous, compared with those of the 45-year-old man (Fig. 2). C, parenchymal capillaries; G, glomeruli; I, terminal end of the interlobular artery. x 190.

FIG. 4. A closer view of a subcapsular glomerulus of the 45-year-old man. Note that there is no capillary directly connecting the afferent and efferent arterioles (A and E) which are leaving the glomerulus through the tight vascular pole. a, afferent rootlets. x 400.

(Murakami, 1971; Murakami et al., 1973). The blood vascular casts of the kidneys thus obtained were dissected with forceps, and the glomeruli were isolated together with their affiliated afferent and efferent arterioles. The isolated glomerular casts were mounted on metal stubs, coated with gold in a vacuum evaporator (IB-3, Eiko) and observed by SEM using an acceleration voltage at 5 kV (JSM-U3, JEOL or HHS-2R, Hitachi). After SEM observation, most of the glomerular casts were microdissected with sharpened forceps or needles under a binocular light microscope (SMZ-10, Nikon). The microdissected glomerular casts were observed again by SEM with or without stretching or unfolding in a hot ethanol bath (Murakami et al., 1971; Murakami, 1972).

Results

Methacrylate media of low viscosity infused through renal arteries gave good castings of blood vascular lumen of glomeruli and their affiliated afferent and efferent arterioles in all specimens including the kidneys of fetus (Figs. 1 – 3). Unexpected leakages of the injected media from the glomerular capillaries occurred rarely (Fig. 5). Microdissections, especially stretching and unfolding in the hot ethanol bath disclosed the internal or hidden parts of the glomerulus with the well-kept vascular connections (Figs. 6 – 10).

The adult kidney glomerulus was formed by a conglomerated tuft of anastomosing capillaries. It was usually connected to a single afferent arteriole from the interlobular artery and a single efferent arteriole linked to the paren-

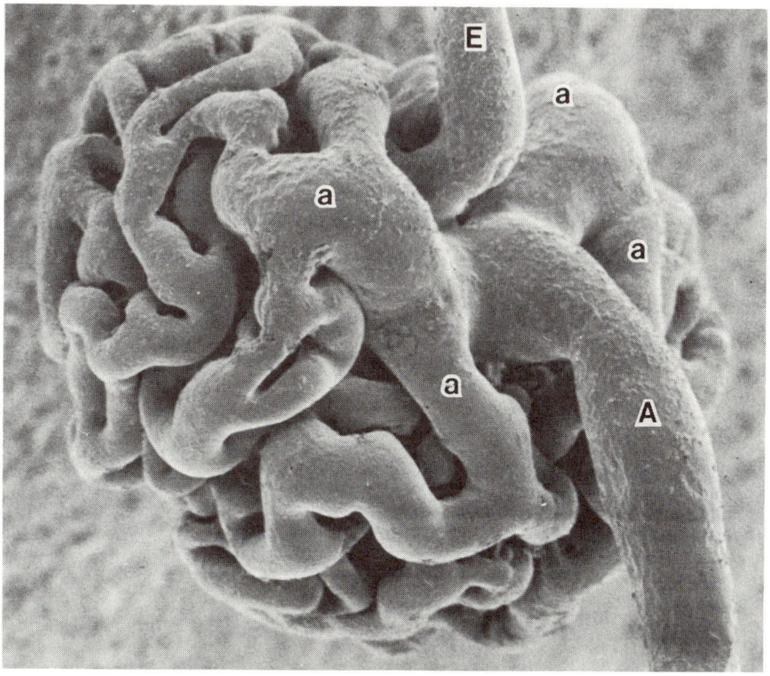

4

chymal capillaries (Figs. 1 — 5). In each kidney, larger glomeruli, which were found in deeper area, were composed of numerous capillaries (Figs. 4, 5). The hilus or vascular pole of the juxtamedullary glomerulus was usually widened by invasion of a part of the well developed capillary tuft between the afferent and efferent arterioles (Fig. 5). Such glomerulus having a markedly widened vascular pole was not found in the superficial or subcapsular area of cortex (Fig. 4). The afferent arteriole was usually thicker than the efferent arteriole (Figs. 1 — 4), but in the juxtamedullary glomerulus the afferent arteriole was almost always thinner than the efferent arteriole which descends into renal medulla (Fig. 5).

The afferent arteriole branches out into several, usually three to five, afferent rootlets at the vascular pole (Fig. 4). Each afferent rootlet further ramifies and constructs its own capillary network (Figs. 4 — 9). The capillary network belonging to each afferent rootlet, now considered as the glomerular capillary lobule, is an independent unit, though it is usually connected to the adjacent capillary lobules with a few translobular capillaries (Fig. 6). The translobular capillaries are always thin and located near the vascular pole. The capillaries constructing the lobules finally converge into the efferent root-

5

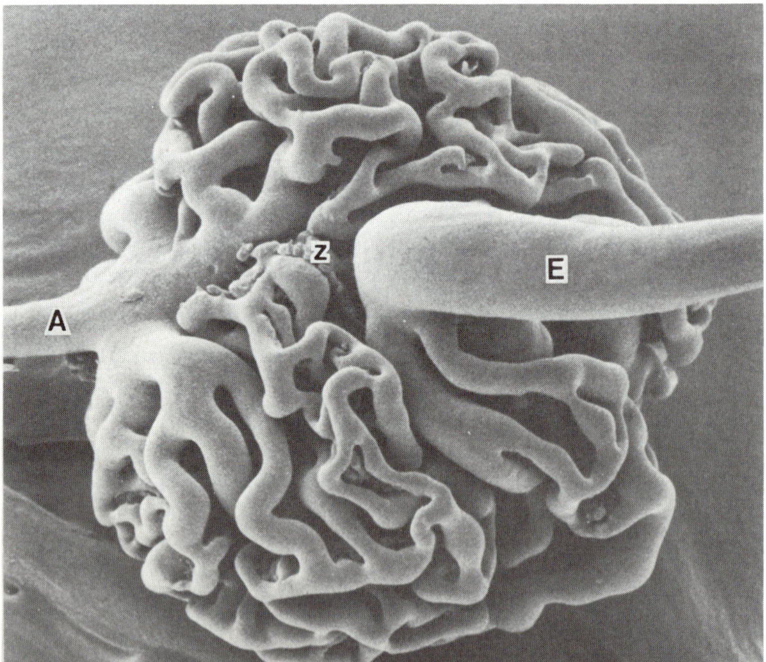

FIG. 5. A closer view of a juxtamedullary glomerulus of the 45-year-old man. Note a capillary cluster occupying the wide space between the afferent and efferent arterioles (A and E). z, leaked resin. x 350.

FIG. 6. A profile of an unfolded and microdissected subcapsular glomerulus of the

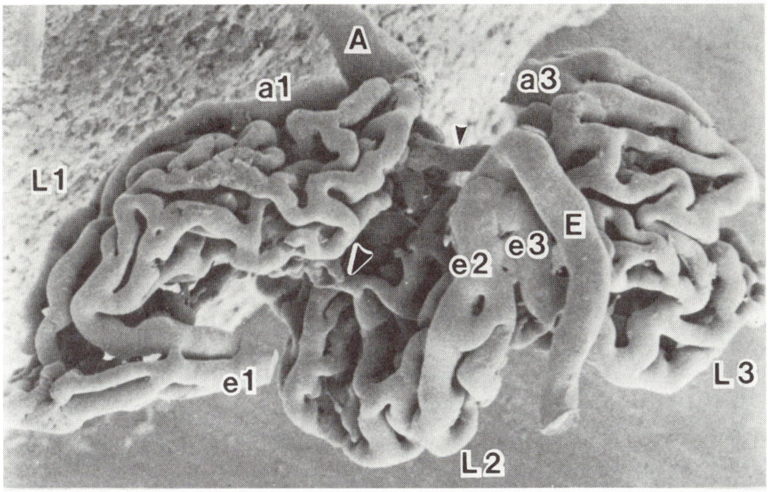

6

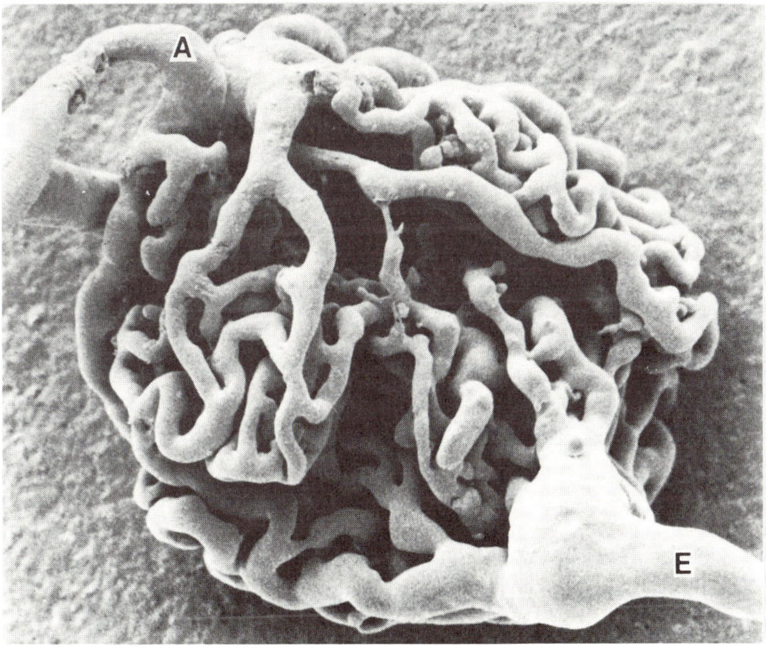

7

45-year-old man. Note the three lobules constructing one glomerular tuft, where the well developed two lateral lobules (L1 and L3) sandwiching a rather flattened and less developed middle lobule (L2). A and E, afferent and efferent arterioles; al and el, afferent and efferent rootlets of the L1 lobule; e2, efferent rootlet of L2 lobule; a3 and e3, afferent and efferent rootlets of L3 lobule; thick arrowhead, translobular capillaries; thin arrowhead, accessory afferent vessel to L3 lobule. x 300.

FIG. 7. A subcapsular glomerulus of the 45-year-old man, stretched and viewed from the vascular pole. Note that there is no short-cut communication between the afferent and efferent arterioles (A and E). x 300.

lets at or beneath the vascular pole and drain into the afferent arteriole. Usually, each glomerular lobule has a single efferent rootlet as well as the single

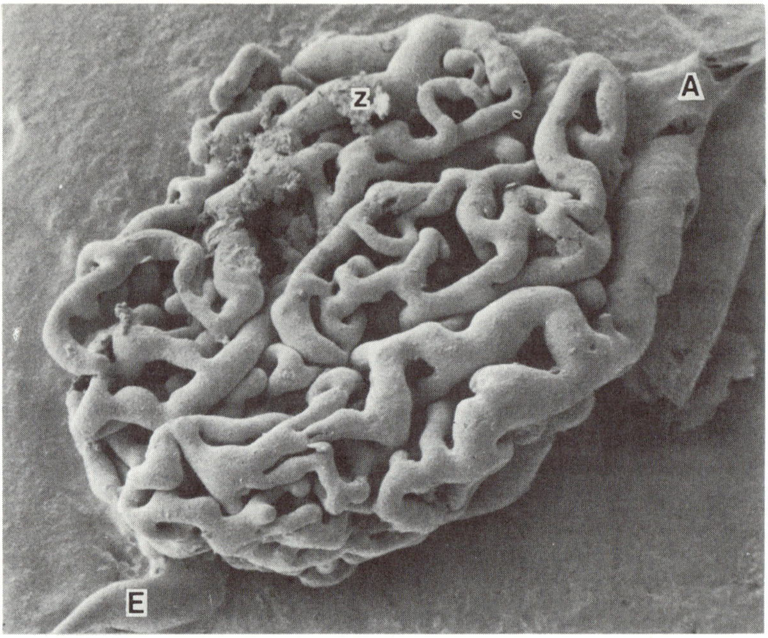

8

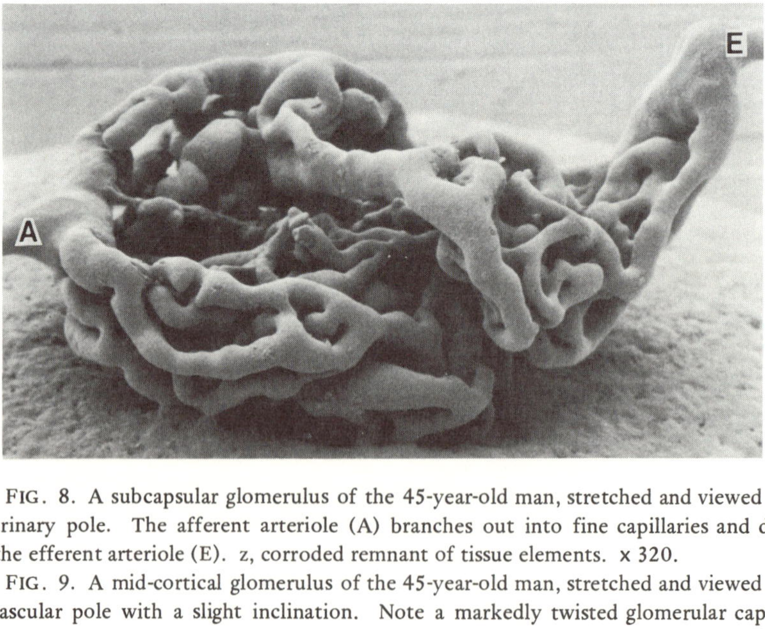

9

FIG. 8. A subcapsular glomerulus of the 45-year-old man, stretched and viewed from the urinary pole. The afferent arteriole (A) branches out into fine capillaries and drains into the efferent arteriole (E). z, corroded remnant of tissue elements. x 320.

FIG. 9. A mid-cortical glomerulus of the 45-year-old man, stretched and viewed from the vascular pole with a slight inclination. Note a markedly twisted glomerular capillary tuft (see text). A and E, afferent and efferent arterioles. x 320.

afferent rootlet (Fig. 6). However, some lobules occasionally receive a few accessory afferent capillaries from the adjacent lobules (Fig. 6) and some others lack in proper efferent rootlets to drain into the distal or efferent segments of the adjacent lobules. The efferent arteriole passes through the spaces in-between the afferent rootlets of the afferent arteriole and leaves the glomerulus, to run in opposite direction to the afferent arteriole (Figs. 1 – 5). It is rather rare that the glomerular capillary tuft shows no lobulation.

Form and size of the glomerular capillary lobules varied widely in each glomerulus. In general, the glomerulus composed of two lobules had fully developed ones occupying equally the hemispheres of the glomerulus, and those having three or more lobules had rather flattened and poorly developed ones sandwiched between the lateral lobules (Fig. 6).

The glomerulus or glomerular capillary tuft sometimes showed a marked twisting or rotation. An unfolded or extended form of a markedly twisted glomerulus is shown in Fig. 9. In this case, the left-sided afferent rootlet crossed the vascular pole and its lobule emptied from the right-sided aspect into the efferent arteriole, and the right-side afferent rootlet ran toward the urinary pole and its lobule emptied from the left-sided aspect into the efferent arteriole (Fig. 9). The twisted glomerulus, thus, had widely opened vascular pole.

The glomerulus having two efferent arterioles was occasionally observed. They leave glomerulus separately, usually at the vascular pole (Fig. 10), though sometimes near the urinary pole. The glomerulus having three efferent arterioles were also observed, though very rarely. In this case, too, each arteriole left glomerulus separately, *viz.* one near the urinary pole and the remainings at or near the vascular pole.

The glomerular capillaries were 10 to 25 μm in diameter, thicker ones in the proximal (afferent) and distal (efferent) segments and thinner ones in the middle segments of the glomerular lobules. Besides, very thin capillaries less than 6 μm in diameter were frequently encountered in some restricted areas

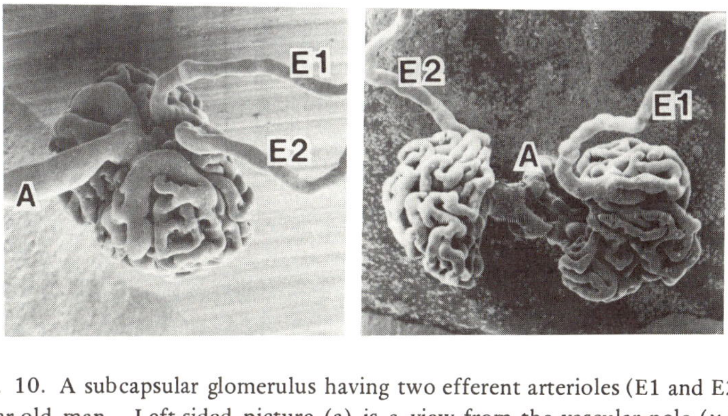

FIG. 10. A subcapsular glomerulus having two efferent arterioles (E1 and E2). From the 45-year-old man. Left-sided picture (a) is a view from the vascular pole (x 200) and right-side one (b) is a microdissected form of this anomaly shown in the picture (a) (x 200). Note that the glomerulus is divided into two parts, each of which has its own efferent arteriole.

close to the vascular pole of the middle segments of the glomerular lobules among the afferent and/or efferent capillary rootlets (Fig. 2).

The 6-month-old fetal kidneys contained many immature glomeruli at varied developmental stages in the subcapsular layer (Fig. 1). The primitive glomeruli appear as straight vessels or terminal branches of the interlobular arteries. Some of these straight vessels have partial dilations or protrusions indicating the initiation of the glomerular development, 1st-stage glomeruli. Some others show the U-shaped loops, more advanced stage, where afferent and efferent arterioles are clearly discernible, second-stage glomeruli (Fig. 1). Some terminal branches have the irregularly winding loops with few anastomoses among them, though small rounded protrusions with free endings were occasionally found on their surfaces or small pits penetrating the loops, the 3rd stage glomeruli (Fig. 1). There can be seen also simplest forms of the conglomerated networks of anastomosing capillaries, 4th stage glomeruli (Fig. 1). With further development, the glomerulus became larger and contained more capillaries. Even in these later development, the glomerular capillaries sometimes had some small protrusions on their surfaces and also small pits penetrating the glomerular capillaries.

The glomerular capillary tufts of the 45-year-old and 76-year-old men were much larger and contained much more capillaries than the well-developed ones of the fetus (Figs. 1 — 3). Furthermore, their glomerular capillaries were more tortuous than those of the fetus (Figs. 1 — 3). The most tortuous capillaries were observed in the glomeruli of the 76-year-old man (Fig. 3). In such aged man, the afferent and efferent arterioles and their parent vessels including the interlobular arteries were also tortuous. The small protrusions and small pits seen in the developing glomeruli were occasionally observed even in the glomeruli of the 45-year-old man near the vascular pole, but rarely in the 76-year-old man.

DISCUSSION

The present study by SEM on vascular casts of human glomeruli confirms our previous findings in man, monkey and rat that the kidney glomerulus is lobulated and each lobule is composed of fine capillary networks. It also confirms that the lobules are fairly independent units for conveying blood from the afferent to efferent arterioles though there are usually some thin translobular capillary communications among them (Murakami, 1972, 1978; Unehira, 1981; Murakami et al., 1985a). The glomeruli are neither the non-anastomosing capillary loops as contended by Vimtrup (1928) nor the sacculated capillaries derived from a wall of an arteriole as claimed by Trabucco and Marquez (1952). Recently, many authors have also investigated the kidney vascular casts of dog, rat and some other animals including bullfrog by SEM, revealing numerous anastomoses of the glomerular capillaries (Lee et al., 1972; Spinelli, 1974; Anderson and Anderson, 1976; Morris and Campbell, 1978; Kazimierczak, 1980; Ohtani and Naito, 1980; Casellas and Mimran, 1981). These authors, however, did not demonstrate the lobulations of the glomerular capillary tuft which can be seen clearly only on microdissected samples. Boyer (1956) and some other authors contended that no area of the glomerular capillary tuft is defined separately. Our findings support those of Hall (1955), who described that each lobule is independent in man, dog and rat. However, he failed to find the translobular capillaries among the lobules, though they are thin and a few in number but occur usually. Recent examination of Yang and Morrison (1980) on the rat glomerulus by reconstruction of ultrathin sections has also confirmed the glomerular lobulations.

Our previous studies in man, monkey and rat have clearly demonstrated occasional occurrence of completely independent glomerular capillary lobules without any interlobular anastomoses (Murakami, 1972, 1978; Unehira, 1981). The present study suggests that the lobulations are differentiated during an early stage of glomerular development, the third stage. Complete failure of transverse anastomoses among the capillary loops in the third stage will lead to the formation of completely independent lobules. If many transverse anastomoses occur in the third stage, this may lead to the formation of non-separable lobules which are interconnected with each other by numerous capillaries.

As described above, the glomerular capillary tuft shows sometimes a marked twisting or rotation. In these cases, the lobulations are not easily defined. However, careful observation of stretched or unfolded samples may make the lobulations clear (Fig. 9). Hall (1955) described in man, dog and rat that some main channels run in the periphery of the lobule near the urinary pole and drain directly into the efferent arteriole. Elias (1957) illustrated some short-cut circuits between the afferent and efferent rootlets. Ljungqvist (1975) also described a connection between the afferent and efferent arterioles at the vascular pole. As seen in Figs. 4 — 10 and also as shown in our previous studies in man, monkey and rat, every branch of the afferent arteriole ramifies into fine capillaries. Furthermore, it should be noted that there exists a deep cleft, which separates completely the afferent and efferent segments of the glomerular capillary lobules and opens to the vascular pole (Murakami, 1972). Therefore, no such main channels or short-cut circuits between the afferent and efferent arterioles can exist. The findings are consistent with those of Spinelli and his associates (1972) who found no shunt between the afferent and efferent arterioles in dog and rat.

It may be of interest that the human glomerulus develops originally from a single vessel. This developing pattern, as preliminarily reported elsewhere (Murakami et al., 1985a), is similar to that of the bullfrog mesonephric glomerulus (Naito, 1984). As is well known, concerning the origin of the glomerular capillary tuft there are two main theories, in-growth and *in situ* ones, as proposed through light microscopic studies of Indian ink-injected samples. The in-growth theory contends the glomerular capillary arising directly from the interstitial vessel (Potter, 1965; Osathanondh and Potter, 1966; Kajimierczak, 1971, 1980), and the *in situ* theory from the lower cleft of the renal vesicle (Suzuki, 1959; Vernier and Birch-Anderson, 1962). Our observation of characteristic U-shaped loop formation from an interstitial single straight vessel suggests the invasion of the interstitial vessel into the renal vesicle, supporting the in-growth theory.

The present study confirms further that the glomerular capillaries increase in number from the initial development to the aged stage. A glomerular capillary proliferation model, in which the luminal capillary endothelial surface protrudes into the capillary lumen and forms septa, splitting the capillary into several daughter capillaries whose lumina communicate at the septal margins, has previously been proposed through light microscopic studies of Indian ink-injected samples (Potter, 1965; Osathanondh and Potter, 1966; Kazimierczak, 1971). The small pits penetrating the glomerular capillaries shown in the present observations should represent the septa. In addition to these small pits, present observations revealed small rounded protrusions of free endings on the developing glomerular capillary surfaces. These blind protrusions or capillary shoots may form anastomoses with the adjacent ones. Thus, our findings also suggest that the glomerular capillaries multiply, at least in part, by sprouting daughter capillaries on their external surfaces. Similar protrusions have been observed in the developing bullfrog glomeruli and also in the mature monkey glomeruli (Unehira, 1981; Naito, 1984). The existence of such small protrusions and pits in the mature glomeruli may indicate that new capillaries are formed even in the adult as well as in developing glomeruli.

As just described, we often found very thin capillaries smaller than 6 μ in diameter near the vascular pole of the adult or mature glomerulus. They will hardly allow the passage of blood cells. Žlábek (1973), who observed the Indian ink-injected adult rat samples by light microscopy, regarded these thin capillaries as preferential and short-cut channels for passage of blood serum. But they may be newly formed capillaries which develop into the usual or thick capillaries in time.

It is also noticeable that the glomerular capillaries were more tortuous in the older man. The increase of capillaries in number and tortuosity may widen the filtration surface of glomerular capillaries and compensate for the decreased functioning of the aged glomerular capillaries. High blood pressure may be needed to keep sufficient blood flow in such a tortuous capillary bed.

Unusual double efferent arterioles in one glomerulus have been reported in man and some other animals by Boenig (1936), Shonyo and Mann (1944), Okano et al. (1959) and Moffat and Fourman (1963). In 1200 rat glomeruli examined in our previous study, 0.9% of them had the double efferent arterioles (Murakami et al., 1971). Casellas and Mimran (1979) proposed that one of the double efferent arterioles would serve as a bypass of the glomerular capillary tuft. But our observation on microdissected samples have shown that each of two efferent arterioles belongs to a different lobule (Murakami et al., 1971) (Fig. 10). The finding is inconsistent with the bypass theory of Casellas and Mimran (1979). As reported elsewhere, unusual glomeruli having double afferent arterioles can be seen in adult man as well as in rat (Murakami, 1976; Murakami et al., 1985a) and the double efferent arterioles occur even in the developing glomeruli (Murakami et al., 1971). Therefore, these appear to be congenital anomalies. Rare occurrence of four or more efferent vessels in one glomerulus has been reported in man by SEM of vascular casts (Murakami et al., 1985b).

Abstract

Blood vascular casts of human fetal, adult and senile kidneys were observed with a scanning electron microscope (SEM) in order to reveal the basic structure, development and aging of the glomerular capillary tufts. The glomerulus starts from a single straight branch of interlobular artery to form a U-shaped loop. Then, the loop multiplies and forms a primitive conglomerated network of anastomosing capillaries. The mature glomerulus contains numerous anastomosing capillaries and shows lobulations. The glomerular capillary lobules are intercommunicated with each other by a few thin translobular capillaries, but regarded as independent functional units for conveying blood from the afferent to efferent arterioles. The glomerular capillaries are more numerous and tortuous in the aged than in the adult. This may compensate for the decreased functioning of the aged glomerular capillaries.

REFERENCES

Anderson, B.G., and Anderson, W.D. (1976). Renal vasculature of the trout demonstrated by scanning electron microscopy, compared with canine glomerular vessels. *Am. J. Anat.* **145**, 443–458.

Boenig, H. (1936). Beiträge zur Kenntnis der Vasa efferentia in der menschlichen Niere. *Z. Mikrosk. Anat. Forsch.* **39**, 105–115.

Bowman, W. (1842). On the structure and use of the Malpighian bodies of the kidney, with observations on the circulation through that gland. *Philos. Trans. R. Soc. London* **1**, 57–80.

Boyer, C.C. (1956). The vascular pattern of the renal glomerulus as revealed by plastic reconstruction from serial sections. *Anat. Rec.* **125**, 433–441.

Casellas, D., and Mimran, A. (1979). Aglomerular pathways in intrarenal microvasculature of aged rats. *Am. J. Anat.* **156**, 293–298.

Casellas, D., and Mimran, A. (1981). Shunting in renal microvasculature of the rat: A scanning electron microscopic study of corrosion casts. *Anat. Rec.* **201**, 237–248.

Elias, H. (1957). De structura glomeruli renalis. *Anat. Anz.* **104**, 26–36.

Hall, B.V. (1955). Further studies of the normal structure of the renal glomerulus. *In* "Proceedings of 6th Ann. Conf. Nephrotic Syndrome", pp. 1–39. Nat. Nephrosis Found., New York.

Johnston, W.B. (1899). A reconstruction of a glomerulus of the human Kidney. *Anat. Anz.* **16**, 260–266.

Kazimierczak, J. (1971). Development of the renal corpuscle and the juxtaglomerular apparatus: A light and electron microscopic study. *Acta Pathol. Microbiol. Scand. Secta A. Suppl.* **218**, 1–115.

Kazimierczak, J. (1980). A study by scanning (SEM) and transmission (TEM) electron microscopy of the glomerular capillaries in developing rat kidney. *Cell Tissue Res.* **212**, 241–255.

Lee, M.L., Purkerson, M.L., Agate, Jr., F.J., and Dempsey, E.W. (1972). Ultrastructural changes in renal glomeruli of rats during experimentally induced hypertension and uremia. *Am. J. Anat.* **135**, 191–204.

Lewis, O.J. (1958). The vascular arrangement of the mammalian renal glomerulus as revealed by a study of its development. *J. Anat.* **92**, 433–440.

Ljungqvist, A. (1975). Ultrastructural demonstration of a connection between afferent and efferent juxtamedullary glomerular arterioles. *Kidney Int.* **8**, 239–244.

Moffat, D.B., and Fourman, J. (1963). The vascular pattern of the rat kidney. *J. Anat.* **97**, 543–553.

Morris, J.L., and Campbell, G. (1978). Renal vascular anatomy of the toad (Bufo marinus). *Cell Tissue Res.* **189**, 501–514.

Murakami, T. (1971). Application of the scanning electron microscope to the study of fine distribution of the blood vessels. *Arch. Histol. Jpn.* **32**, 445–454.

Murakami, T. (1972). Vascular arrangement of the rat renal glomerulus. A scanning electron microscope study of corrosion casts. *Arch. Histol. Jpn.* **34**, 87–107.

Murakami, T. (1976). Double afferent arterioles of the rat renal glomerulus as studied by the injection replica scanning electron microscope method. *Arch. Histol. Jpn.* **39**, 327–332.

Murakami, T. (1978). Methyl methacrylate injection replica method. *In* "Principles and Techniques of Scanning Electron Microscopy. Vol. 6" (M.A. Hayat, ed.), pp. 159–169. Van Nostrand Reinhold, New York.

Murakami, T., Miyoshi, M., and Fujita, T. (1971). Glomerular vessels of the rat kidney with special reference to double efferent arterioles. A scanning electron microscope study of corrosion casts. *Arch. Histol. Jpn.* **33**, 179–198.

Murakami, T., Unehira, M., Kawakami, H., and Kubotsu, A. (1973). Osmium impregnation of methyl methacrylate vascular casts for scanning electron microscopy. *Arch. Histol. Jpn.* **36**, 119–124.

Murakami, T., Kikuta, A., Ohtsuka, A., and Kaneshige, T. (1985a). Renal vasculature as observed by SEM of vascular casts. Basic architecture, development and aging of glomerular capillary beds. *In* "Basic Clinical, Surgical Nephrology" (L.J.A. DiDio and P.M. Motta, eds.), pp. 83–98. Martinus Nijhoff, Boston.

Murakami, T., Kikuta, A., Shinji, S., and Sano, T. (1985b). Multiple efferent arterioles of the human kidney glomerulus as observed by scanning electron microscopy of vascular casts. *Arch. Histol. Jpn.* **48**, in press.

Naito, I. (1984). The development of glomerular capillary tufts of the bullfrog kidney from a straight interstitial vessel to an anastomosed network. A scanning electron microscopic study of vascular casts. *Arch. Histol. Jpn.* **47**, 441–456.

Ohtani, O., and Naito, I. (1980). Renal microcirculation of the bullfrog, *Rana catesbeiana*: a scanning electron microscope study of vascular casts. *Arch. Histol. Jpn.* **43**, 319–330.

Okano, H., Ohta, Y., Fujimoto, T., and Ohtani, Y. (1959). Cubical anatomy of several ducts and vessels by injection method of acrylic resin. VI. On the vascular system of the kidney in Macacus cynomolgus. *Okajimas Folia Anat. Jpn.* **34**, 27–41.

Osathanondh, V., and Potter, E.L. (1966). Development of human kidney as shown by microdissection. *Arch. Pathol.* **82**, 403–411.

Potter, E.L. (1965). Development of the human glomerulus. *Arch. Pathol.* **80**, 241–255.

Shonyo, E.S., and Mann, F.C. (1944). An experimental investigation of renal circulation. *Arch. Pathol.* **38**, 287–296.

Spinelli, F. (1974). Structure and development of the renal glomerulus as revealed by scanning electron microscopy. *In* "International Rev. Cytol. Vol. 139" (G.H. Bourne and J.F. Danielli, eds.), pp. 345–381. Academic Press, New York.

Spinelli, F., Wirtz, H., Brücher, C., and Pehling, G. (1972). Non-existence of shunts between afferent and efferent arterioles of juxtamedullary glomeruli in dog and rat kidneys. *Nephron* **9**, 123–128.

Suzuki, Y. (1959). An electron microscopy of the renal differentiation: II. glomerulus. *Keio J. Med.* **8**, 129–142.

Trabucco, A., and Marquez, F. (1952). Structure of the glomeruli tuft. *J. Urol.* **67**, 235–255.

Unehira, M. (1981). Blood vascular architecture of the rhesus monkey kidney glomerulus. A scanning electron microscope study of corrosion casts. *Okayama Igakkai Zasshi* **93**, 951–961 (in Japanese).

Vernier, R.L., and Birch-Andersen, A. (1962). Studies of the human fetal kidney: I. Development of the glomerulus. *J. Pediatr.* **60**, 754–768.

Vimtrup, B.J. (1928). On the number, shape, structure, and surface area of the glomeruli in the kidneys of man and mammals. *Am. J. Anat.* **41**, 123–151.

Wilmer, H.A. (1941). The arrangement of the capillary tuft of the human glomerulus. *Anat. Rec.* **80**, 507–518.

Yang, G.C.H., and Morrison, A.B. (1980). Three large dissectable rat glomerular models reconstructed from wide-field electron micrographs. *Anat. Rec.* **196**, 431–440.

Žlábek, K. (1973). Über dünne interkapillare Anastomosen im Nierenglomerulus der Ratte. *Acta Anat.* **85**, 177–189.

III. Physiology and Pathology of Glomerulus

A. Role of Size- and Charge-Selective Properties of Glomerular Wall

Work done in the past two decades has resulted in increased understanding of the mechanisms whereby the glomerular capillary wall functions *in vivo* as an efficient ultrafilter. Investigations using functional, morphological, and biochemical approaches have shown that the filtering mechanism is complex, and depends for its efficiency on several factors. Importantly, the filter discriminates between macromolecules not only on the basis of their size, but their electrical charge as well. Thus, the capillary wall has a net negative charge, owing to the presence in its extracellular matrix of a number of negatively charged moieties. By virtue of electrical interactions with these anionic moieties, negatively charged proteins are retarded from entry into the filter, relative to less charged or positively charged molecules.

Increasing understanding of these normal interactions has spurred interest in their possible roles in various aspects of glomerular pathology and pathophysiology. Decrease of or perturbation of the anionic moieties is a cause for proteinuria of glomerular origin. Even more importantly, electrical charge interactions may determine the glomerular localization of macromolecules or macromolecular aggregates, such as immune complexes.

The articles in this section describe the normal interactions of macromolecules with the glomerular capillary wall and highlight some mechanisms whereby these interactions may be disturbed by disease.

Manjeri A. Venkatachalam

PROTEIN LEAKAGE THROUGH GLOMERULAR CAPILLARIES HAVING THE FUNCTIONING AND DYSFUNCTIONING ANIONIC BARRIER

Tadashi Tsujii, Toshiro Ono and Satimaru Seno

Division of Ultrastructure Research and Pathology,
Shigei Medical Research Institute, Okayama

As is well known, the leakage of plasma proteins from the blood vessels is strictly controlled under physiological conditions to maintain the colloid osmotic pressure of blood which serves to keep the blood volume at a certain fixed level. The endothelial cells of glomerular capillaries are largely fenestrated with gross pores, approximately 70 nm in mean size, and the glomerular basement membrane (GBM) is of fibrous structure porous enough to make some macromolecules permeate (Tisher, 1976). Therefore, the anionic groups of glycoproteins, glycolipids, and sialoproteins (Latta et al., 1975; Kerjaschki et al., 1984) on the cell surface, and heparan sulfate proteoglycan in the GBM (Kanwar and Farquhar, 1979a; Kanwar et al., 1980; Klein et al., 1983; Kanwar, 1984; Mynderse et al., 1983; Vernier et al., 1983; Laurie et al., 1984; Parthasarathy and Spiro, 1984; Cavallo et al., 1984) have been suspected to contribute largely to the prevention of the leakage of anionic plasma proteins from capillaries.

Recent experiments using tracer macromolecules of different electrical charge have indicated that the negative electric charges of the glomerular capillary wall is an important factor for the functional filtration barrier against polyanionic macromolecules or serum proteins (Bohrer et al., 1978; Brenner et al., 1977; Kanwar et al., 1980; Kelley and Cavallo, 1978; Rennke and Venkatachalam, 1977; Rosenzweig and Kanwar, 1982; Simionescu et al., 1982a; Venkatachalam and Rennke, 1978).

The anionic groups on the cell surface and those in GBM can be visualized under light microscope (LM) by staining with cationic dyes and under electron microscope (EM) by staining with cationic metal compounds (Latta et al., 1975; Schurer et al., 1977; Kanwar and Farquhar, 1979b; Alcorn and Ryan 1981; Reale et al., 1983; Seno et al., 1983a, b; Rollason and Brewer, 1984). By using such techniques it has been shown that the ionized anionic groups of glomerular wall reduce in density in some renal diseases accompanying proteinuria (Caulfield and Farquhar, 1978; Brenner et al., 1978; Caulfield, 1979; Kreisberg et al., 1979; Kelley and Cavallo, 1980; Hirsch et al., 1981; Melnick et al., 1981; Olson et al., 1981; Cotran and Rennke, 1983; Mynderse et al., 1983; Schneeberger et al., 1983; Tsujii et al., 1983; Vernier et al., 1983; Weening and Rennke 1983; Barnes et al., 1984). Recently, Assel et al. (1984) and Sonnenburg-Hatzopoulos (1984) also demonstrated that the reduction of glomerular anionic sites caused pronounced proteinuria prior to the detectable morphological alterations of podocytes (Blau and Hass, 1973; Bennet et al.,

1976; Caulfield, 1979; Camussi et al., 1982). However, it was also shown that there was no change in the density of the anionic sites of the GBM in experimental aminonucleoside nephrosis (Kanwar and Jakubowski, 1984) and in some patients with nephrotic syndrome (Faraggiana et al., 1982).

The inconsistency of the results may be due to factors related to the electric charge of serum proteins. Cationic molecules perfused *via* the arteries will be adsorbed directly on to the anionic sites of the endothelial cell surfaces, but those injected intravenously may bind with anionic serum proteins reducing their electric charge. Therefore, the results of experiments when cationic probes are either perfused or injected intravenously may need to be interpreted in the what of these factors. Electrically neutralized serum protein-cationic probe complexes may penetrate the healthy anionic barrier of endothelial cells and form deposits in the GBM or be excreted into the urinary space after passing through the capillary walls.

With these considerations in mind, we have perfused normal rat kidneys with poly-L-lysine—human serum albumin conjugate (PLL-HA) or cationized ferritin—human serum albumin conjugate (CF-HA), and in another series of studies, injected the same tracers intravenously in normal rats.

In this paper it is demonstrated that PLL-HA and CF-HA introduced into the renal artery by perfusion and also those injected intravenously deposit in the subendothelial spaces, indicating that the negative electric charge of serum proteins as well as that of capillary walls is essential to keep serum proteins in circulation.

Materials and Methods

Experimental design: One hundred and eight adult female Wistar rats weighing 210 — 250 g were used. They were kept on standard diet and water *ad libitum*. The animals were divided into 3 groups: 60 for perfusion tests (1st group), 42 for intravenous injection tests (2nd group) and 6 as nontreated controls (3rd group) (Table 1). The animals in the 1st group were divided further into 10 subgroups; 1A, 1B, 1C, 1D, 1E, 1F, 1G, 1H, 1I, 1J, and those in the 2nd group into 7 subgroups, 2A, 2B, 2C, 2D, 2E, 2F, 2G, 6 animals in each subgroup.

1) *For perfusion*: The animals were anesthesized with sodium pentobarbital (Pitman-Moore Inc., Washington Crossing, NJ, USA), 50 mg per Kg of body weight, the abdominal cavity was opened and the abdominal aorta was cannulated according to the method described by Elling et al. (1977) for the perfusion fixation of pig kidney and modified by us for rat. All the animals were perfused first with 5 ml of pure Krebs-Ringer's bicarbonate buffer solution (KRB) or Hanks' balanced salt solution (HBSS), pH 7.4, 37 ℃, to wash out blood, and then with 10 ml of KRB solution containing various tracers (anionic ferritin (AF) for 1A, CF for 1B, CF-HA for 1C, PLL-HA for 1D, HA for 1E, PLL for 1F, KRB alone for 1I, and HBSS alone for 1J). Animals in groups 1G and 1H were perfused using a 2 step procedure after the wash out the blood. The first step was with 5 ml of KRB containing either 0.1 mg/ml poly-L-lysine (PLL) (1G) or protamine sulfate (PS) (1H); the second step was with 10 ml of AF just as in 1A. In all cases perfusion was made at 110 mm Hg

TABLE 1 EXPERIMENTAL DESIGN

Groups	Subgroups	No. of animals	Renal perfusion
Perfusion test group 1	1A	6	KRB → AF → KRB
	1B	6	KRB → CF → KRB
	1C	6	KRB → CF-HA → KRB
	1D	6	HS → PLL-HA → HS
	1E	6	HS → HA → HS
	1F	6	KRB → PLL → KRB
	1G	6	KRB → PLL → AF → KRB
	1H	6	KRB → PS → AF → KRB
	1I	6	KRB → KRB → KRB
	1J	6	HS → HS → HS
Intravenous injection test group 2			Intravenous injection
	2A	6	CF (single inj.)
	2B	6	CF-HA (4 inj.)
	2C	6	PLL-HA (single inj.)
	2D	6	PLL-HA (4 inj.)
	2E	6	PLL (single inj.)
	2F	6	HA (4 inj.)
	2G	6	HS (4 inj.)
Control group 3			Control
		6	non treated

by a cylinder pump (Model STC-521, Termo Co., Tokyo, Japan).

2) *For intravenous injection*: Intravenous injection was made *via* the jugular vein. The animals in group 2A received single injections of 3 ml of 1% cationized ferritin (CF) in KRB (10 mg CF/100 g body weight), and those in group 2C received PLL-HA instead of CF. The animals in group 2B received 2 ml of CF-HA conjugate daily for 4 days, and those in group 2D had PLL-HA instead of CF-HA conjugate.

The animals in group 2E received a single injection of 3 ml of PLL solution and those in group 2F 3 ml of human serum albumin (HA) solution daily for 4 days. Those in group 2G served as controls and received 3 ml of HBSS daily for 4 days, respectively.

All the animals which received PLL (2E) died a few min after injection.

The animals in groups 2A, 2B, 2C, 2D, 2F and 2G, were sacrificed 1, 14 and 24 hr after the last injection, 12 animals at one time, 2 in each subgroup. Those allowed to survive for 24 hr after the last injection were kept in metabolic cages, urine was collected for 15 hr before sacrifice, and total urinary proteins were estimated by turbidimetry at 450 nm adding 3% sulfosalicilic acid (Kingsbury, 1926).

Six untreated animals served as healthy controls and were sacrificed by decapitation at the end of this experiment.

After sacrifice or death, kidneys were taken out in all the animals of groups 1, 2 and 3 and fixed for morphologic observations.

Tissue processing for morphologic observations: For general histologic studies the tissues were fixed in 10% formol in phosphate buffer solution (pH 7.3), dehydrated, embedded in paraffin, sectioned and stained with hematoxylin-eosin (HE). Some tissues were fixed in Dubosq-Brazil fixative (Zollinger and Mihatsch, 1978) for silver methenamine stain (PAM) (De Martino and Zamboni, 1967) and PAS staining.

For histochemical detection of HA, the immunofluorescent method was used. Small pieces of fresh tissues were frozen in liquid nitrogen, frozen-sectioned, fixed in chilled acetone and stained with fluorescein isothiocyanate-conjugated anti-human serum albumin rabbit IgG fraction (FITC-IgG) (Cappel Lab. Inc., Cochranville, PA, USA) and observed by fluorescent microscope (FM). Before use the FITC-IgG was treated with crystallized rat serum albumin (Sigma, St. Louis, MO. USA) to reduce nonspecific binding. Thus, the FITC-IgG reacted specifically with HA but not with rat albumin as confirmed by immunoelectrophoresis.

For general EM observations, small pieces of the kidney tissues were fixed with ice cold Karnovsky's fixative (Karnovsky, 1965) for 2 hr, post fixed with ice cold 2% OsO_4 in 0.05 M sodium cacodylate buffer (pH 7.3) containing 0.2 M sucrose for 3 hr, dehydrated through ethanol to acetone and embedded in TAAB embedding resin (Taab Lab., Reading, England). Ultrathin sections were obtained with a diamond knife on a Reichert OmU-3 ultramicrotome (Reichert-Jung, Wien, Austria), stained with uranyl acetate and lead citrate, and examined under a Hitachi H-700 transmission electron microscope (Hitachi, Tokyo, Japan) at an accelerating voltage of 75 kV.

For detection of ionized anionic groups, the method of Seno et al. (1983b) "Fe-Cac" was used.

For immuno-cytochemical-EM observation of HA, small pieces of kidney tissues were fixed in 4% paraformaldehyde in 0.05 M citric acid buffer (pH 4.5) for 6 hr at −5 ℃, and washed in 0.05 M citric acid buffer solution (pH 4.5), containing glucose to adjust the osmolarity to 300 milliosmoles. The tissues were sectioned using a Vibratome tissue sectioner (Model G, Oxford Lab., Foster City, Calif. USA), 50 μm thick, and the HA was stained by the method of Ryan and Karnovsky (1976).

To observe the structure of PLL-HA by EM, negative staining was used; a drop of PLL-HA solution was mixed with a drop of phosphotungstic acid staining solution (Thomas, 1978), put on surface of the collodion-coated grid, dried in air and examined by EM.

Reagents: All the macromolecules used in this experiment were from Sigma, St. Louis, MO, USA. Both anionic ferritin (AF) and cationized ferritin (CF) were horse-spleen ferritins. Human serum albumin (HA) was of crystallized and lyophilized one, poly-L-lysine (PLL) was HBr salt of Type 1-B, 350,000 MW and protamine sulfate (PS) was of Grade X from salmon.

To prepare solutions for perfusion and injection, these were dissolved in Hanks' balanced salt solution (HBSS), 0.8 mg/ml for HA and 0.4 mg/ml for

PLL·HBr, and the pH of the solutions was adjusted to pH 7.3 by using sodium bicarbonate and the osmolarity to 300 milliosmols with glucose. PLL-HA conjugate solution was prepared by adding 2 volumes of 0.16% HA in HBSS solution to 1 volume of 0.08% PLL in HBSS solution drop by drop with constant stirring. CF-HA conjugate was prepared by adding 1 volume of 1% CF solution in Krebs-Ringer's bicarbonate buffer solution (KRB) to 2 volumes of 2% HA solution in KRB drop by drop with constant stirring. The pH of these solutions was adjusted to 7.3 and the osmolarity to 300 milliosmols. All the solutions were prepared just before use.

The electrical mobility of the solutes tested were checked by electrophoresis on cellulose acetate membranes (Separax, Joko Sangyo Co. Ltd., Tokyo) at 0.6 mA/cm for 45 min in 0.06 M Veronal buffer, pH 8.6.

Results

Electrophoresis revealed the positive electric charge of CF and PLL and the negative charge of HA and AF. All of them were completely soluble in aqueous solution. The PLL-HA and CF-HA gave somewhat cloudy solutions (Fig. 1C) and had no measurable electric charge. EM observation of PLL-HA conjugate revealed its bead-necklace-like fibrous profiles by negative staining (Fig. 2).

Perfusion test: Macroscopically, all the kidneys perfused with AF, CF, PLL, HA and their conjugates appeared pale and showed no specific change to distinguish them from each other.

LM observations of HE-stained sections of kidney tissue from all subgroups in group 1 and 2 showed slight swelling of the glomerular tufts and the mesangial matrix in all cases but no distinct pathologic changes (Fig. 3A, B). GBM did not show any specific changes in all cases as revealed by observing PAM- and PAS-stained sections. Immunofluorescence of HA was detected only in glomeruli perfused with PLL-HA (Fig. 4A, B and 5).

EM observations of glomeruli of the kidney perfused with CF revealed the CF molecules adhering heavily to the luminal and abluminal surfaces of endothelial cells and some in GBM (Fig. 6A). The perfused CF-HA were also adherent to the endothelial surface but only slightly. Most of the agglomerated particles infiltrated into the *lamina rara interna* of GBM passing through the fenestrae of the glomerular capillary endothelium and some in *lamina rara externa* (Fig. 6B). The perfused AF neither adhered to the endothelial surface nor infiltrated into the GBM (Fig. 6C). But, in kidneys perfused first with PLL solution and subsequently with AF, some AF molecules penetrated into the subendothelial space (Fig. 6D). EM observations of the Fe-Cac-stained sections of PLL-perfused kidney revealed much less anionic sites of the glomeruli on the surfaces of endothelial cells and also within the GBM (Fig. 7A), as compared to those of controls whose glomeruli had heavy deposition of the colloidal iron particles on both luminal and abluminal surfaces of endothelial cells (Fig. 7B), though the surfaces of podocytes showed nearly equal heavy deposition of Fe-Cac in both cases. The Fe-Cac staining intensity of the glomeruli of the animals perfused with PLL-HA (Fig. 7C) and HA (Fig. 7D) was nearly the same as that of controls.

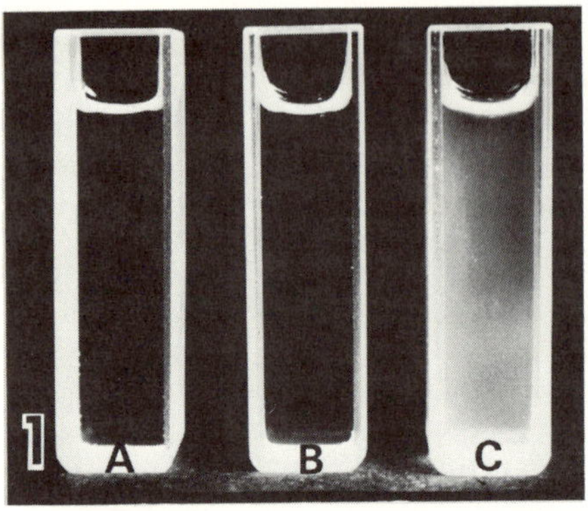
1
A
B
C

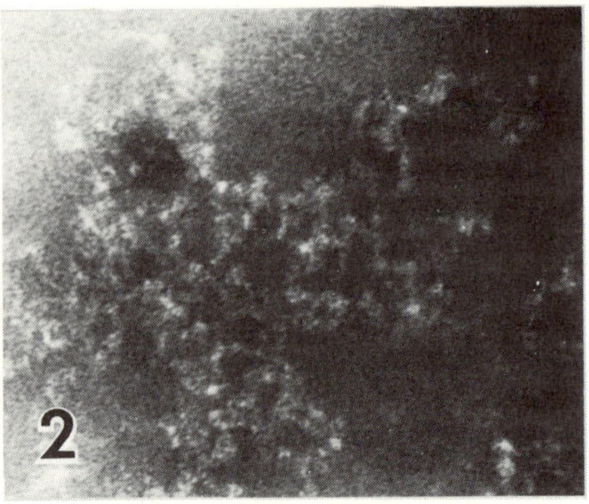
2

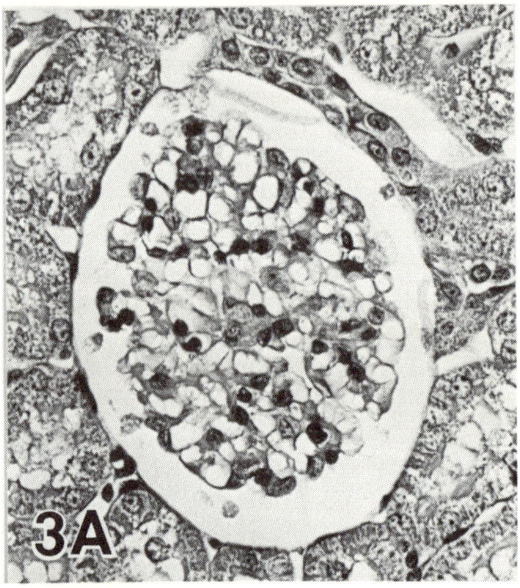
3A

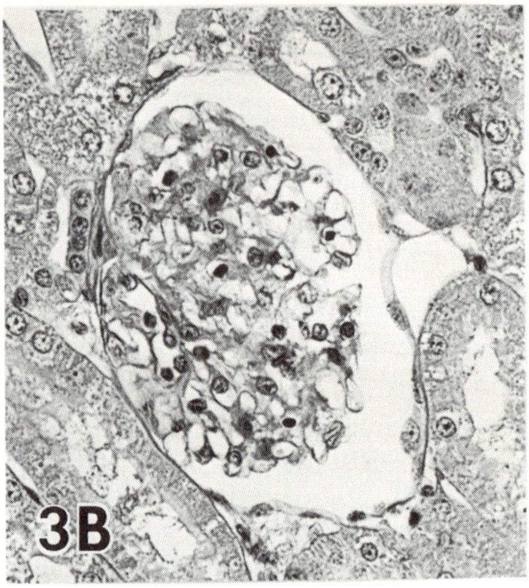
3B

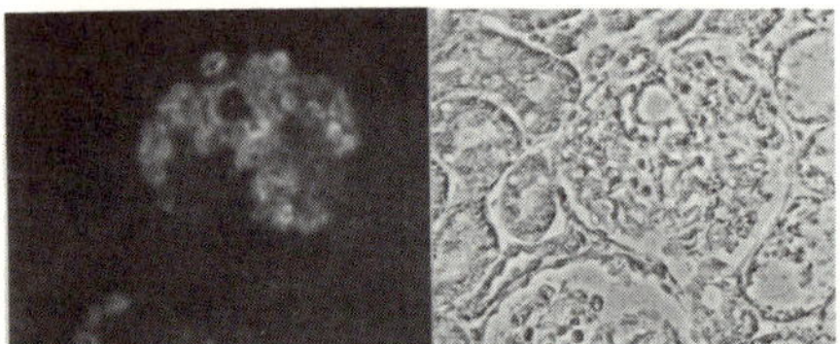
4A

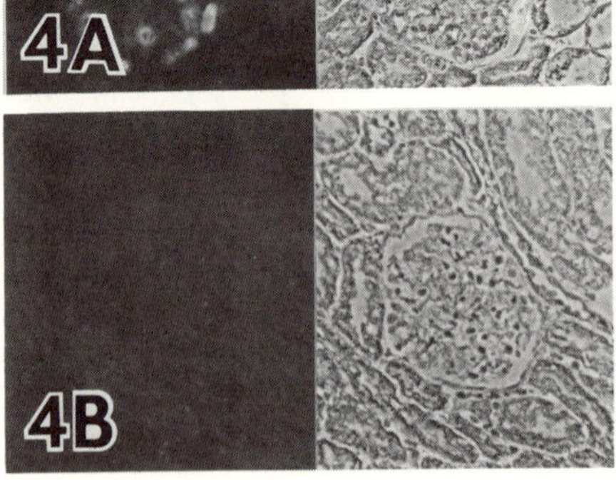
4B

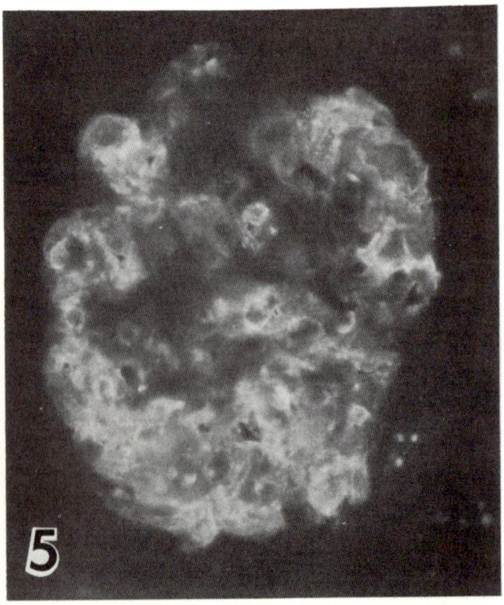
5

The glomeruli perfused with PLL-HA showed some focal amorphous subendothelial deposits (Fig. 8).

Perfusion with PLL or PS induced the "fusion" of foot processes of podocytes (Fig. 9). These morphologic changes were never found in the kidney perfused with HA (Fig. 10) and KRB, and those sacrificed without any treatment.

Intravenous injection test: The animals injected with PLL solution died with shock syndromes within a few min after the injection. The autopsy revealed the petechial bleeding in the lung. The animals which received intravenous injections of CF, CF-HA, PLL-HA, HBSS and HS solutions survived the injections. The urinary protein contents of these animals were found to be in the physiologic range, 2.79 $\pm$ 0.04 mg/15 hr per animal. Autopsy revealed no remarkable macroscopic changes. Observations of HE-stained kidney tissue sections showed no pathological changes of the glomeruli in all cases injected with CF, CF-HA, PLL-HA (Fig. 3B), HA, PLL, KRB and HBSS as compared to the untreated controls, though some hyaline droplets appeared in convoluted tubules of those which received 1 and 4 injections of PLL-HA. No hyaline droplets were observed in the animals received HA, PLL and HBSS. The PAM and PAS staining of these tissue sections revealed no structural changes in GBM of glomeruli in all the animals which received the injection of CF, CF-HA, PLL, PLL-HA and HA. Immunofluorescence staining for HA revealed fluorescence in glomeruli of animals which received PLL-HA and CF-HA injections, but the fluorescence intensity was rather weak compared to that seen in the PLL-HA-perfused animals. No fluorescence was observed on the glomeruli of those injected with HA, PLL and PS.

EM observations of the glomeruli from animals injected with CF revealed the massive CF infiltration into subendothelial area with only a slight adhesion of CF molecules on the surfaces of endothelial cells (Fig. 6E). In the animals which received PLL-HA conjugates some subendothelial deposits were observed (Fig. 11). The deposits appeared amorphous similar to those found in the glomeruli of PLL-HA perfused animals. The subendothelial deposits were not

---

FIG. 1A, B, C. Pictures of macromolecular solutions of HA (A), PLL (B) and PLL-HA (C). The "cloudiness" can be observed in PLL-HA, and signifies the formation of poly-L-lysine–human serum albumin conjugate having no electric charges.

FIG. 2. Transmission electron micrograph of HA-PLL. The complex shows the bead-necklace like fibrous profiles by negative stain. x 180,000.

FIG. 3A, B. Two Light micrographs of the glomeruli of the animal received the perfusion (A) or intravenous injection (B) with HA-PLL. The pictures show the slight swelling of the glomerular tufts. HE stain. x 390.

FIG. 4A, B. The immunofluorescence microscope pictures of glomeruli of the kidney perfused with HA-PLL (A) and HA (B). Pictures on the left show the same glomerulus taken under phase contrast microscope. x 110.

FIG. 5. Fluorescent microscopic picture of a glomerulus from the rat kidney perfused with HA-PLL and shows the heavy deposition of HA in the capillary walls. FITC-IgG stain. x 410.

increased in both mass and number by the repeated injections of PLL-HA, though some thickening of the mesangial matrix and the partial detachment of endothelium became more distinct in those received 4 injections than those received single injection. The so-called "fusion" of foot processes of podocyte was often encountered and some platelet aggregates were found in the capillary lumen of the corresponding area. Detachment of capillary endothelial cells and cytoplasmic projections of mesangial cells were often found in the area of deposits. The mesangial cell projections occasionally reached the capillary lumen through the deposits (Fig. 12). No subepithelial deposits were found but the so-called "fusion" of foot processes of podocytes was often met

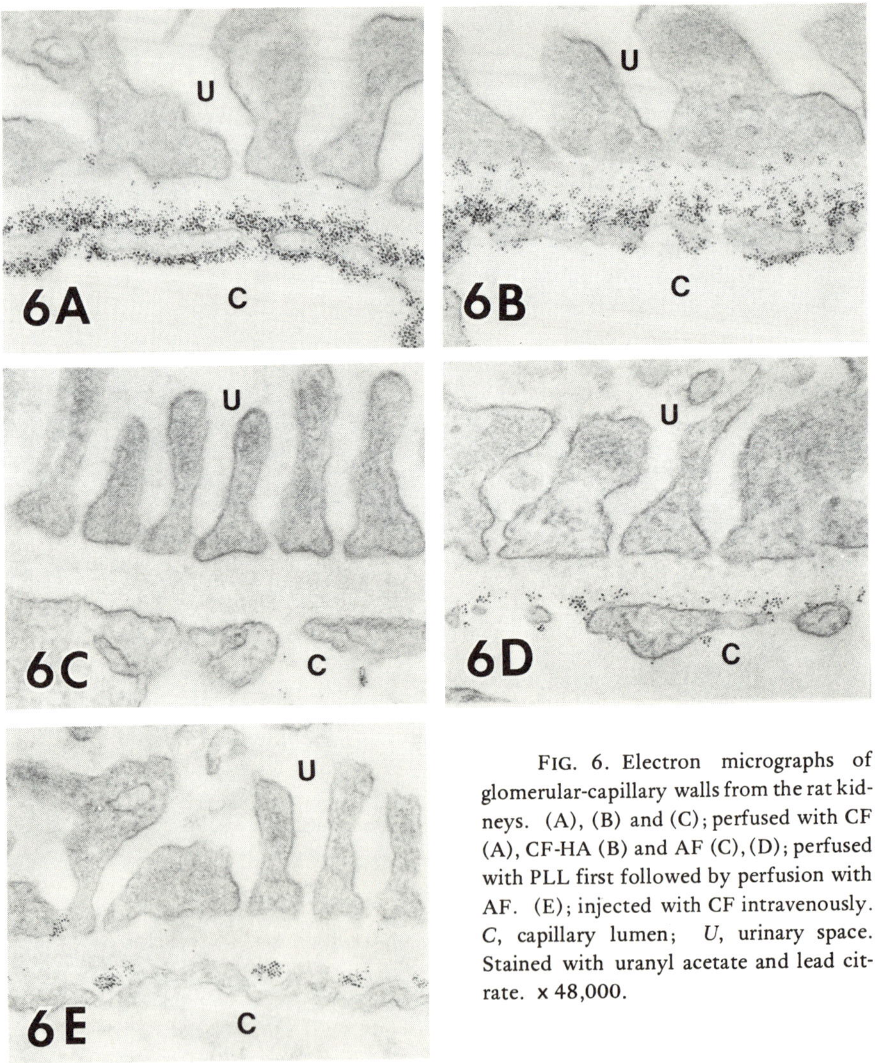

FIG. 6. Electron micrographs of glomerular-capillary walls from the rat kidneys. (A), (B) and (C); perfused with CF (A), CF-HA (B) and AF (C), (D); perfused with PLL first followed by perfusion with AF. (E); injected with CF intravenously. *C*, capillary lumen; *U*, urinary space. Stained with uranyl acetate and lead citrate. x 48,000.

with. No such changes were observed in all the animals received HA and HBSS injections.

By immuno-peroxidase EM method, HA appeared as electron dense reaction product in subendothelial spaces and in the luminal surface of capillary endothelial cells of glomeruli in the animals which received PLL-HA injections (Fig. 13). No such reaction products were found in those which received HA, PLL and HBSS injections, though some reaction product was occasionally found in the capillary lumen of glomeruli of the animals which received HA injection.

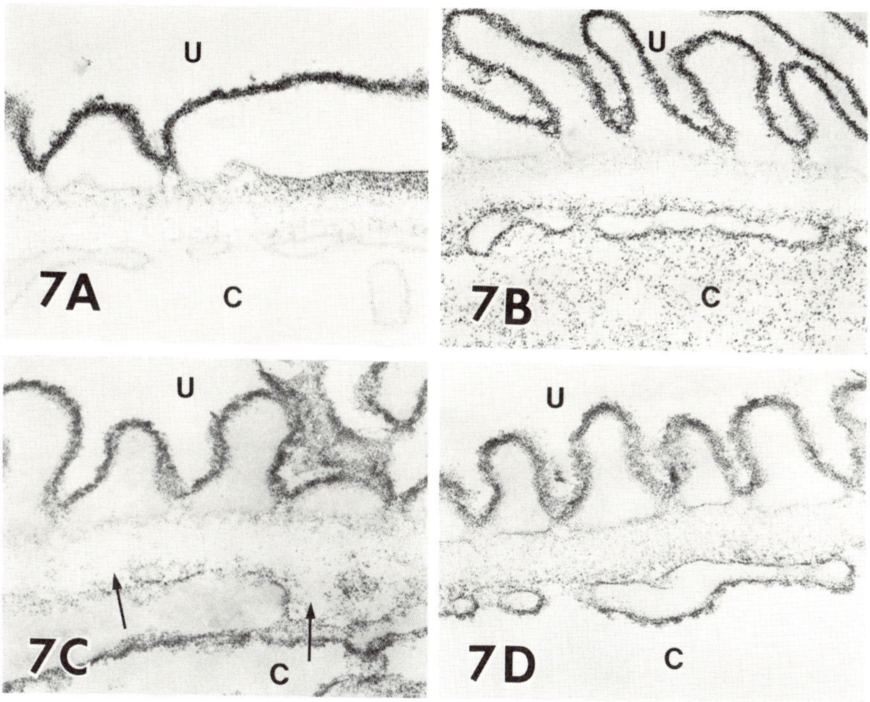

FIG. 7. Electron micrographs showing the distribution of ionized anionic groups on the capillary walls. The glomerulus fixed and stained with cationic colloidal iron method by Seno et al. (1983b). Arrows, deposition of PLL-HA; C, U, see the legend of Fig. 6. x 60,200. (A) A picture of the glomerular wall of the rat received PLL perfusion. Note the decrease of colloidal iron density on the endothelial cell surface and in IRI of GBM. (B) The picture of the glomerular capillary wall of a healthy rat incubated with cationic Fe-Cac (pH 4) for 5 hr and shows heavy deposition of the iron colloid particles on both endothelial cell surfaces facing to capillary lumen and GBM and also the podocyte surface facing to urinary spaces. Slight deposition of colloidal iron particles in GBM. (C) The picture of the glomerular wall of the rat perfused with PLL-HA complex. Note there is no abnormalities in distribution of the iron colloid particles as compared to Fig. 7B. (D) A picture of the glomerular capillary wall of the rat received HA perfusion, and shows no abnormalities in distribution of the iron colloid particles.

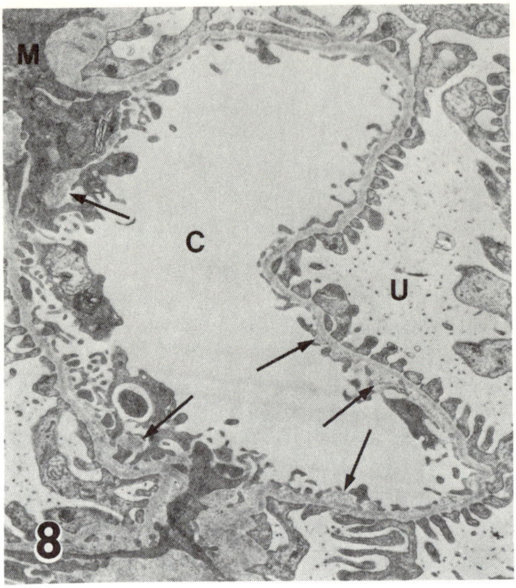

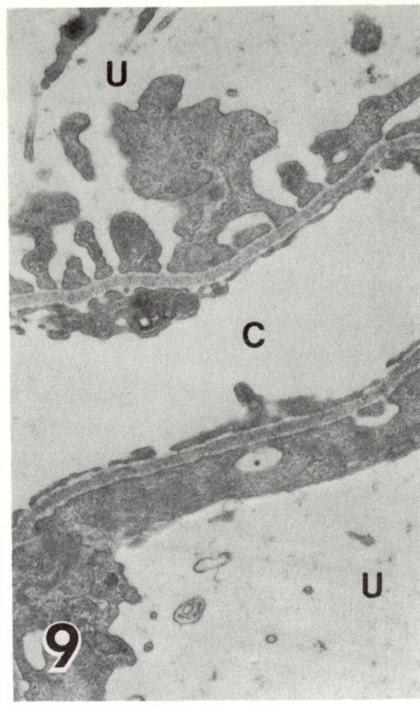

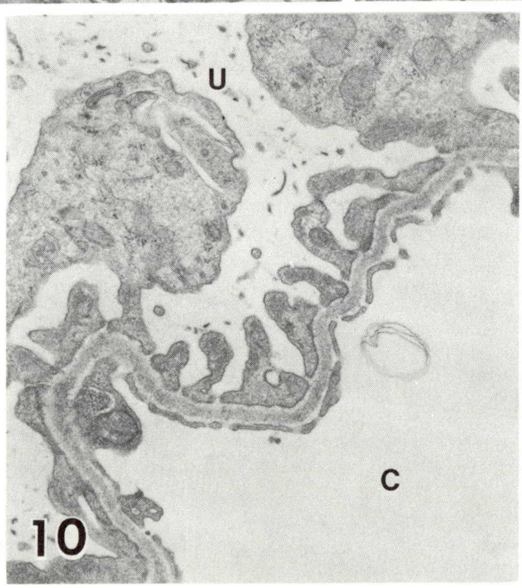

FIG. 8. Low power electron micrograph of a glomerular capillary wall from the rat kidney perfused with PLL-HA. Note that the gross subendothelial and paramesangial deposits with the partial detachment of endothelial cells. Arrows, deposits; C, M, U, see the legends of Fig. 6. Stained with uranyl acetate and lead citrate. x 9,000.

FIG. 9. Electron micrograph of a glomerular capillary wall from the rat kidney perfused with PLL. Note the so-called "fusion" of the foot processes of podocytes. C, U, see the legends of Fig. 6. Stained with uranyl acetate and lead citrate. x 9,000.

FIG. 10. Electron micrograph of a glomerular capillary wall from the rat kidney per-

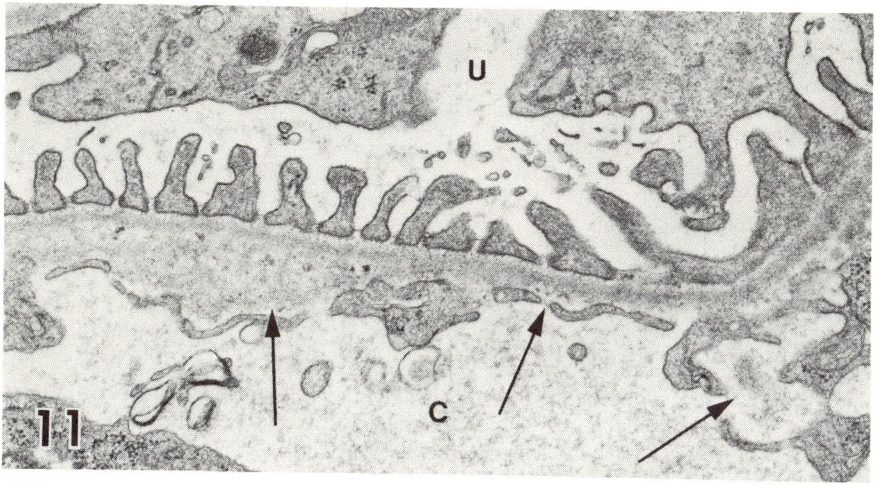

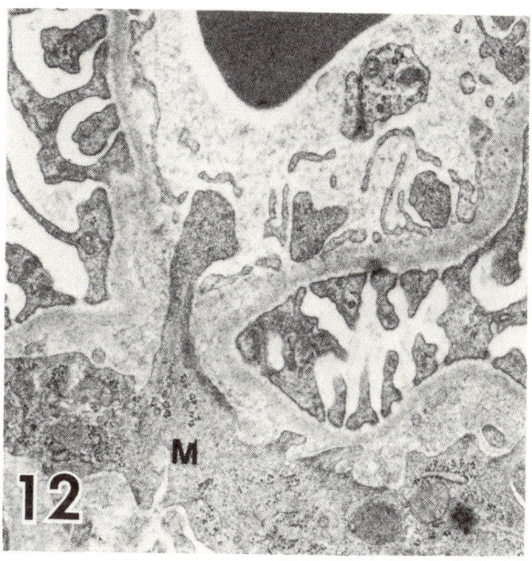

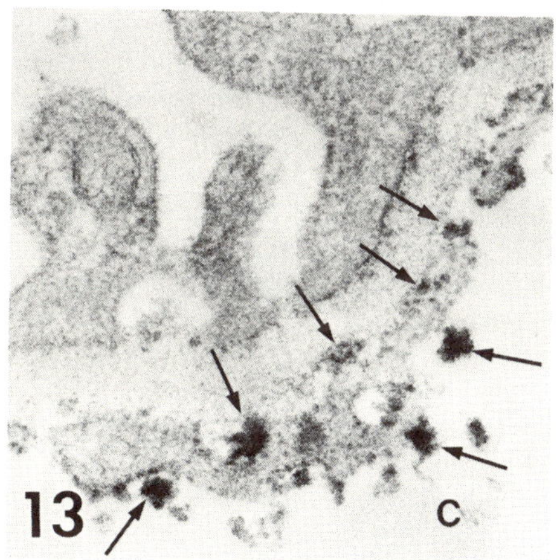

FIG. 11. Electron micrograph of a glomerular capillary wall from a rat received 4 intravenous injections of PLL-HA complex. Note the complex seen in subendothelial space. Arrows, HA-PLL; C, U, see the legend of Fig. 6. x 25,300.

FIG. 12. An electron-microscope picture of a part of glomerular capillary wall and mesangium of rat kidney received 4 intravenous injections of PLL-HA, and shows the desquamated endothelial cells with the elongated cytoplasmic projections of mesangial cells in to the capillary lumen through the subendothelial deposits. M, see the legend of Fig. 6. Stained with uranyl acetate and lead citrate. x 10,000.

FIG. 13. An immune-electron micrograph of a glomerular capillary wall from the rat received 4 intravenous injections of PLL-HA. Note the electron dense reaction products in subendothelial spaces and on the luminal surface of the glomerular capillary (arrows). C, U, see the legend of Fig. 6. x 43,800.

---

fused with HA. The picture shows no pathologic changes. C, U, see the legends of Fig. 6. Stained with uranyl acetate and lead citrate. x 16,000.

Distribution and density of ionized anionic groups of polysaccharides and proteins in glomeruli, which were revealed by staining with Fe-Cac at pH 1.8, 4.0 and 7.0, appeared nearly the same in all animals which received PLL-HA, HA and HBSS injections.

Discussion

As shown above, PLL-HA and CF-HA perfused through aorta or injected into vein of rat did not adhere to the endothelial cell surfaces of glomeruli, but deposited in the subendothelial spaces penetrating the endothelial fenestrae of glomerular capillaries having undamaged anionic groups on their surfaces, though the deposits appeared somewhat heavier after perfusion than after intravenous injection. The results indicate that macromolecules losing their negative electric charge pass through the healthy endothelial cell layer having intact ionized anionic groups and deposit in subendothelial spaces, if the molecules are too large in size to pass through GBM.

CF perfused through aorta adhered to the surface of endothelial cells of glomeruli. Intravenously injected CF also adhered to the luminal surface of endothelial cells, but some CF invaded into the subendothelial spaces and mesangial matrix of glomeruli. The findings seems to show that free CF molecules adhere to endothelial cell surface but those conjugated with serum albumin infiltrate into subendothelial spaces.

Thus, the present experiment shows clearly that cationic macromolecules introduced into vessels and bound firmly to anionic serum albumin do not have a significant net charge, and are removed from the blood stream forming deposits in subendothelial spaces and in the mesangial matrix.

The formation of stable hydrophobic complexes by conjugation of polycationic macromolecules with polyanionic serum proteins as understood from the principle of colloid titration (Ono et al., 1979; Toei and Kohara, 1976; Henck et al., 1983) and the segregation of the complexes from blood vessels may be one of the mechanisms to remove the foreign substances from blood stream. The penetration appeared focal, but not uniform, suggesting that the endothelial layer is not uniform for macromolecule penetration. The pictures were similar to that of the deposits of the aggregated HA (Lee and Vernier, 1980) and mimic those seen in some cases of immune complex glomerulonephritis.

Leakage of macromolecules can occur by the loss of repulsive force between the macromolecules and the endothelial surfaces by the loss of negative charge of either endothelium or the macromolecules. The findings are consistent with those of Shen et al. (1978) who elucidated the dramatic increase of cellular transport of human serum albumin and horseradish peroxidase when they were linked to a small fragment of PLL. The results also support the view of those stressing the important contribution of immune complexes formed with cationic antigens or antibodies to the glomerular depositions (Border et al., 1981, Gallo et al., 1981, 1982; Gauthier et al., 1982; Isaacs and Miller, 1982, Vogt et al., 1982; Cavallo et al., 1983).

Our present experiments also proved that intravenous injection of 3 ml of PLL solution, 0.4 mg/ml, is lethal. It has been reported by many authors that the structural alterations of glomeruli can be induced by various polycations at a very dilute solution (Caulfield, 1979; Caulfield and Farquhar, 1978; Kerjaschki, 1978; Melnick et al., 1981; Seiler et al., 1977; Hunsicker et al., 1981; Coimbra et al., 1983). The results do not necessarily mean that specific damage of kidney has occurred. Rather, they indicate a reversible functional and structural change in the capillary wall. Integrity of the capillary walls is necessary to keep the circulatory blood volume at a certain level (Eppinger, 1935; Seno, et al., 1983a). Perfusion of animals with PLL induced patchy desquamation of capillary endothelial cells of glomeruli with a distinct reduction in the density of ionized anionic groups. This should be the general picture of damage in glomerular capillaries exposed directly to cationic macromolecules which will react specifically with anionic cell surfaces (Seiler et al., 1977).

Injection of PLL-HA, however, induced neither any ill symptoms nor severe capillary damage, though some endothelial deposits were formed. The phenomenon is very similar to the results after CF-HA perfusion of CF intravenous injection, and shows again that serum albumin, an anionic macromolecule, will serve to neutralize cationic macromolecules and facilitate their excretion into the urine through the healthy anionic barrier of glomeruli, though some gross agglomerates may stay in the subendothelial spaces similar to PLL-HA or protamine-heparin complexes (Hoyer et al., 1982; Seiler et al., 1980; Sharon et al., 1978). Gauthier et al. (1982) indicated that large latticed immune complexes formed with cationic antibodies deposited rapidly and persisted in renal glomeruli as electron dense masses, however, small-latticed ones deposited only transitorily without persistence in glomeruli.

Prior observations support our view regarding the glomerular deposition of the deionized proteins. In studies using CF molecules with pI >8.8 perfused through the renal arteries of mice adheres to the endothelial cell surface and some reaches GBM (Rennke and Venkatachalam, 1977). CF (pI >10.0) injected into rats intravenously did not adhere to the endothelial cell surface of glomeruli at all, but penetrated into GBM through the endothelial fenestrae, and was found in *lamina rara externa* (Vogt et al., 1982). Similar results were obtained by Simionescu et al. (1982b), who injected CF into mice intravenously (*in vivo*) or perfused the animals with CF through aorta. These findings seem to suggest that the CF introduced into blood vessels should conjugate with negatively charged macromolecules in blood, serum albumin and globulin, lose their electric charge and penetrate into subendothelial spaces of GBM.

Hoyer et al. (1982), Seiler et al. (1977, 1980) and Sharon et al. (1977) showed that alternative perfusions or injections of protamine and heparin led to the deposition of electron dense aggregates along GBM. Kelley and Cavallo (1978) reported that injection of the preformed protamine-heparin complexes did not lead to deposition in GBM. But they injected centrifuged precipitates from suspended protamine-heparin complexes, and might have selected for aggregates that are too large to pass through the endothelial fenestrae.

It has been reported that rats receiving injections of cationic bovine serum albumin (Purtell et al., 1979, Border, et al., 1981), heparin-protamine complexes (Fiedel et al., 1976) and polyvinyl alcohol-bovine serum albumin (Suzuki, 1980) developed much more granular mesangial deposits of IgG, C3 than in those treated with native anionic bovine serum albumin. In another series of our experiments where we injected PLL-HA daily for 9 days, however, no activation in antibody formation and complement fixation were observed (unpublished data).

In the present study, "hyaline droplets" (reabsorption protein droplets) were observed in proximal convoluted tubules in the PLL-HA injected animals, suggesting glomerular penetration by PLL-HA and its reabsorption at the tubules. But the animals were not proteinuric, probably because of complete reabsorption.

In conclusion, ionized anionic groups of the glomerular capillary wall form a barrier indispensable for the prevention of the serum protein leakage. But, serum protein leakage can occur due to penetration by proteins losing their surface anionic charge through healthy capillary walls. This will explain the mechanism of subendothelial deposits of denaturated proteins and excretion in urine, at least in some cases.

Acknowledgments

The aid of Dr. H. Shigei, Chairman of the Board of Shigei Medical Research Institute, that made this work possible is gratefully acknowledged. Thanks are also due to Dr. H. Takamiya, Shigei Medical Research Hospital, for his valuable discussions.

References

Alcorn, D., and Ryan, G.B. (1981). Distribution of anionic groups in the glomerular capillary wall in rat nephrotoxic nephritis and aminonucleoside nephrosis. *Pathology* **13**, 37–50.

Assel, E., Neuman, K-H., Schurek, H-J., Sonnenburg, C., and Stolte, H. (1984). Glomerular albumin leakage and morphology after neutralization of polyanions. 1. Albumin clearance and sieving coefficient in the isolated perfused rat kidney. *Renal Physiol.* **7**, 357–364.

Barnes, J.L., Radnik, R.A., Gilchrist, E.P., and Venkatachalam, M.A. (1984). Size and charge selective permeability defects induced in glomerular basement membrane by a polycation. *Kidney Int.* **25**, 11–19.

Bennett, C.M., Glassock, R.J., Chang, R.L.S., Deen, W.M., Robertson, C.R., and Brenner, B.M. (1976). Permselectivity of the glomerular capillary wall. Studies of experimental glomerulonephritis in the rat using dextran sulfate. *J. Clin. Invest.* **57**, 1287–1294.

Blau, E.B., and Haas, J.E. (1973). Glomerular sialic acid and proteinuria in human renal disease. *Lab. Invest.* **28**, 477–481.

Bohrer, M.P., Baylis, C., Humes, H.D., Glassock, R.J., Robertson, C.R., and Brenner B.M. (1978). Permselectivity of the glomerular capillary wall. Facilitated filtration of circulating polycations. *J. Clin. Invest.* **61**, 72–78.

Border, W.A., Kamil, E.S., Ward, H.J., and Cohen, A.H. (1981). Antigenic charge as a determinant of immune complex localization in the rat glomerulus. *Lab. Invest.* **40**, 442–449.

Brenner, B.M., Bohrer, M.P., Baylis, C., and Deen, W.M. (1977). Determinants of glomerular permselectivity: Insights derived from observation *in vivo*. *Kidney Int.* **12**, 229–237.

Brenner, B.M., Hostetter, T.H., and Humes, H.D. (1978). Molecular basis of proteinuria of glomerular origin. *Physiol. Med.* **298**, 826–833.

Camussi, G., Tetta, C., Segoloni, G., Coda, R., and Vercellone, A. (1982). Localization of neutrophil cationic proteins and loss of anionic changes in glomeruli of patients with systemic lupus erythematosus glomerulonephritis. *Clin. Immunol. Immunopathol.* **24**, 299–314.

Caulfield, J.C. (1979). Alterations in the distribution of Alcian blue-staining fibrillar anionic sites in the glomerular basement in aminonucleoside nephrosis. *Lab. Invest.* **40**, 503–511.

Caulfield, J.P., and Farquhar, M.G. (1978). Loss of anionic sites from the glomerular basement membrane in aminonucleoside nephrosis. *Lab. Invest.* **39**, 505–512.

Cavallo, T., Graves, K., and Granholm, N. (1984). Murine lupus nephritis. Effects of glucocorticoid on glomerular permeability. *Lab. Invest.* **50**, 378–384.

Cavallo, T., Goldman, M., Graves, K., and Lambert, P-H. (1983). Altered permeability in the early phase of immune complex nephritis. *Kidney Int.* **24**, 632–637.

Coimbra, T.M., Furtado, M.R., Lachat, J.J., and de Carvalho, I.F. (1983). Effects of administration of cationic and native homologous albumin on the kidney. *Nephron* 33, 208–215.

Cotran, R.S., and Rennke, H.G. (1983). Anionic sites and mechanisms of proteinuria. *N. Engl. J. Med.* **309**, 1050–1052.

Elling, F., Hasselager, E., and Friis, C. (1977). Perfusion fixation of kidneys in adult pigs for electron microscopy. *Acta Anat.* **98**, 340–342.

De Martino, C., and Zamboni, L.C. (1967). Silver methenamine stain for electron microscopy. *J. Ultrastruct. Res.* **19**, 273–282.

Eppinger, H. (1935). Serose Entzung, Eine Permeabilitats-Pathologie. pp. 1–299. Verlag von Julius Spriger, Wien.

Faraggiana, T., Grishaman, E., and Churg, J. (1982). Cell coat of podocytes in patients with nephrotic syndrome. *Histopathology* **6**, 299–307.

Fiedel, B.A., Rent, R., Myhrman, R., and Gewurz, H. (1976). Complement activation by interaction of polyanions and polycations. II. Precipitation and role of IgG, Clq and C1-INH during heparin-protamine-induced consumption of complement. *Immunology* **30**, 161–169.

Gallo, G.R., Caulin-Glaser, T., and Lamm, M.E. (1981). Charge of circulating immune complexes as a factor in glomerular basement membrane localization in mice. *J. Clin. Invest.* **67**, 1305–1313.

Gallo, G.R., Caulin-Glaser, T., Steven, M.S., Emancipator, S.N., and Lamm, M.E. (1983). Nephritogenecity and differential distribution of glomerular immune complexes related to immunogen charge. *Lab. Invest.* **48**, 353–362.

Gauthier, V.J., Mannik, M., and Striker, G.E. (1982). Effect of cationized antibodies in performed immune complexes on deposition and persistence in renal glomeruli. *J. Exp. Med.* **156**, 766–777.

Henck, C.C., Daerr, W., Haberbosch, W., Horn, O., and Luddecke, E. (1983). The surface charge of apolipoproteins, phospholipid liposomes, and human very low density lipoproteins. *J. Biol. Chem.* **258**, 8317–8322.

Hirsch, H. Z., Ainsworth, S.K., Spicer, S.S., Kurtz, E.H., and Brissie, R.M. (1981). Ultrastructural assessment by colloidal iron of anionic sites in human glomerulonephritis. *Am. J. Pathol.* **102**, 99–107.

Hoyer, J.R., Krueger, T.E., and Seiler, M.W. (1982). Kinetics of protamine-heparin complex formation in rat glomeruli during renal perfusion. *Kidney Int.* **21**, 102–104.

Hunsicker, L.G., Shearer, T.P., and Shaffer, S.J. (1981). Acute reversible proteinuria induced by infusion of the polycation hexadimethrine. *Kidney Int.* **20**, 7–17.

Isaacs, K.L., and Miller, F. (1982). Role of antigen size and charges in immune complex glomerulonephritis. I. Active induction of disease with dextran and its derivatives. *Lab. Invest.* **47**, 198–205.

Kanwar, Y.S. (1984). Biology of disease, biophysiology of glomerular filtration and proteinuria. *Lab. Invest.* **51**, 7–21.

Kanwar, Y.S., and Farquhar, M.G. (1979a). Presence of heparan sulfate in the glomerular basement membrane. *Proc. Natl. Acad. Sci. U.S.A.* **76**, 1303–1307.

Kanwar, Y.S., and Farquhar, M.G. (1979b). Anionic sites in the glomerular basement membrane. In vivo and in vitro localization to the laminae rarae by cationic probes. *J. Cell Biol.* **81**, 137–153.

Kanwar, Y.S., and Jakubowski, M.L. (1984). Unaltered anionic sites of glomerular basement membrane in aminonucleoside nephritis. *Kidney Int.* **25**, 613–618.

Kanwar, Y.S., Linker, A., and Farquhar, M.G. (1980). Increased permeability of the glomerular basement membrane to ferritin after removal of glycosaminoglycans (heparan sulfate) by enzyme digestion. *J. Cell Biol.* **86**, 688–693.

Karnovsky, M.J. (1965). A formaldehyde-glutaraldehyde fixative of high osmolarity for use in electron microscopy (abstr). *J. Cell Biol.* **27**, 137A.

Kelley, V.E., and Cavallo, T. (1978). Glomerular permeability. Transfer of native ferritin in glomeruli with decreased anionic sites. *Lab. Invest.* **39**, 547–553.

Kelley, V.E., and Cavallo, T. (1980). Glomerular permeability. Focal loss of anionic sites in glomeruli of proteinuric mice with lupus nephritis. *Lab. Invest.* **42**, 59–64.

Kerjaschki, D. (1978). Polycation-induced dislocation of slit diaphragms and formation of cell junctions in rat kidney glomeruli. The effects of low temperature, divalent cations, colchicine, and cytochalasin B. *Lab. Invest.* **39**, 430–440.

Kerjaschki, D., Sharkey, D.J., and Farquhar, M.G. (1984). Identification and characterization of podocalyxin—the major sialoprotein the renal glomerular epithelial cell. *J. Cell Biol.* **98**, 1591–1596.

Kingsbury, F.B., Clark, C.C., Williams, G., and Post A.L. (1926). Rapid determination of albumin in urine. *J. Lab. Med.* **11**, 981–989.

Klein, D.V., Oegema, T.H., Eisenstein, F., Furcht, L., Michael, A.F., and

Brown, D.M. (1983). Renal localization of heparan sulfate proteoglycan by immunohistochemistry. *Am. J. Pathol.* **111**, 323–330.

Kreisberg, J.I., Wayne, D.B., and Karnovsky, M.J. (1979). Rapid and focal loss of negative charge associated with mononuclear cell infiltration early in nephrotoxic serum nephritis. *Kidney Int.* **16**, 290–300.

Latta, H., Johnston, W.H., and Stanley, T.M. (1975). Sialoglycoproteins and filtration barriers in the glomerular capillary wall. *J. Ultrastruct. Res.* **51**, 354–376.

Laurie, G.W., Leblond, C.P., Inoue, S., Martin, G.R., and Chung, A. (1984). Fine structure of the glomerular basement membrane and immunolocalization of fine basement membrane components to the lamina densa (Basal lamina) and its extensions in both glomeruli and tubules of the rat kidney. *Am. J. Anat.* **169**, 463–481.

Lee, S., and Vernier, R.L. (1980). Immunoelectron microscopy of the glomerular mesangial uptake and transport of aggregated human albumin in the mouse. *Lab. Invest.* **42**, 44–58.

Melnick, G.F., Ladoulis, C.T., and Cavallo, T. (1981). Decreased anionic groups and increased permeability precedes deposition of immune complexes in the glomerular capillary wall. *Am. J. Pathol.* **105**, 114–120.

Mynderse, L.A., Hassell, J.R., Kleinman, H.K., Martin, G. R., and Martinez-Hernandez, A. (1983). Loss of heparan sulfate proteoglycan from glomerular basement membrane of nephrotic rats. *Lab. Invest.* **48**, 292–302.

Olson, J.L., Rennke, H.G., and Venkatachalam, M.A. (1981). Alterations in the charge and size selectivity barrier of the glomerular filter in aminonucleoside nephrosis in rats. *Lab. Invest.* **44**, 271–279.

Ono, T., Miyata, H., and Toei, K. (1979). Polysoap as a new titrant for the determination of sodium dodecylbenzensulfonate by colloid titration. *Bull. Chem. Soc. Jpn.* 52, 425–427.

Parthasarathy, N., and Spiro, R.G. (1984). Isolation and characterization of the heparan sulfate proteoglycan of the bovine glomerular basement membrane. *J. Biol. Chem.* **259**, 12749–12756.

Purtell, J.N., Pesce, A.J., Clyne, D.H., Miller, W.C., and Pollak, V.E. (1979). Isoelectric point of albumin: Effect of renal handling of albumin. *Kidney Int.* **16**, 366–376.

Real, E., Luciano, L., and Kühn, K. (1983). Ultrastructural architecture of proteoglycans in the glomerular basement membrane: A cytochemical approach. *J. Histochem. Cytochem.* **31**, 662–668.

Rennke, H.G., and Venkatachalam, M.A. (1977). Structural determinants of glomerular permselectivity. *Fed. Proc., Fed. Am. Soc. Exp. Biol.* **36**, 2619–2626.

Rollason, T.P., and Brewer, D.B. (1984). Study of glomerular basement membrane anionic sites and glomerular visceral epithelial cell coat in protein overload proteinuria in the rat. *J. Pathol.* **142**, 301–316.

Rosenzweig, L.J., and Kanwar, Y. (1982). Removal of sulfated (heparan sulfate) or nonsulfated (hyaluronic acid) glycosaminoglycans results in increased permeability of the glomerular basement membrane to ^{125}I-bovine serum albumin. *Lab. Invest.* **47**, 177–184.

Ryan, G.B., and Karnovsky, M.J. (1976). Distribution of endogenous albumin in the rat glomerulus: Role of hemodynamic factors in glomerular barrier function. *Kidney Int.* **9**, 36–45.

Schneeberger, E.E., Stavrakis, G., and McCarthy, K. (1983). Alterations in glomerular anionic sites in autologous immune complex nephritis. *Lab. Invest.* **49**, 445–452.

Schurer, J.W., Haedemaeker, PH. J., and Molenaar, I. (1977). Polyethyleneimine as tracer particle for (immuno) electron microscopy. *J. Histochem. Cytochem.* **25**, 384–387.

Seiler M.W., Rennke H.G., Venkatachalam, M.A., and Cotran, R.S. (1977). Pathogenesis of polycation-induced alterations ("Fusion") of glomerular epithelium. *Lab. Invest.* **36**, 48–81.

Seiler M.W., Hoyer, J.R., Kureger, T.E. (1980). Altered localization of protamine-heparin complexes in aminonucleoside nephrosis. *Lab. Invest.* **43**, 9–17.

Seno, S., Ono, T., and Tsujii, T. (1983a). Macromolecular charge and cellular surface charge in adhesion, ingestion and blood vessel leakage. *Ann. N.Y. Acad. Sci.* **416**, 410–425.

Seno, S., Tsujii, T., Ono, T., and Ukita, S. (1983b). Cationic cacodylate iron colloid for the detection of anionic sites on cell surface and the histochemical stain of acid mucopolysaccharides. *Histochemistry* **78**, 27–31.

Sharon, Z., Schwarts, M.M., and Lewis, E.J. (1977). The glomerular localization and transport of aggregated protamine-heparin complexes. *Lab. Invest.* **37**, 43–52.

Shen, W.-C., and Ryser, H.J.-P. (1978). Conjugation of poly-L-lysine to albumin and horseradish peroxidase: A novel method of enhancing the cellular uptake of proteins. *Proc. Natl. Acad. Sci. U.S.A.* **75**, 1872–1875.

Simionescu, M., Simionescu, N., and Palade, G.E. (1982). Preferential distribution of anionic sites on the basement membrane and the abluminal aspect of the endothelium in fenestrated capillaries. *J. Cell Biol.* **95**, 425–443.

Simionescu, M., Simionescu, N., and Palade, G.E. (1982b). Biochemically differentiated microdomains of the cell surface of capillary endothelium. *Ann. N.Y. Acad. Sci.* **401**, 9–24.

Sonnenburg-Hatzopoulos, C., Assel, E., Schurek, H.J., and Stolte, H. (1984). Glomerular albumin leakage and morphology after neutralization of polyanions. II. Discrepancy of protamine induced albuminuria and fine structure of the glomerular filtration barrier. *J. Submicrosc. Cytol.* **16**, 741–751.

Suzuki, Y. (1980). Acute glomerular lesions induced by polyvinyl alcohol-bovine serum albumin (PVA-BSA) complex in the rat. A possible mechanism of local immune complex formation. *Jpn. J. Exp. Med.* **50**, 395–401.

Tisher, C.C. (1976). Anatomy of the kidney. *In* "The Kidney" (B.M. Brenner, F.C. Rector, eds.), Vol. 1, pp. 11–64. W.B. Saunders, Philadelphia.

Thomas, J.D. (1978). Electron microscopy of DNA. *In* "Principles and Techniques of Electronmicroscopy" p. 68. van Nostrand Reinhold, New

York.

Toei, K., and Kohara, T. (1976). A conductmetric method for colloid titrations. *Anal. Chim. Acta* **83**, 59–65.

Tsujii, T., Ono, T., Ukita, S., Inoue, S., Takamiya, H., and Seno, S. (1983). Ionized anionic groups of glomerular capillaries in human glomerulonephritis and aminonucleoside nephrosis in rat. *J. Clin. Electron Microsc.* **16**, 711–712.

Venkatachalam, M.A., and Rennke, H.G. (1978). The structural and molecular basis of glomerular filtration. *Circ. Res.* **43**, 337–347.

Vernier, R.L., Klein, D.J., Sisson, S.P., Mahan, J.D., Oegema, T.R., and Brown, D.M. (1983). Heparan sulfate-rich anionic sites in the human glomerular basement membrane. *N. Engl. J. Med.* **309**, 1001–1009.

Vogt, A., Rohrbach, R., Shimizu, F., Takamiya, H., and Batsford, S. (1982). Interaction of cationized antigen with rat glomerular basement membrane: *In situ* immune complex formation. *Kidney Int.* **22**, 27–35.

Weening, J.J., and Rennke, H.G. (1983). Glomerular permeability and polyanion in adriamycin nephrosis in the rat. *Kidney Int.* **24**, 152–159.

Zoolinger, H.U., and Mihatsch, M.J. (1978). *In* "Renal Pathology in Biopsy" p. 8. Springer-Verlag, Berlin.

A BIOCHEMICAL APPROACH TO GLOMERULAR PERMEABILITY

Hikaru Koide, Susumu Hanzawa, and Isao Shirato

Division of Nephrology, Department of Medicine,
Juntendo University School of Medicine, Tokyo

The enhancement of glomerular permeability in glomerulonephritis is associated with alterations in size-selective barrier of the glomerular filter due to the molecular changes of collagenous and non-collagenous glycoproteins (Koide et al., 1981).

Recently, the fixed anionic sites of the glomerular capillary walls have been considered to influence its permeability to plasma macromolecules. This charge-based barrier to macromolecules is dependent on negatively charged components of glomerular basement membrane (GBM).

The purpose of this study is to determine the chemical properties of anionic sites in the GBM and the alterations of these anionic sites in the GBM in glomerulonephritic rats or in the patients with different glomerulonephritides.

Chemical Properties of Anionic Sites in the Glomerular Basement Membranes

The kidneys were exposed and perfused with physiological saline at a rate of 3 – 4 ml/min to wash out the blood, after which enzyme solutions were perfused. Perfusion conditions were as follows; chondroitinase ABC 0.5 units/ml, neuraminidase 0.5 units/ml, heparitinase 0.2 mg/ml, collagenase 200 units/ml, and pronase 3 mg/ml. At the end of perfusion, the anionic sites of the kidney were stained by perfusion with 0.1% polyethyleneimine (PEI) for 10 min (Schurer et al., 1977).

As described by Kanwar and Farquhar (1979), the distribution of anionic sites in the *lamina rara externa* and *interna* of the GBM can be visualized *in situ* by using the cationic PEI. These sites are distributed at regular intervals (Fig. 1A). Perfusion with chondroitinase ABC did not affect the distribution of PEI-stained anionic sites in the GBM (Fig. 1B). The PEI-stained sites were also unaffected by treatment with neuraminidase. Specimen perfused with PEI showed no staining of the epithelial cell coat due to the removal of sialic acid. In addition, the detachment of epithelial and endothelial cells from the GBM was observed in neuraminidase-treated glomeruli, suggesting changes in laminin, a sialic acid-rich glycoprotein in the GBM (Fig. 1C).

In contrast to the negative results obtained with the enzymes mentioned above, heparitinase caused a loss of the PEI-stained GBM sites as shown in Fig. 1D. However, the anionic sites on the epithelial cell coats were not affected by heparitinase treatment.

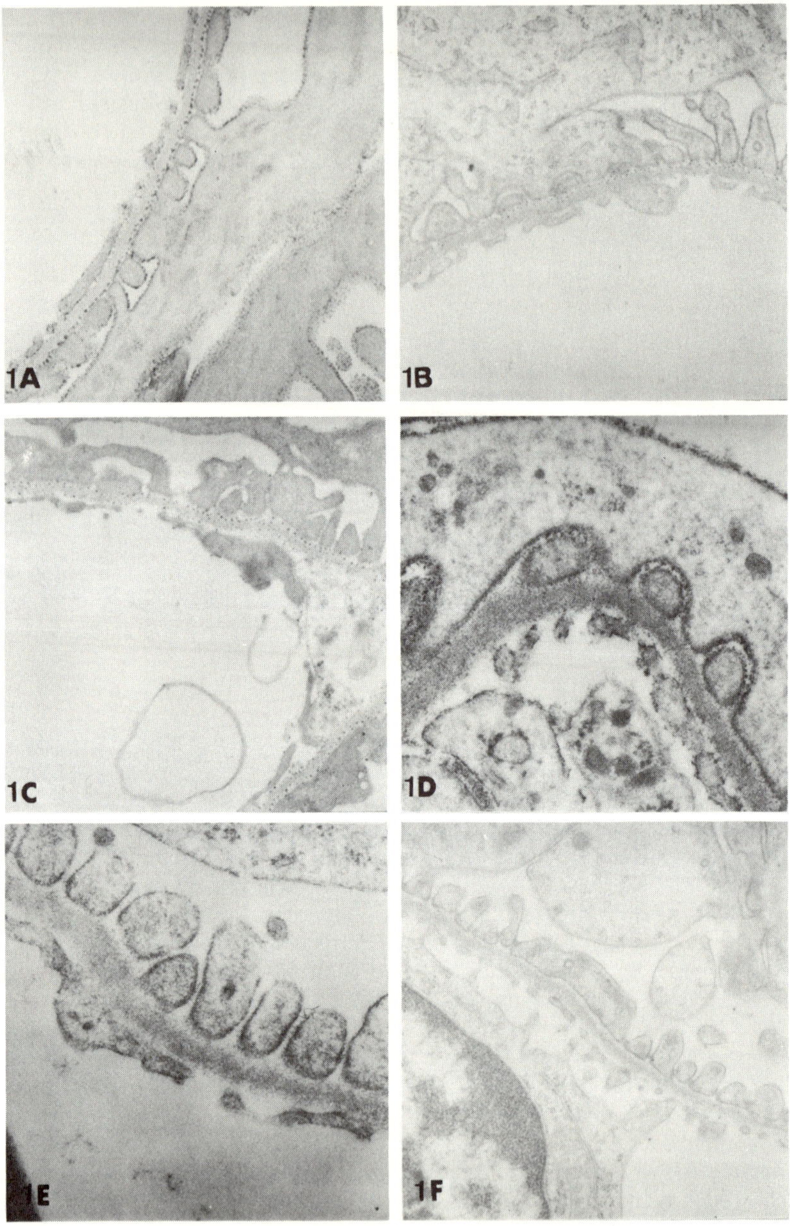

FIG. 1. Effects of various enzymes on the anionic sites of glomerular basement membrane. (A) Control, (B) Chondroitinase ABC, (C) Neuraminidase, (D) Heparitinase, (E) Collagenase, (F) Pronase.

The anionic sites were also susceptible to collagenase. In animals perfused with collagenase, the GBM exhibited a heterogenous *lamina densa* and disrupted slit membranes. The anionic sites of the *lamina rara externa* could not be detected. Both endothelium and epithelium were detached and lifted off the GBM (Fig. 1E).

Pronase treatment also removed all anionic sites of the GBM, suggesting that the protein component of glycoproteins or proteoglycans plays an important role in the support of anionic sites on the GBM (Fig. 1F).

Furthermore, we studied the effect of urea and dithiothreitol on the anionic sites in the isolated GBM. Glomeruli were isolated from human kidneys by sieving technique and the basement membranes were prepared therefrom by sonication. The isolated GBM were then incubated by suspension in 2.0 M urea or 0.1 M dithiothreitol solution for 30 min. At the end of incubation, they were washed and then incubated with 0.5% PEI solution for 30 min to stain the anionic sites. Fig. 2 shows the results obtained on the isolated GBM. Cationic PEI molecules are seen binding at the sites on both sides of the GBM (Fig. 2A). The anionic sites of GBM were removed by treatment with urea (Fig. 2B). Treatment with 0.1 M dithiothreitol also caused a virtually complete elimination of PEI-binding.

These results suggest that the anionic sites of GBM consist of heparan sulfate proteoglycans and other glycoproteins which would be connected with type IV collagen molecules by hydrogen bonds and disulfide linkages.

The Anionic Sites of Glomerular Basement Membrane in Experimental Glomerulonephritic Rats

In control rat kidneys, the anionic sites of GBM can be seen in clusters by using the cationic dye PEI. These PEI-stained particles are seen predominantly along the *lamina rara externa* and *interna* in rows distributed at regular intervals (Fig. 3A).

In daunomycin nephrosis, an experimental model of lipoid nephrosis, the PEI-stained particles were not detected in the GBM and the epithelial cell coats (Fig. 3B).

The anionic sites of the GBM were markedly decreased and dispersed in nephrotoxic serum nephritis (Fig. 3C) and in glycoprotein nephritis, an experimental model of membranous nephropathy (Fig. 3D). These anionic sites were not observed within the immune deposits (Shibata et al., 1972).

Table 1 shows the concentration of glycosaminoglycans in the GBM of daunomycin nephrotic rats and nephrotoxic nephritic rats.

In nephrotoxic nephritic rats, the content of acidic glycosaminoglycans was significantly decreased in the GBM, while unchanged in daunomycin nephrosis.

What is the cause of contradiction between the results obtained from chemical determinations of glycosaminoglycans and those obtained from the PEI staining of anionic sites in the GBM? To obtain an answer for this question, we perfused rat kidneys with normal rat serum or with the rat serum

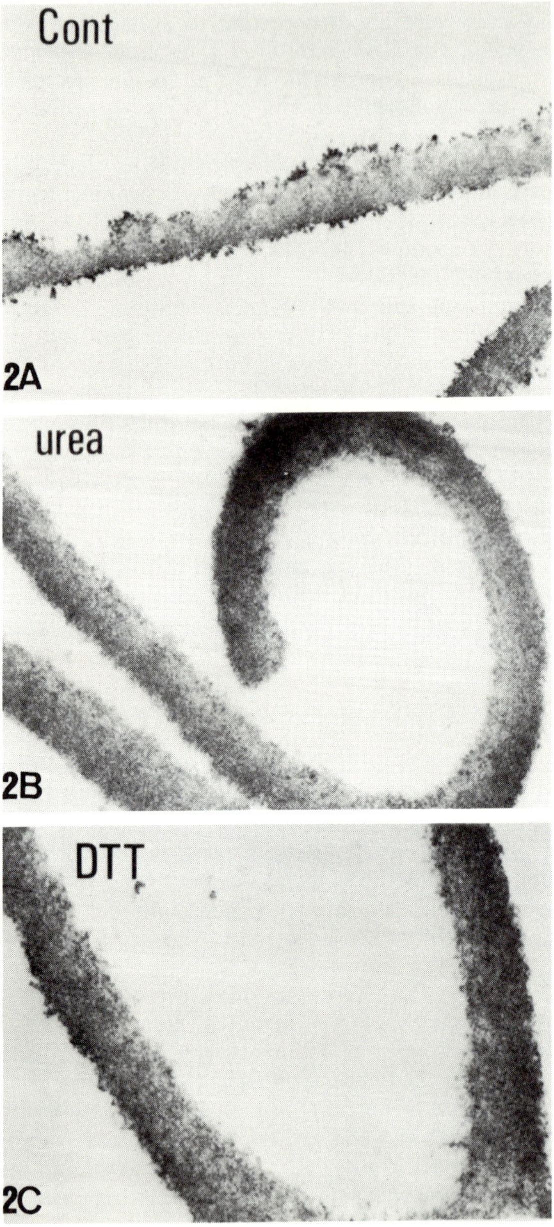

FIG. 2. Effects of urea and dithiothreitol on the anionic sites of glomerular basement membrane. (A) Control, (B) Urea, (C) Dithiothreitol.

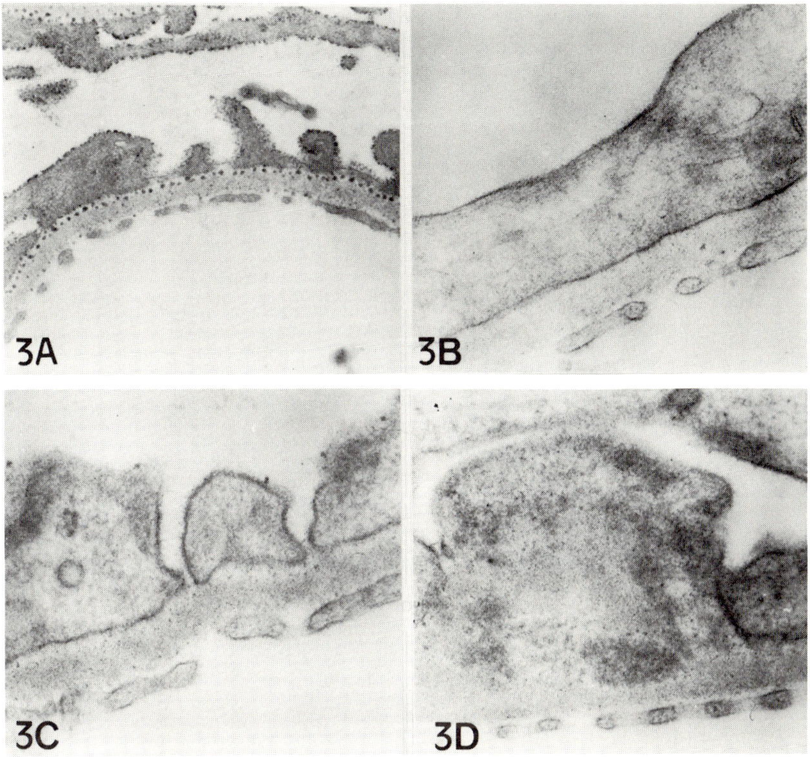

FIG. 3. The anionic sites of glomerular basement membrane in daunomycin nephrosis, nephrotoxic nephritis and glycoprotein nephritis. (A) Control, (B) Daunomycin nephrosis, (C) Nephrotoxic nephritis, (D) Glycoprotein nephritis.

TABLE 1

ACIDIC GLYCOSAMINOGLYCANS IN GLOMERULAR BASEMENT MEMBRANE OF DAUNOMYCIN NEPHROTIC RATS AND NEPHROTOXIC NEPHRITIC RATS

	N	Acidic Glycosaminoglycan (ug/mg)	P
Control	5	2.57±0.21	
D M N	5	2.73±0.43	N.S.
N T N	5	1.89±0.36	<0.05

DMN, daunomycin nephrosis; NTN, nephrotoxic nephritis; N.S., not significant

from daunomycin nephrosis (Fig. 4). Perfusion with sera obtained from rat with daunomycin nephrosis showed a loss of PEI-staining particles in the GBM as well as epithelial and endothelial cell coats.

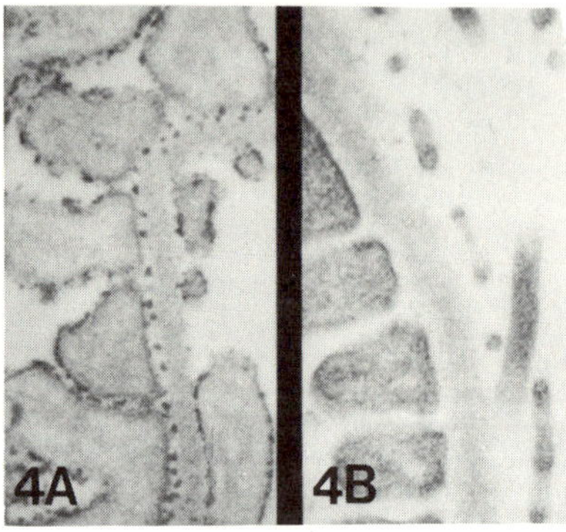

FIG. 4. Effect of the serum obtained from daunomycin nephrosis on the anionic sites of glomerular basement membrane. Perfusion of the rat kidney with the serum from normal rat (A) and with the serum from daunomycin nephrotic rat (B).

The same cationic effect was observed in the human serum. Perfusion of rat kidneys with serum obtained from a patient with minimal change nephrotic syndrome (lipoid nephrosis) showed the disappearance of the anionic sites of the GBM, whereas the normal serum had no influences on the anionic sites, indicating that a certain cationic substance occurs in the serum of this disease (Fig. 5).

Interleukin 2 produced by stimulated human lymphocytes was considered the most likely candidate responsible for this cationic substance since perfusion of the rat kidneys with this substance showed a loss of fixed negative charge from the GBM (Fig. 6).

Alterations of the Anionic Sites of Glomerular Basement Membrane in Glomerulonephritides

We studied the anionic sites of the GBM in patients with glomerulonephritis with heavy proteinuria to evaluate the role of the charge in the GBM in the pathogenesis of proteinuria.

In a patient with benign reccurrent hematuria, the PEI-stained particles were seen predominantly along the *lamina rara externa* at regular intervals. These particles were also seen in the *lamina rara interna* and the cell coat (Fig. 7A).

In lipoid nephrosis, the anionic sites of the GBM were markedly decreased or completely disappeared (Fig. 7B).

In membranous nephropathy, the PEI positive particles were decreased and dispersed in the *lamina rara externa* of the GBM. They were present around the immune deposits on the epithelial side of the GBM, but not detected within the immune deposits (Fig. 7C).

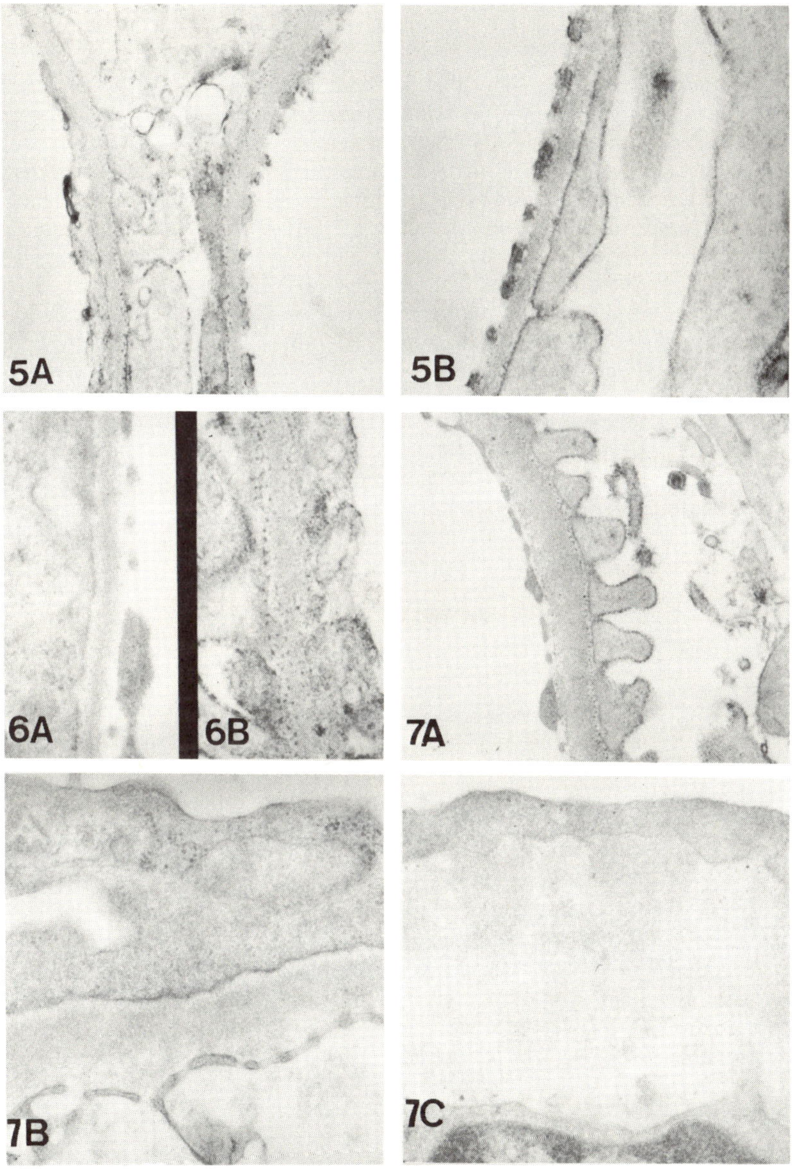

FIG. 5. Effect of the serum from lipoid nephrosis on the anionic sites of glomerular basement membrane. (A) Perfusion of the rat kidney with normal human serum, (B) Perfusion of the rat kidney with the serum obtained from a patient with lipoid nephrosis.

FIG. 6. Effect of interleukin 2 on the anionic sites of glomerular basement membrane. (A) Perfusion of the rat kidney with interleukin 2, (B) Perfusion of the rat kidney with physiological saline.

FIG. 7. The anionic sites of glomerular basement membrane in glomerulonephritides. (A) Benign reccurrent hematuria, (B) Lipoid nephrosis, (C) Membranous nephropathy.

Abstract

The anionic sites of glomerular basement membrane consist of heparan sulfate proteoglycan and glycoproteins connected with type IV collagen molecules by hydrogen bonds and disulfide linkages.

In nephrotoxic serum nephritis, the anionic sites of glomerular basement membrane were decreased due to a decrease of heparan sulfate content. In daunomycin nephrosis, the anionic sites of glomerular basement membrane were decreased in spite of unchanged concentration of heparan sulfate in the glomerular basement membrane. Perfusion with human serum obtained from patients with minimal change nephrotic syndrome showed the disappearance of the anionic sites of glomerular basement membrane, indicating that a certain cationic substance occurs in the serum of this disease. Interleukin 2 was considered the most likely candidate responsible for the cationic substance because the perfusion of the rat kidney with interleukin 2 showed a loss of anionic sites from the glomerular basement membrane.

In IgA nephropathy with nephrotic syndrome, the anionic sites of glomerular basement membrane were not detected. In membranous nephropathy, the number of clusters of anionic sites in glomerular basement membrane were decreased and dispersed.

References

Kanwar, Y.S., and Farquhar, M.G. (1979). Anionic sites in the glomerular basement membrane. In vivo and in vitro localization to the laminae rarae by cationic probes. *J. Cell Biol.* **81**, 137–153.

Koide, H., Soeda, N., and Ohno, J. (1981). Biochemical properties of glomerular basement membrane in daunomycin nephrosis and nephrotoxic serum nephritis. *Renal Physiol.* **4**, 102–107.

Schurer, J.W., Hoedemaeker, PH. J., and Molenaar, I. (1977). Polyethyleneimine as tracer particle for (immuno)electron microscopy. *J. Histochem. Cytochem.* **25**, 384–387.

Shibata, S., Sakaguchi, H., Nagasawa, T., and Naruse, T. (1972). Nephritogenic glycoprotein. II. Experimental production of membranous glomerulonephritis in rats by a single injection of homologous renal glycopeptide. *Lab. Invest.* **27**, 457–465.

PATHOGENIC POTENTIAL OF THE GLOMERULAR BINDING OF POLYCATIONS

Jeffrey L. Barnes and Manjeri A. Venkatachalam

Departments of Pathology and Medicine
The University of Texas, Health Science Center at San Antonio
San Antonio, Texas

Glomerular permeability to macromolecules is influenced by molecule-filter interactions with respect to charge, size and shape (Brenner et al., 1978; Venkatachalam and Rennke, 1978). The glomerular basement membrane (GBM) is richly endowed with a number of polyanionic substances including the N-sulfated glycosaminoglycan heparan sulfate (Kanwar and Farquhar, 1979), the sialic acid containing glycoproteins laminin (Scheinman et al., 1980) and fibronectin (Courtoy et al., 1980) and the sulfated glycoprotein entactin (Bender et al., 1981). These fixed polyanions form a charge barrier to circulating anionic macromolecules but not to cationic species of the same molecules as indicated by clearance and ultrastructural studies (Brenner et al., 1978; Venkatachalam and Rennke, 1978).

Studies to date have focused on the role of net charge of tracer macromolecules (Brenner et al., 1978; Venkatachalam and Rennke, 1978) and immune reactants (Border et al., 1982; Gallo et al., 1981; Oite et al., 1982) as determinants of increased permeability and enhancement of immune complex deposition in an intact glomerular capillary wall. Conversely, pathological changes in the permeability or affinity of the glomerular capillary wall itself to antigens, antibodies or their complexes would also increase the likelihood of immune complex deposition. Indeed, loss or neutralization of glomerular polyanion may result in increased permeability to circulating anionic macromolecules (Barnes et al., 1984a; Caulfield and Farquhar, 1978; Hunsicker et al., 1981; Kanwar et al., 1980; Kelley and Cavallo, 1978; Olson et al., 1981; Vehaskari et al., 1982).

We hypothesize that positively charged proteins upon local release from activated inflammatory cells and/or platelets during disease processes might penetrate the GBM and bind to glomerular polyanions, thus effectively neutralizing the electrostatic barrier to circulating native anionic proteins, including antigens and antibodies or immune complexes of suitable size and influence their glomerular localization.

To examine this hypothesis, a synthetic exogenous polycation, polyethyleneimine (PEI), was used as a prototype molecule for endogenous cationic proteins to study: (1) the effect of neutralization of glomerular polyanion on glomerular permeability to macromolecules, and (2) the influence of neutralization of glomerular polyanions by PEI on the glomerular deposition of immune complexes. In addition, platelet factor 4 (PF4), a platelet specific cationic protein, was tested for its ability to bind to GBM.

SIZE AND CHARGE SELECTIVE PERMEABILITY DEFECTS INDUCED IN THE GLOMERULAR BASEMENT MEMBRANE BY A POLYCATION (PEI)

Recent studies have indicated that circulating exogenous synthetic polycations can bind to glomerular polyanion and neutralize the electrostatic barrier to circulating anionic macromolecules. To define *in vivo* the sites of PEI induced enhancement of glomerular permeability and the roles played by the charge and steric interactions of polycation induced permeability defects, ultrastructural tracer studies were performed utilizing an electron dense tracer, ferritin. By using native (anionic) and cationic ferritins, PEI-induced alterations in both charge and size selective barriers were examined (Barnes et al., 1984a). If an alteration in charge selective permeability is the sole defect induced by PEI, one would expect an increase in penetration of native anionic ferritin with respect to controls. However, if a size defect is superimposed on a charge defect, then no change or an increase in penetration of the number of cationic ferritin particles in the GBM can be expected with respect to controls.

Two groups of rats were anesthetized with ether and treated in the following fashion: Group I, a control group, was injected with 0.05 M phosphate buffered saline (PBS) pH 7.35 *via* a tail vein. Group II received an equal volume of PBS containing 0.5% PEI to deliver 15 μg per g body weight. Fifteen min following PBS alone or PEI, the rats received native ferritin (isoelectric point (pI) of 4.5 to 4.8) or one of three cationic ferritins with pIs of 7.5 –8.2, 8.0 – 8.7 and 8.7 – 9.0 at a dose of 0.1 mg per g body weight, i.v. The rats were sacrificed 15 min later and kidney tissue was fixed and processed for light and electron microscopy. Penetration of ferritin into the GBM was assessed by counting the number of ferritin particles in enlarged micrographs and expressed as the number of tracer molecules per μm^2 within the inner and/or outer aspect of the GBM. PEI-induced permeability change was measured as the ratio of counted ferritin particles within the GBM in the corresponding PEI and control groups.

This index, PEI/control, represents the degree of increase in the quantity of ferritin particles in the GBM following PEI relative to controls for each ferritin species in all groups of experiments. The results showed that rats given PBS without PEI had few native (anionic) ferritin molecules within the GBM (Fig. 1a), indicating that the electrostatic barrier to anionic molecules

---

FIG. 1. Glomerular capillary walls of rats given 0.1 mg/g body weight of native ferritin (NF, 4.5 – 4.8) following (A) phosphate-buffered saline or (B) polyethyleneimine, 15 μg/g body weight. The number of ferritin particles within the GBM following PEI is substantially increased (>100-fold) when compared to the PBS-control. (From *Kidney Int.* **25**:11 –19, 1984)

FIG. 2. Glomerular capillary walls of rats given 0.1 mg/g body weight of weakly cationic ferritin (CF, 7.5 – 8.2) following (A) phosphate-buffered saline or (B) polyethyleneimine, 15 μg/g body weight. The number of ferritin molecules within the GBM following PEI is three to four times greater than in the GBM of the PBS-control. (From *Kidney Int.* **25**:11 –19, 1984)

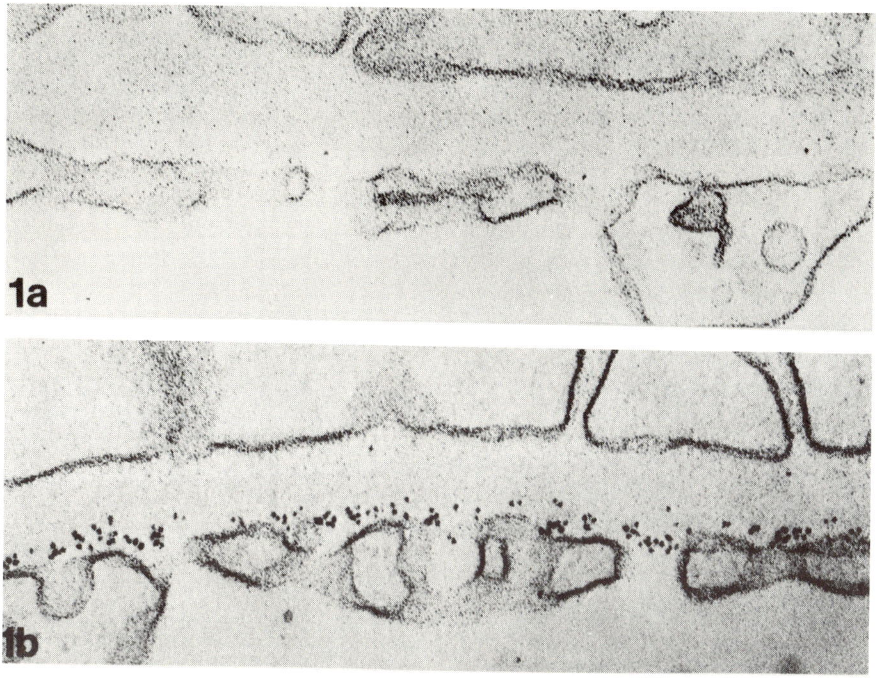
1a
1b

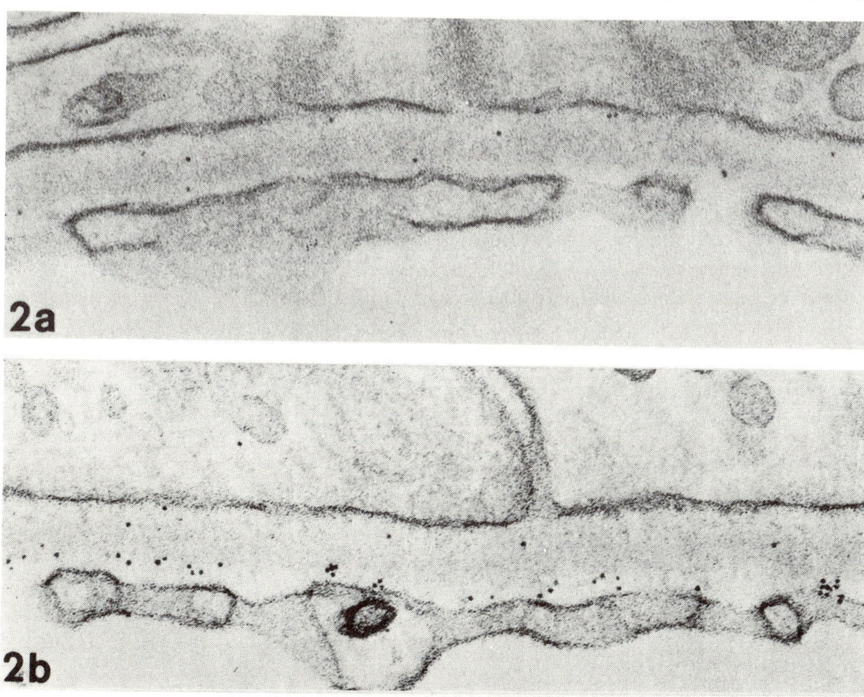
2a
2b

was intact. However, PEI markedly enhanced glomerular permeability to native ferritin as indicated by a greater than 100-fold increase in the number of tracer molecules in the GBM when compared to PBS controls (Fig. 1b, Table 1). The majority of tracer molecules localized within the internal aspect of the GBM; however, the number of molecules was also increased in the external aspect of the GBM.

Penetration of cationic ferritin 7.5 – 8.2 into the GBM was also increased 3 – 4 times by PEI when compared to controls (Figs. 2a, 2b) (Table 1) despite neutralization of the glomerular polyanions. Similarly, PEI increased the permeability of the GBM to cationic ferritins 8.0 – 8.7. Penetration of CF 8.7 – 9.0 was increased only into the inner aspect of the GBM (Table 1).

TABLE 1

PERMEABILITY RATIOS (PEI/C) OF COUNTED FERRITIN MOLECULES WITHIN THE GLOMERULAR BASEMENT MEMBRANE IN CORRESPONDING POLYETHYLENEIMINE AND CONTROL GROUPS

		PEI/C	
Ferritin (pI)	GBM	Inner Aspect	External Aspect
NF (4.5 – 4.8)	107	146	16.4
CF (7.5 – 8.2)	3.3	4.3	1.3
CF (8.0 – 8.7)	1.7	1.9	1.0
CF (8.7 – 9.0)	0.9	1.2	0.4

NF, native ferritin; CF, cationic ferritin; pI, isoelectric point; PEI, polyethyleneimine; C, control; GBM, glomerular basement membrane.

PEI increased glomerular permeability to both native and cationic tracers; however, an inverse relationship between the ratio PEI/control and the charge of the tracer was observed at all levels of the GBM. That is, as the isoelectric point of the ferritin species increased, the ratio between the PEI and control groups approached one. This effect is best explained if polycations *including* cationic ferritins alter the porosity of the GBM.

Hemodynamic effects as a factor in PEI's effect on glomerular permeability to ferritin were ruled out by the examination of renal blood flow (RBF) and glomerular filtration rates (GFR) in an additional 13 rats following PBS or PEI. Clearance of inulin and ^{3}H-paraminohippurate showed that PEI reduced GFR by approximately 50% when compared to controls. PEI-induced reductions in renal plasma flow and RBF were proportionate to decrements in GFR. Thus, filtration fractions were unchanged compared to controls. In additional studies, lowering kidney perfusion pressure to 40 mm of Hg had no effect on penetration of ferritin. Since filtration fractions were unchanged following PEI and low perfusion pressure did not alter ferritin penetration, the observed increases in ferritin penetration into the GBM cannot be attributed to hemodynamic effects. Thus, PEI-induced alterations in

GBM penetration of ferritin are the product of alterations in both charge and size selective barriers independent of hemodynamic effects.

Influence of PEI on Glomerular Deposition of Passively Administered Preformed Immune Complexes

A number of recent studies have indicated that the net charge of an antigen, antibody or of the immune complex influences glomerular localization of immune deposits (Border et al., 1982; Gallo et al., 1981; Oite et al., 1982). Immunization with cationic antigens and/or passive administration of cationic immune complexes have been shown to lead to localization of immune deposits within the GBM whereas anionic species of these same molecules leads to localization of deposits exclusively within the mesangium.

The objective of the next series of experiments was the reverse. Experiments were designed to examine the potential of PEI to bind to and neutralize glomerular polyanions and alter glomerular permeability to circulating immune complexes. These experiments were performed by using a model in which preformed immune complexes were passively administered to rats following PBS-alone or PEI (Barnes and Venkatachalam, 1984).

Immune complexes were prepared by adding the equivalence amount of BSA to pooled IgG rich fractions of rabbit anti-BSA followed by washing and subsequent incubation in 40x antigen excess. In some of the paired experiments ^{125}I-labelled anti-BSA antibody was added to unlabelled immunoglobulin fractions prior to preparation of the soluble immune complexes. Measurement of serum concentration of complexes and the distribution of size of immune complexes in serum of controls and experimentals was performed.

Twelve rats were paired according to age and size, then divided into two groups. The rats were briefly anesthetized with ether then injected with PEI at a dose of 10 μg/g body weight *via* a tail vein followed 5 min later with an injection of preformed immune complexes to deliver 30 mg of anti-BSA antibody. Controls received PBS without PEI followed by administration of immune complexes. In both groups all injections were repeated two additional times 4 hr apart. After each series of injections the rats were placed in metabolic cages and urine was collected for subsequent protein analysis. One hr after the last injection, the rats were anesthetized and kidney tissue obtained for subsequent light and electron microscopy and immunofluorescence. To assess any toxic effect of PEI, an additional group of rats was given PEI, but without subsequent injections of preformed immune complexes.

Sections of renal cortex were assessed for glomerular localization of BSA and rabbit IgG by immunofluorescence microscopy. The intensity of glomerular immunofluorescence of localized BSA and rabbit IgG was quantitated by photometric analysis.

Administration of PEI-alone produced no untoward effects. Administration of PEI followed by preformed immune complexes enhanced glomerular deposition of immune deposits when compared to PBS controls. In glomeruli of rats given PEI, numerous small deposits were observed primarily in the subendothelium and to a lesser extent in the subepithelium of the glomerular

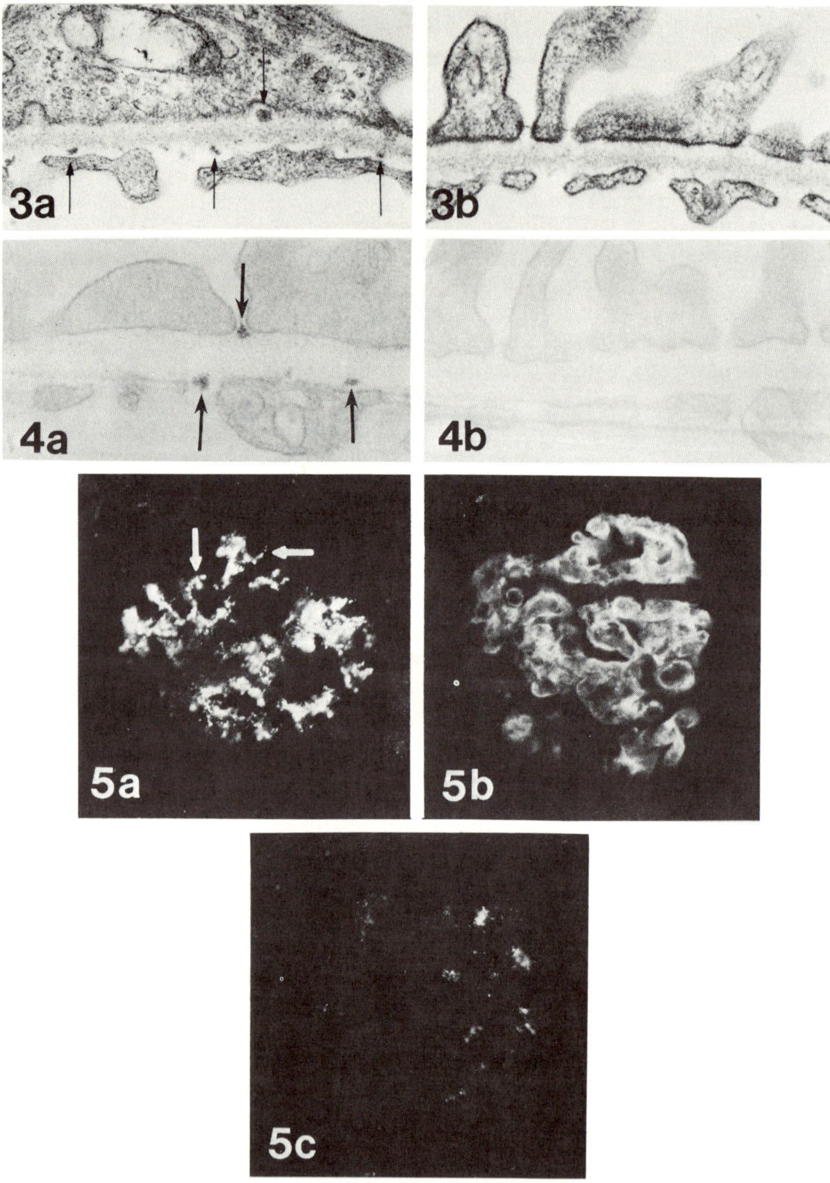

FIG. 3. Electron micrographs of glomerular capillary walls of (a) Group I (PEI plus immune complexes) and (b) Group II (control, diluent plus immune complexes). Electron-dense deposits (arrows) are localized in the subendothelial and subepithelial aspects of the GBM of Group I (a), but absent in the GBM of Group II (b). (From *J. Exp. Med.* **160**: 286 – 293, 1984)

FIG. 4. Glomerular localization of rabbit IgG by immunoperoxidase electron microcapillary wall (Fig. 3a). In PBS controls, peripheral capillary wall deposits were absent (Fig. 3b). The immune nature of these deposits was verified by immunoperoxidase electron microscopy (Figs. 4a, 4b). The mesangial matrix in both groups was expanded and rarefied but deposits were infrequently observed. Intensity of fluorescence of localized rabbit IgG and BSA was greater in PEI treated rats when compared to PBS controls by quantitative fluorescence microscopy. Localization of rabbit IgG (Figs. 5a, 5b) and BSA in rats treated with PEI plus immune complexes revealed a granular but irregular pattern in peripheral capillary walls and mesangium. Localization of rabbit IgG (Fig. 5c) and BSA in peripheral capillary walls in PBS controls was negligible.

Serum concentrations of ^{125}I-anti-BSA-BSA immune complexes at the first collection period were not significantly different between PBS and PEI groups. Serum concentration of immune complexes in blood samples taken at the termination of the experiment was significantly greater in rats given PEI (4.50 ± 0.27 mg/ml) when compared with PBS controls (3.66 ± 0.17 mg/ml, $P < 0.05$). However, reduction of the dose of immune complexes administered to PEI rats lowered serum levels of immune complexes to the same level as PBS rats but had no effect on the difference in localization and distribution of immune deposits as examined by immunofluorescence and electron microscopy. In all serum samples immune complexes were heterogenous in size; however, the peak counts occurred in collection fractions corresponding to thyroglobulin standard with a molecular weight of 669,000 daltons.

These experiments indicate that PEI not only enhances glomerular permeability to circulating tracer macromolecules (ferritin) but also enhances the glomerular deposition of immune complexes.

Binding of Platelet Factor Four to Glomerular Polyanions

The objective of the next series of experiments was to examine the potential of a platelet derived cationic secretory protein, platelet factor 4 (PF4), to bind to glomerular polyanions. If endogenous polycations released from inflammatory cells can enhance glomerular permeability and influence glomerular permeability and influence glomerular deposition of immune complexes obviously they must first interact with glomerular polyanions. Although

---

scopy. In glomeruli of Group I (a), reaction product (arrows) is localized in an identical distribution as the dense deposits observed by routine staining methods (see Fig. 3a). Reaction product (rabbit IgG) is absent in the GBM of Group II controls (b). (From *J. Exp. Med.* **160**:286 –293, 1984)

FIG. 5. Glomerular immunofluorescence localization of rabbit IgG of Group I (a and b) and Group II (c) rats. In Group I, staining is predominantly mesangial but some peripheral capillary loops (arrows) also show IgG localization (a). In some rats localization of rabbit IgG was observed in peripheral capillary loops (b). Group II controls showed only mesangial localization of rabbit IgG in a segmental distribution (c). (From *J. Exp. Med.* **160**:286 – 293, 1984)

its isoelectric point is close to neutral (pI 7.6), PF4 behaves like a strong polycation due to a unique polar region containing numerous cationic amino acid residues. The following experimental protocol was used to assess binding of human PF4 to glomerular polyanions (Barnes et al., 1984b):

(1) PF4 ($590 - 720$ μg/ml) was layered onto sections of human or rat kidney cortex, washed with barbital buffer containing 0.15 M NaCl, then followed by indirect immunofluorescence. To examine an ionic interaction of PF4 with glomerular polyanion, sections were washed after layering with PF4, with buffers containing progressively increasing concentrations of NaCl from 0.15 to 3.0 M. In addition, heparin, which has a strong affinity for PF4, was layered onto sections previously treated with PF4. Following subsequent washes and incubations with immunoreagents, all sections were examined by fluorescence microscopy and assessed for PF4 binding; (2) To further assess the ability of PF4 to bind to GBM *in vitro*, ^{125}I-labelled PF4 was added at increasing concentrations from 10 to 100 μg to separate tubes containing isolated GBM suspensions; (3) To assess PF4 binding to glomerular polyanions *in vivo* male Sprague Dawley rats were divided into three groups, and lightly anesthetized with ether. The first group was given 125 or 250 μg of PF4 in 0.5 ml of barbital buffer *via* a tail vein. A control group received barbital buffer alone. Five min later, the animals were sacrificed. To examine an ionic interaction between PF4 and glomerular polyanion, a second group of rats was given PEI, at a dose of 15 μg per g BW, to bind to glomerular polyanions and block subsequent PF4 binding. Controls received PBS without PEI. Five min later, the rats were given 125 μg of PF4 and were sacrificed 5 min later. Similarly, treatment with heparin should displace the platelet protein from glomerular polyanions. Thus, a third group of rats received PF4, followed 5 min later by 500 μg of heparin, i.v. Controls received PF4 followed by vehicle alone. Rats were sacrificed 5 min later. Immediately after sacrifice, kidney tissue was obtained from all groups of rats, and frozen and processed for immunofluorescence microscopy as already described; (4) An additional series of experiments were performed to examine the ultrastructural localization of PF4 binding sites by immunocytochemical procedures utilizing immunoperoxidase on tissue sections obtained from kidneys perfused *ex vivo* with PF4.

Rats were anesthetized with sodium pentobarbital and surgically prepared for perfusion of the left kidney. The kidney was washed free of blood by perfusion of oxygenated Krebs-Henseleit saline (KHS) followed by perfusion of $500 - 600$ μg of PF4 in saline containing 1% BSA. Controls received diluent without PF4. After perfusion of PF4 or diluent the kidneys were washed with KHS followed by perfusion of fixative solution. Kidney cortex was sliced and prepared for immunoperoxidase procedures for light and electron microscopic localization of PF4.

All sections of rat and human kidney cortex incubated with PF4 showed a strong binding of the platelet protein to the walls of peripheral capillary loops and to the mesangium. Also, peritubular capillaries and/or tubular basement membranes showed strong staining for PF4. PF4 was readily removed from the sections by washing with barbital buffer containing 1.0 or 3.0 M NaCl. Also, treatment of sections with heparin removed PF4 from glomerular polyanions.

A linear relationship between amount of ^{125}I-PF4 added to GBM suspensions and amount bound was shown to occur between 10 and 40 μg of added ^{125}I-PF4. This relationship diminished when greater than 40 μg of ^{125}I-PF4 was added to the GBM suspension indicating saturation of PF4 binding sites. Addition of heparin to the suspension following PF4 almost completely abolished PF4 binding.

In vivo, an avid binding of PF4 to GBM and the mesangium was observed (Fig. 6). Controls receiving diluent or non-immune serum in place of primary anti-PF4 serum showed negligible background staining. Prior administration of PEI blocked PF4 binding (Fig. 7) and post treatment with heparin following injection of PF4 eliminated staining (not shown).

Light microscopical immunoperoxidase localization of PF4 following perfusion revealed intense staining of the GBM in a linear pattern similar to that observed by immunofluorescence following intravenous injection. Ultrastructural localization of PF4 by immunoperoxidase staining revealed that the platelet protein was bound to multiple sites throughout the glomerular capillary wall (Fig. 8). Reaction product was observed throughout the GBM but tended to localize in small punctate sites in both *lamina rarae* especially in the *lamina rara externa*. Reaction product was also observed on the surfaces of endothelial and epithelial cells; but, the strongest staining was observed just beneath epithelial cells adjacent to the GBM.

These studies allow for the following conclusions with regard to the interaction of PF4 with glomerular polyanions: (1) Purified human PF4 avidly binds to human and rat GBM and epithelial and endothelial cell surfaces; (2) PF4's interaction with glomerular structures is ionic in that binding can be blocked by prior exposure of glomerular polyanions with a synthetic polycation PEI and can be removed by post treatment with heparin or high ionic strength buffer; (3) PF4 binding sites in rat GBM, revealed by immunoperoxidase cytochemistry, are heterogenous in distribution and show a similar pattern as described for glomerular anionic sites stained by cationic dyes.

Discussion

Synthetic polycations, including PEI, bind to glomerular polyanions and alter glomerular permeability to circulating macromolecules (Barnes et al., 1984a; Hunsicker et al., 1981; Kelley and Cavallo, 1978; Vehaskari et al., 1982). The electrostatic interaction between the polycation and glomerular polyanions has been shown not only to alter the charge selective barrier to negatively charged molecules but also alter the porosity of the GBM. A theoretical basis for polycation induced structural changes in synthetic polyanionic gel matrices has been proposed by Tanaka (1981). Polyacrylamide-polyacrylic acid gels consist of polymers of negatively charged chain molecules cross-linked to create a tangled network with a uniform population of pores (analogous to GBM). Collapse of the gel and separation of gel components into domains of high and low density concomitant with an increase in porosity can be brought about by small alterations in the charge of the gel by changing the pH, ionic strength of the buffer or exposure to an electrical field. A similar collapse or precipitation of proteoglycans has been shown to occur in biological

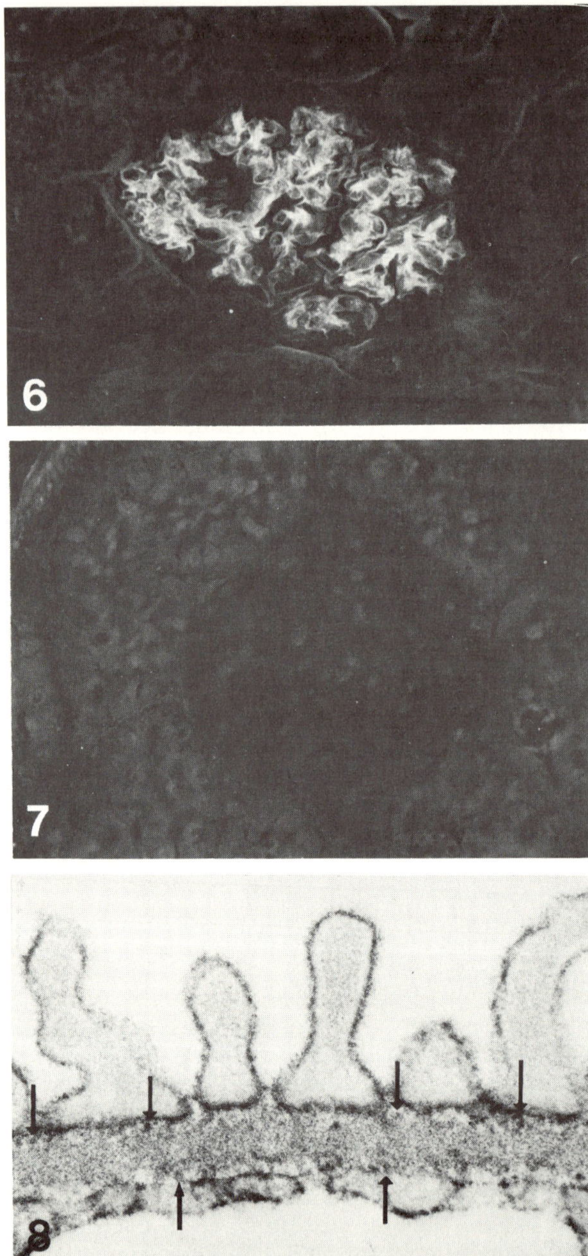

FIG. 6. Glomerular immunofluorescence localization of human PF4 after intravenous injection into a rat. Strong staining of peripheral capillary loops and the mesangium is apparent. (From *Kidney Int.* **25**:759 – 765, 1984)

FIG. 7. Rat glomerulus stained for PF4 5 min after an injection of polyethylene-

tissues (including GBM) following staining with cationic dyes (Coltoff-Schiller and Goldfischer, 1981; Hunzicker and Schenk, 1984; Reale et al., 1983; Shepard and Mitchell, 1976). Thus, binding of circulating polycations to glomerular polyanions *in vivo* may alter the electrostatic barrier and also alter the porosity of the filter by altering the conformation of anionic polymers in a similar fashion as demonstrated for synthetic gels.

PEI also increased glomerular permeability to preformed immune complexes leading to enhanced deposition of complexes in the GBM and mesangium. This study did not address the mode in which immune complexes deposit in glomerular structures (trapping of intact immune complexes *vs.* formation of deposits *in situ*). However, both modes of the enhanced localization of complexes can conceivably be implied. The size distribution of complexes is heterogenous (most about 669,000 dalton); thus, one may infer alterations in porosity of the GBM in addition to alterations in charge selectivity, particularly with reference to the large subepithelial complexes observed by electron microscopy.

Alteration of GBM charge and structure by polycation binding might also influence the deposition of immune complexes during natural disease processes. For example, like PEI, positively charged proteins released by activated inflammatory cells and/or platelets, may bind to polyanions in the GBM and cause permeability defects that could affect the localization of antigens, antibodies, or their complexes in the capillary wall (Fig. 9).

Indeed, our studies show that a platelet cationic secretory protein, PF4, is capable of binding to the glomerular polyanions. Whether or not PF4 or other platelet secretory proteins can alter glomerular permeability remains to be determined. However, evidence exists implicating a role for polycations in glomerular disease processes. For example, in experimental models of Lupus glomerulonephritis, losses of polyanion in the GBM have been shown to precede increased permeability to anionic proteins prior to deposition of immune complexes (Cavallo et al., 1983a; Cavallo et al., 1983b; Kelley and Cavallo, 1977; Kelley and Cavallo, 1980; Melnick et al., 1981). Similar losses of polyanion have been reported by Camussi et al. in human cases of lupus nephritis (Camussi et al., 1982). In addition to loss of polyanion, Camussi et al. described glomerular localization of neutrophil and platelet cationic proteins in affected glomeruli, further implicating a role for polycations in glomerular immune complex disease (Barnes and Venkatachalam, 1985; Camussi, et al., 1982).

A number of polycationic proteins have been isolated from platelets and are known to have biologic activity (i.e., are chemotactic or mitogenic); thus their localization in glomerular structures may have broader implications other

---

imine (PEI) followed by PF4. Pre-treatment with PEI blocked PF4 binding as indicated by the absence of glomerular staining when compared to Fig. 6. (From *Kidney Int.* **25**: 759 – 765, 1984)

FIG. 8. Immunoperoxidase cytochemical localization of PF4 following intrarenal perfusion. Reaction product is present throughout the GBM but particularly at small punctate sites in the *laminae rarae* (arrows). Also, surfaces of endothelial and epithelial cells stain for PF4. (From *Kidney Int.* **25**: 759 – 765, 1984)

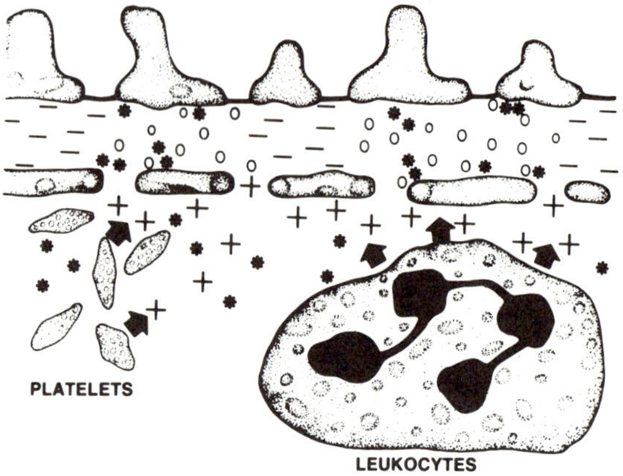

FIG. 9. Schematic representation of hypothetical events leading to enhanced glomerular permeability during glomerulonephritis. Positively charged proteins (+) upon local release from activated platelets and/or leukocytes, penetrate the glomerular basement membrane and bind to glomerular polyanions (–); thus effectively perturbing (o) the electrostatic and size barriers to circulating immune reactants and their complexes (asterisks).

than their capillary permeability enhancing potential. These considerations have been discussed at length in a recent review on platelet polycations in glomerular disease (Barnes and Venkatachalam, 1985).

Abstract

Polycations may bind to glomerular polyanion and lead to permeability alterations. We have shown that glomerular binding of polyethyleneimine (PEI), after i.v. injection, results in 100x increase in glomerular basement membrane (GBM) penetration by the large protein tracer, anionic ferritin (pI = 4.5 – 4.8). Paradoxically, GBM penetration by cationic ferritins (pI = 7.5 – 8.2; 8.0 – 8.7; 8.7 – 8.9) was also increased, indicating that perturbation of the charge barrier was accompanied by changes in porosity. Polycations may collapse and distort the gel structure of GBM, similar to the interactions of counterions with synthetic gels. Polycations may also enhance glomerular permeability to antigens, antibodies or immune complexes. Therefore, we examined the effect of PEI on glomerular localization of bovine serum albumin (BSA)-anti-BSA complexes. By quantitative immunofluorescence, and immunoperoxidase electron microscopy, PEI caused dramatic alterations both in the quantity and sites of localization of immune complexes in glomeruli compared to controls. In rats given PEI, deposits were within the GBM, and mesangium. In controls not given PEI, deposits localized only in the mesangium, in smaller amounts than after PEI. Thus, neutralization of glomerular polyanion by a polycation enhançes the deposition and alters the distribution of immune complexes in glomeruli. Because endogenous polycations may also influence glomerular permeability, we examined the potential of platelet factor four (PF4), a secretory protein with polycationic properties, to bind to glomerular polyanion. *In vivo* or *in vitro*, PF4 or ^{125}I-PF4 bound to glomerular structures in a saturable manner. Binding was prevented or reversed by heparin, high ionic strength buffers, or by prior treatment with PEI. These studies show that an endogenous cationic protein is capable of ionic interactions with glomerular polyanion. By virtue of their affinity for glomerular polyanion, PF4 and/or other endogenous cationic proteins may affect glomerular permeability and play an important role in disease.

References

Barnes, J.L., Radnik, R.A., and Venkatachalam, M.A. (1984a). Size and charge selective permeability defects induced in glomerular basement membrane by a polycation. *Kidney Int.* **25**, 11–19.

Barnes, J.L., Levine, S.P., and Venkatachalam, M.A. (1984b). Binding of platelet factor four (PF4) to glomerular polyanion. *Kidney Int.* **25**, 759–765.

Barnes, J.L., and Venkatachalam, M.A. (1984). Enhancement of glomerular immune complex deposition by a circulating polycation. *J. Exp. Med.* **160**, 286–293.

Barnes, J.L., and Venkatachalam, M.A. (1985). Role of platelets and polycationic mediators in glomerular vascular injury. *Seminars in Nephrol.*

Bender, B.L., Jaffe, R., Carlin, B., and Chung, A.E. (1981). Immunolocalization of entactin, a sulfated basement component, in rodent tissues, and comparison with GP-2 (laminin). *Am. J. Pathol.* **103**, 419–426.

Border, W.A., Ward, H.J., Kamil, E.S., and Cohen, A.H. (1982). Induction of membranous nephropathy in rabbits by administration of an exogenous cationic antigen. Demonstration of a pathogenic role for electrical charge. *J. Clin. Invest.* **69**, 451–461.

Brenner, B.M., Hostetter, T.H., and Humes, H.D. (1978). Molecular basis of proteinuria of glomerular origin. *N. Engl. J. Med.* **298**, 826–833.

Camussi, G., Tetta, C., Segoloni, G., Coda, R., and Vercellone, A. (1982). Localization of neutrophil cationic proteins and loss of anionic charges in glomeruli of patients with systemic lupus erythematosus glomerulonephritis. *Clin. Immunol. Immunopathol.* **24**, 299–314.

Caulfield, J.P., and Farquhar, M.G. (1978). Loss of anionic sites from the glomerular basement membrane in aminonucleoside nephrosis. *Lab. Invest.* **39**, 505–512.

Cavallo, T., Goldman, M., Graves, K., and Lambert, P-H. (1983a). Altered glomerular permeability in the early phase of immune complex nephritis. *Kidney Int.* **24**, 632–637.

Cavallo, T., Goldman, M., and Lambert, P-H. (1983b). Proliferative glomerulonephritis associated with polyclonal B-cell activation. *Am. J. Pathol.* **114**, 346–348.

Coltoff-Schiller, B., and Goldfischer, S. (1981). Glycosaminoglycans in the rat aorta. Ultrastructural localization with toluidine blue 0 and osmium-ferrocyanide procedures. *Am. J. Pathol.* **105**, 232–240.

Courtoy, P.J., Kanwar, Y.S., Hynes, R.O., and Farquhar, M.G. (1980). Fibronectin localization in the rat glomerulus. *J. Cell Biol.* **87**, 691–696.

Gallo, G.R., Caulin-Glaser, T., and Lamm, M.E. (1981). Charge of circulating immune complexes as a factor in glomerular basement membrane localization in mice. *J. Clin. Invest.* **67**, 1305–1313.

Hunsicker, L.G., Shearer, T.P., and Shaffer, S.J. (1981). Acute reversible proteinuria induced by infusion of the polycation hexadimethrine. *Kidney Int.* **20**, 7–17.

Hunzicker, E.B., and Schenk, R.K. (1984). Cartilage ultrastructure after high pressure freezing, freeze substitution, and low temperature embedding. II. Intercellular matrix ultrastructure-preservation of proteoglycans in their native state. *J. Cell Biol.* **98**, 277–282.

Kanwar, Y.S., and Farquhar, M.G. (1979). Presence of heparan sulfate in the glomerular basement membrane. *Proc. Natl. Acad. Sci. U.S.A.* **76**, 1303–1307.

Kanwar, Y.S., Linker, A., and Farquhar, M.G. (1980). Increased permeability of the glomerular basement membrane to ferritin after removal of glycosaminoglycans (Heparan Sulfate) by enzyme digestion. *J. Cell Biol.* **86**, 688–693.

Kelley, V.E., and Cavallo, T. (1977). Glomerular permeability. Ultrastructural studies in New Zealand Black/White mice using polyanionic ferritin as a molecular probe. *Lab. Invest.* **37**, 265–275.

Kelley, V.E., and Cavallo, T. (1978). Glomerular permeability. Transfer of native ferritin in glomeruli with decreased anionic sites. *Lab. Invest.* **39**, 547–553.

Kelley, V.E., and Cavallo, T. (1980). Glomerular permeability. Focal loss of anionic sites in glomeruli of proteinuric mice with lupus nephritis. *Lab. Invest.* **42**, 59–64.

Melnick, G.F., Ladoulis, M.D., and Cavallo, T. (1981). Decreased anionic groups and increased permeability precedes deposition of immune complexes in the glomerular capillary wall. *Am. J. Pathol.* **105**, 114–120.

Oite, T., Batsford, S.R., Mihatsch, M.J., Takamiya, H., and Vogt, R.J. (1982). Quantitative studies of *in situ* immune complex glomerulonephritis in the rat induced by planted antigen. *J. Exp. Med.* **155**, 460–474.

Olson, J.L., Rennke, H.G., and Venkatachalam, M.A. (1981). Alterations in the charge and size selectivity barrier of the glomerular filter in aminonucleoside nephrosis in rats. *Lab. Invest.* **44**, 271–279.

Reale, E., Luciano, L., and Kühn, K.W. (1983). Ultrastructural architecture of proteoglycans in the glomerular basement membrane. *J. Histochem. Cytochem.* **31**, 662–668.

Scheinman, J.I., Foidart, J.M., Gehron-Robey, P., Fish, A.J., and Michael, A.F. (1980). The immunohistology of glomerular antigens. IV. Laminin, a defined noncollagen basement membrane glycoprotein. *Clin. Immunol. Immunopathol.* **15**,175–189.

Shepard, N., and Mitchell, N. (1976). Simultaneous localization of proteoglycan by light and electron microscopy using toluidine blue 0. A study of epiphyseal cartilage. *J. Histochem. Cytochem.* **24**, 621–629.

Tanaka, T. (1981). Gels. *Sci. Am.* **244**, 124–138.

Vehaskari, V.M., Root, E.R., Germuth, F.G., and Robson, A.M. (1982). Glomerular charge and urinary protein excretion: Effects of systemic and intrarenal polycation infusion in the rat. *Kidney Int.* **22**, 127–135.

Venkatachalam, M.A., and Rennke, H.G. (1978). The structural and molecular basis of glomerular filtration. *Circ. Res.* **43**, 337–347.

MECHANISM OF PROTEINURIA IN RATS WITH CHRONIC SERUM SICKNESS

Zensuke Ota, Hirofumi Makino, Michio Takaoka
Kenji Soda and Shinya Suzuki

Third Department of Internal Medicine, Okayama University Medical School
Okayama

The exact mechanism of proteinuria in glomerulonephritis is not fully understood, although it is a common manifestation. We have recently demonstrated under electron microscopy after negative staining (Ota et al., 1979, 1980) that the glomerular basement membrane (GBM) is a three-dimensional molecular sieve composed of numerous *pores and strands.* The GBM pores were slightly smaller than albumin molecules, and GBM was thus considered to be the main filtration barrier of the glomerulus. We have also observed *in vitro* destruction of GBM after lysosomal enzyme digestion (Makino et al., 1980). It was presumed that enlargement of the GBM sieve pores caused proteinuria in glomerulonephritis.

This chapter deals with ultrastructural changes of the isolated GBM in rats with chronic serum sickness (CSS) in addition to the ultrastructures of normal GBM and the tubular basement membrane (TBM).

Electron Microscopy of Normal Glomerular and Tubular Basement Membrane

Bovine glomerular basement membrane: Glomerular capillaries with epithelial cells, basement membrane and endothelial cells are thought to function as a mechanical filter. In normal glomerular capillaries, the GBM is the only continuous layer between blood and urine. Using tracer molecules of different size and charge, many investigators have concluded that it is the main filter (Ryan and Karnovsky, 1976; Farquhar et al., 1961; Rennke and Venkatachalam, 1977; Brenner et al., 1978). There could be two regulatory factors that determine glomerular filtration, i.e. the charge barrier and sizc barrier. The former refers to the electric charge difference between GBM and molecules, and the latter refers to a size of the molecules.

GBM does not show pores when conventional methods of fixation and embedding are used. By transmission electron microscopy, the *lamina densa* appears as a felt-work of 30 to 40 Å fibrils which appear to be embedded in an amorphous matrix (Kurtz and McManus, 1960; Farquhar et al., 1961). We have recently demonstrated the existence of numerous pores (about 4 nm in diameter) in purified bovine GBM, with negatively stained material (Ota et al., 1977, 1979, 1980). Briefly, fresh bovine kidneys obtained from cattle were transported in ice to our laboratory, where they were kept frozen at

-10 ℃ until used. The isolation procedure used to obtain renal GBM was mainly a modification of Spiro's method (Spiro, 1967). The pellet consisting of glomeruli was examined for purity under a phase microscope. The same specimen used for negative staining was also processed in the final step for the ultrathin-sectioning to check for purity.

Under negatively staining, bovine GBM had a characteristic appearance. The fragments of GBM varied in diameter from several micrometers to about 50 nm. The larger fragments resembled torn paper pieces or folded paper with linear contours and angular ends (Fig. 1). The smaller fragments were round, oval or occasionally polygonal shaped. The membrane surface appeared felt-like or spongy at lower magnifications, whereas GBM was composed of fine strands and pores at higher magnification (Fig. 2). The strands were approximately equal in diameter. The pores were round, oval or polygonal shaped. Some pores were elongated forming short straight or bent channels.

These observations led us to conclude that GBM had a three-dimensional meshwork structure, resembling a crystal lattice which was penetrated throughout by numerous tortous, branched channels. Fifty pores and strands were measured. The mean long dimension of the pores was 3.1 ± 0.6 nm ($\pm$SD) and the short, 2.5 ± 0.3 nm, and mean strand was 1.8 ± 0.3 nm in diameter. The mean density of the pores was $36 \pm 2/1{,}000$ nm^2. Purified GBM storaged at -70 ℃ appeared the same as those described here.

Bovine albumin has a molecular weight of 66,248 and has a shape close to a prolate ellipsoid with axes of 14.0×4.0 nm (Peter, 1975). Rat albumin has a molecular weight of 64,616 and therefore, is considered to have a shape and axes fairly similar to those of bovine albumin. The diameter of the pores in our bovine GBM was much smaller than the axes of bovine albumin. Therefore, it is unlikely that albumin could pass through GBM, although the albumin molecule has a very flexible consistency. This is also consistent with the well-known finding that glomerular filtrate contains hardly any protein. It thus appears that GBM could be a molecular sieve in the glomeruli.

Bovine and rat tubular basement membrane:

1) *TBM prepared by sonic disruption*: The method described by Krisco et al. (1977) was used to isolate and purify the bovine and rat TBM immediately after animal sacrifice. TBM was broken by sonic disruption into pieces measuring a few hundred nanometers in diameter. Under negative staining, a fragment of bovine and rat TBM looked like paper with angular ends (Ota et al., 1980; Makino, 1981). At low magnifications, the TBM surface was rough and appeared as a piece of felt. The basement membrane showed a characteristic linear contour and angular shape and could be easily distinguished from contaminants. Higher magnification of the basement membrane fragment (Fig. 3) revealed a fine meshwork. TBM was composed of numerous small pores and strands. The pores were round, oval or polygonal in shape. Some pores were elongated to form a channel. The strands were almost equal in diameter and formed a three-dimensional lattice work. The count of 50 pores and strands indicated that the long and short dimensions were 3.8 ± 1.2 and 2.5 ± 0.7 nm in bovine TBM, and 4.9 ± 1.5 and 2.8 ± 0.6 nm in rat TBM. The diameter of the strands was 2.5 ± 0.6 nm in bovine TBM and 3.7 ± 0.7 nm in rat TBM. The density of the pores was $22 \pm 2/1{,}000$ nm^2 in bovine

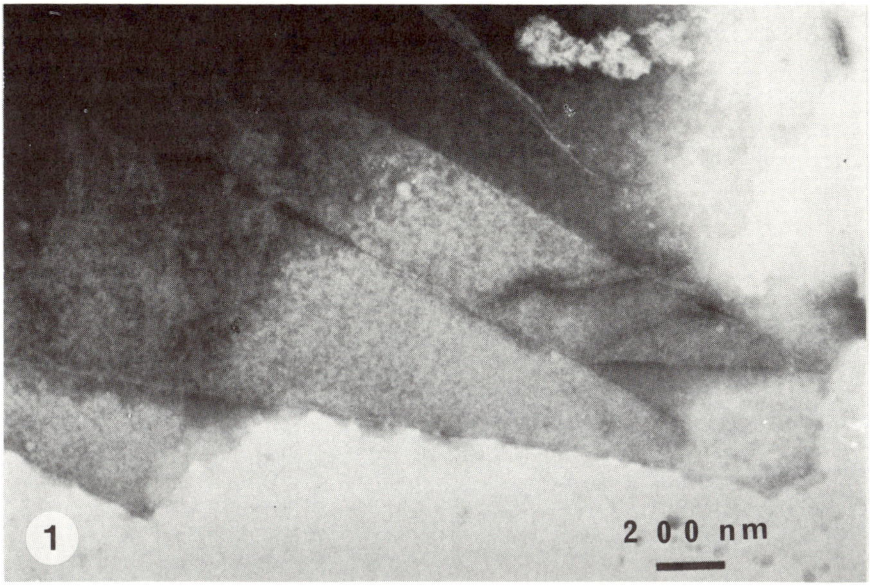

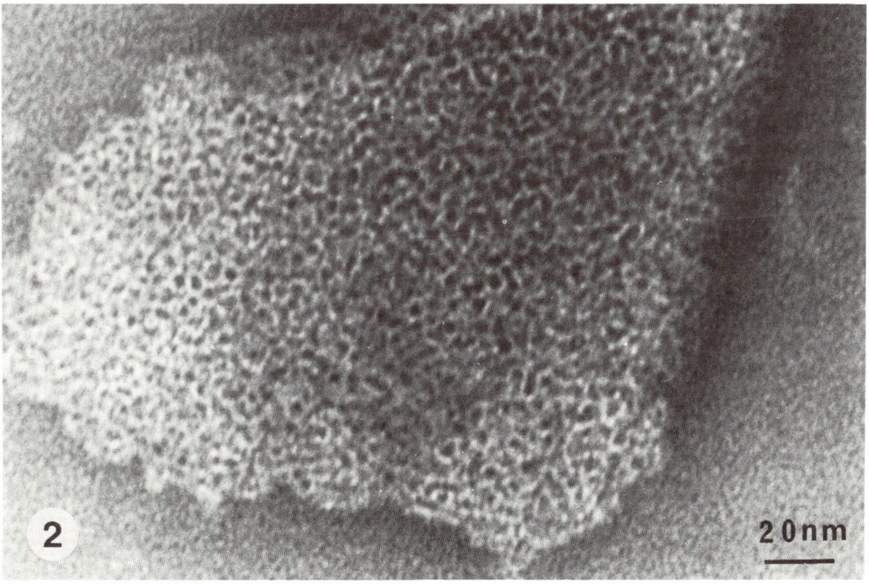

FIG. 1. Negative staining of unfixed bovine GBM, isolated by sonication, with 1% PTA at low magnification. Note the characteristic felt-like surface, linear contour and angular ends. x 45,000.

FIG. 2. An unfixed fragment of bovine GBM. Pores are round, oval, or polygonal in shape. Negative staining with 1% PTA. x 450,000.

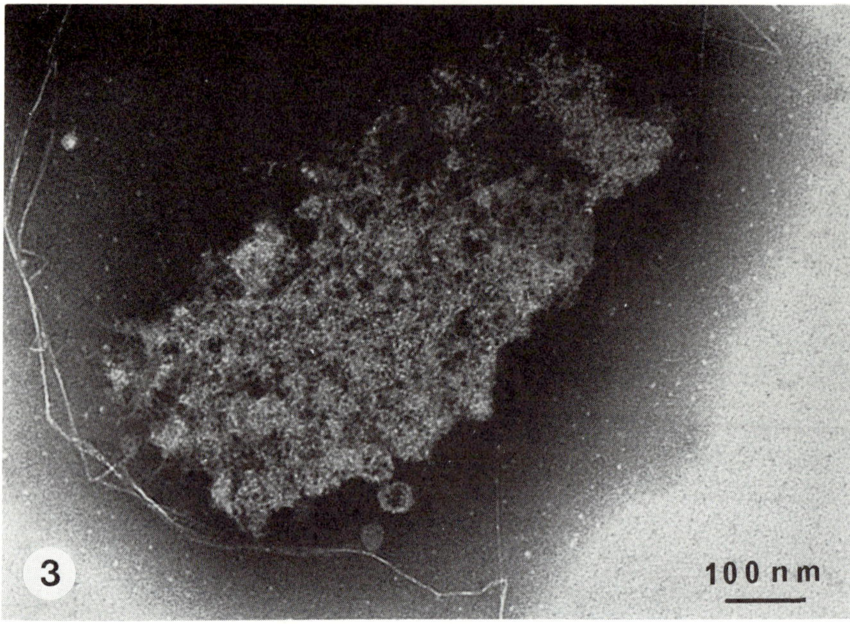

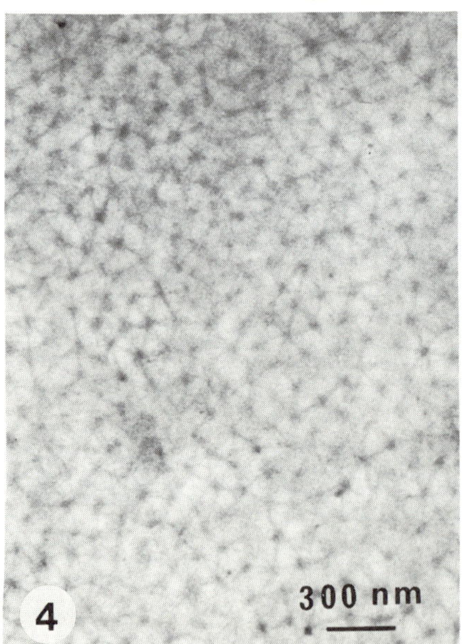

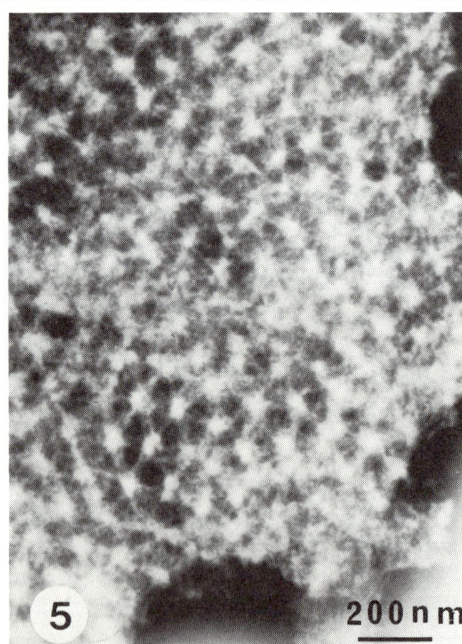

FIG. 3. An unfixed fragment of rat TBM shows a fine meshwork. A few fine strands appear coming out from the margin of the fragment. Negative staining with 1% PTA. x 110,000.

FIG. 4. Ultrathin section of fixed bovine Descemet's membrane. x 32,000.

FIG. 5. Negative staining of unfixed bovine Descemet's membrane with 1% PTA. x 43,000.

TBM and 15 ± 3/1,000 nm^2 in rat TBM.

2) *TBM prepared by the method of Carlson et al. (1978)*: The results were almost the same as those by sonic disruption (Ota et al., 1980), however, in some fragments the TBM appeared rough, and the fragments were loosened and even destroyed. At higher magnification, the meshwork showed the same morphologic features and the pore size was the same.

Comparison of Bovine Descemet's Membrane in Ultrathin Sections and Negatively Stained Preparations in Ultrastructure

Fig. 4 shows in a conventional ultrathin section that the bovine Descemet's membrane has a unique microstructure. For negative staining, the Descemet's membrane was stripped from the cornea; a part of the membrane was fixed and embedded for conventional ultrathin sectioning for observations by transmission electron microscopy, and the remainder was sonicated in 1 M NaCl and washed in distilled water. The pellet from the centrifugation was examined by electron microscopy using negative staining with 1% phosphotungstic acid, pH 7.3. The surface of the small fragment had a very regular hexagonal pattern composed of nodes and thin internodal filaments. The filaments connected each node with the six others around it to form a hexagon (Fig. 5). The mean distance between the nodes was approximately 110 nm; the diameter of the nodes was approximately 30 nm; and the width of the connecting filaments was approximately 10 nm.

Our observations of negatively staining material were very similar in ultrastructure to material prepared by ultrathin sectioning (Makino et al., 1982). Therefore, our technique of negative staining appeared valid.

Permeability and Ultrastructure of GBM of Rats with Chronic Serum Sickness

Chronic serum sickness (CSS) rats: Experimental animals were treated according to the method of Arisz et al. (1979): 3 mg of BSA (Sigma Laboratory) with complete Freund's adjuvant (CFA, Difco Lab.) was injected subcutaneously every 2 weeks (SC phase) for 6 weeks. In the 7th week, 1 mg of BSA was administered intraperitoneally 3 times a week (IP phase). From the 8th week, 2 mg of BSA were injected intravenously 6 times a week for 6 weeks (IV phase).

Fig. 6 shows that CSS rats had proteinuria at the late phase (phase IV) but not in the early phase (phase SC and IP). The proteinuria increased progressively from the 11th week to 13th week, namely from 129 ± 203 mg/day to 472 ± 222 mg/day (Fig. 6). All rats had proteinuria. In CSS rats at the 12th week total serum protein level was significantly decreased to 5.4 ± 1.2 g/dl (n = 13).

Permeability of ferritin particles in GBM: Three rats with nephrotic syndromes and their controls were given an intravenous injection of anionic ferritin (Sigma Lab. pI 4.3 – 4.4) at 0.5 mg/g body weight through the tail vein. There-

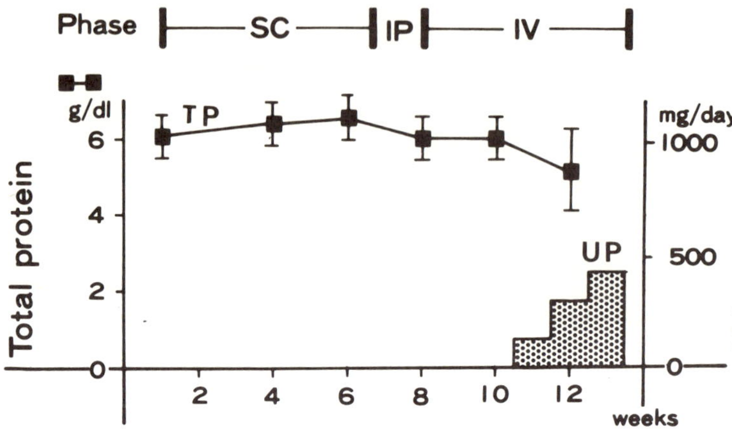

FIG. 6. Total protein and urinary protein in rats with CSS.

after, the renal cortices were biopsied, and the specimens processed for electron microscopy. In controls 20 min after ferritin injection most ferritin molecules were limited to the *lamina rara interna* of the GBM (Fig. 7). However, in CSS rats at 15 min after ferritin injection, the ferritin had already permeated the full width of the GBM with subepithelial deposits and general thickening (Fig. 8). Even hours later, ferritin showed the same distribution. These observations indicated that permeability was increased in GBM of CSS rats.

Ultrastructure of GBM in normal and CSS rats: Rat GBM was isolated from 20 normal rats and 20 CSS rats according to the method of Spiro (1967). The purity of GBM of CSS rats was demonstrated by ultrathin sectioning technique (Fig. 9). Figs. 10 and 11 are micrographs of negative staining with 1% PTA. It was more difficult to get a clearer result on rat GBM than bovine GBM. Either rat or bovine GBM showed the characteristic meshwork, i.e. a molecular sieve with strands and many pores. The pore diameter size of CSS rats was larger and more variable than in normal rats. In control rats (Fig. 10), the mean long dimension of the pore was 4 nm and the short dimension, 3 nm. In CSS rats (Fig. 11), the long mean dimension was 9 nm and short dimension, 6 nm. The long and short dimensions of pores from CSS rats differed significantly from those of control rats. The albumin molecule appeared to be about 14.0 x 4.0 nm in size, so that it could not pass through the GBM of normal rats. However, an enlarged molecular sieve in CSS would allow albumin molecules to pass very easily through GBM. Thus, enlargement of the pores of GBM is probably responsible for the proteinuria in CSS rats (Fig. 12).

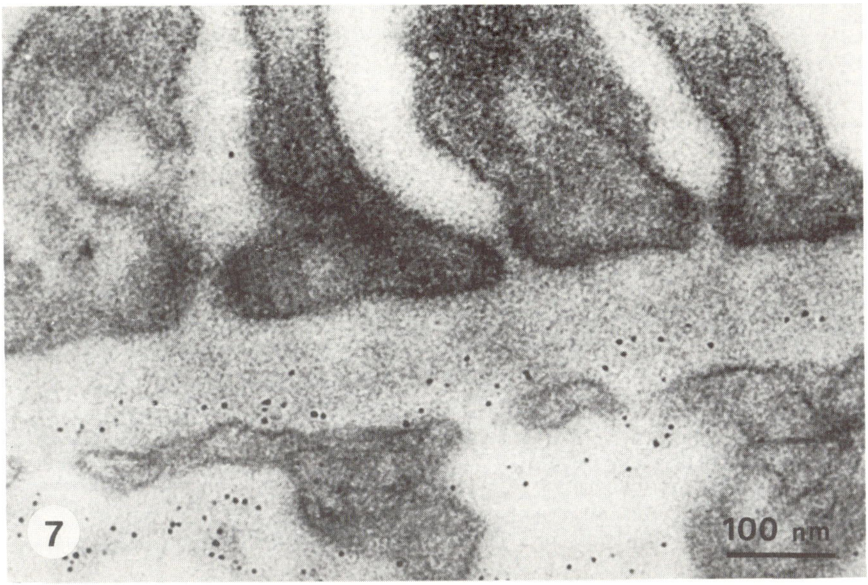

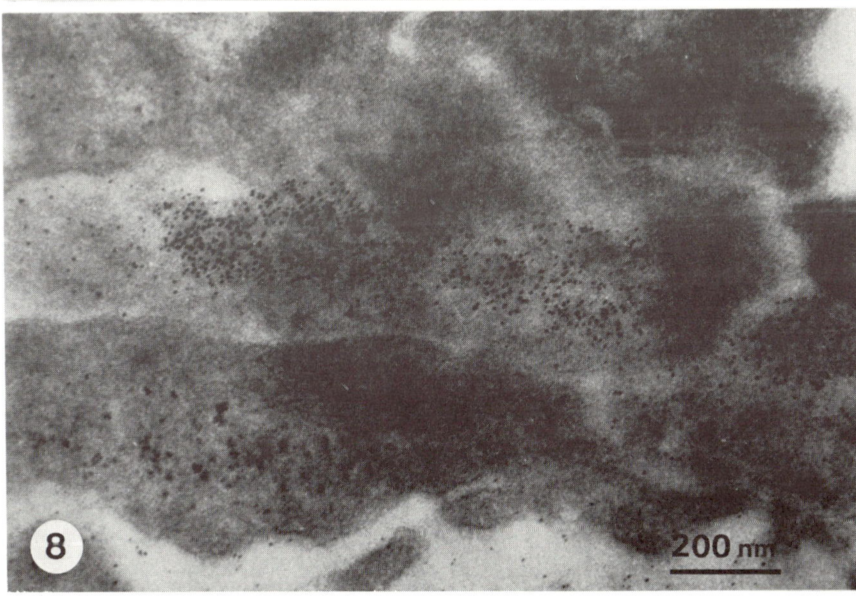

FIG. 7. In controls 20 min after ferritin injection most ferritin molecules were limited to the *lamina rara interna* of the rat GBM. x 136,000.

FIG. 8. In CSS rats at 15 min after ferritin injection, the ferritin had already permeated the full width of the GBM with subepithelial deposits and general thickening. x 82,000.

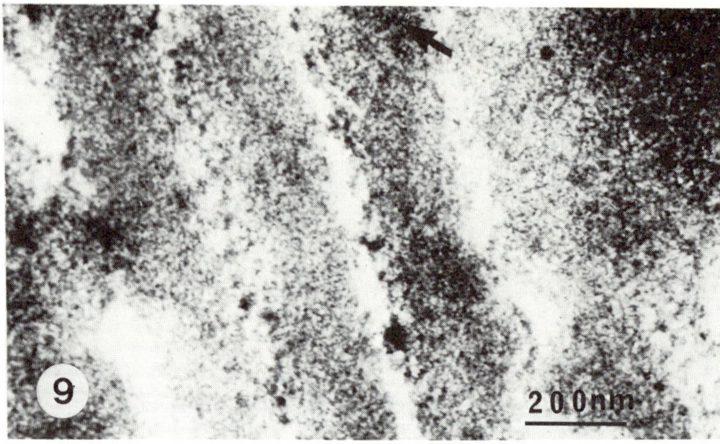
9
200nm

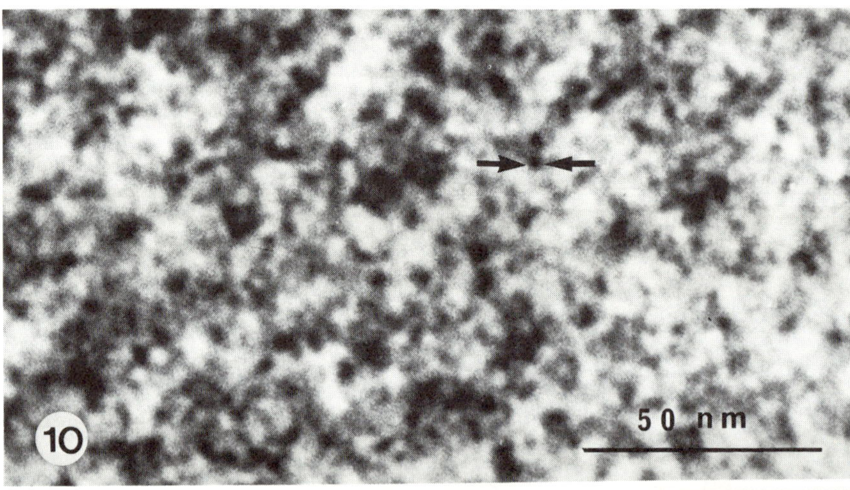
10
50 nm

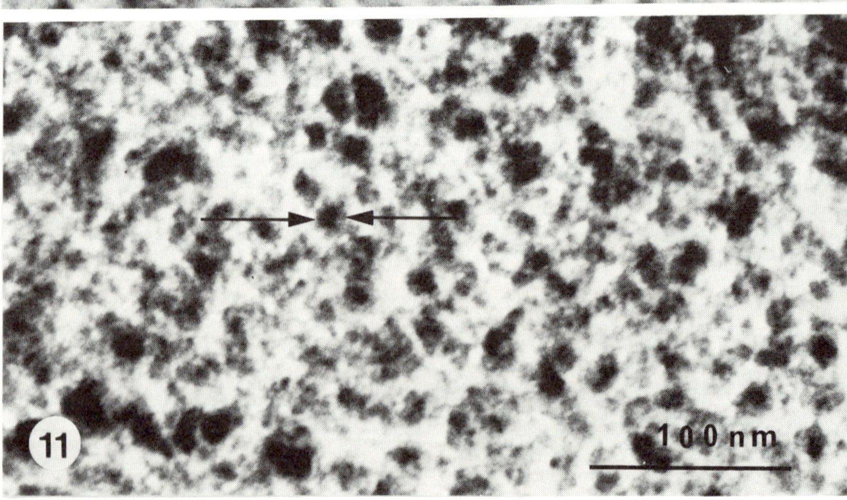
11
100nm

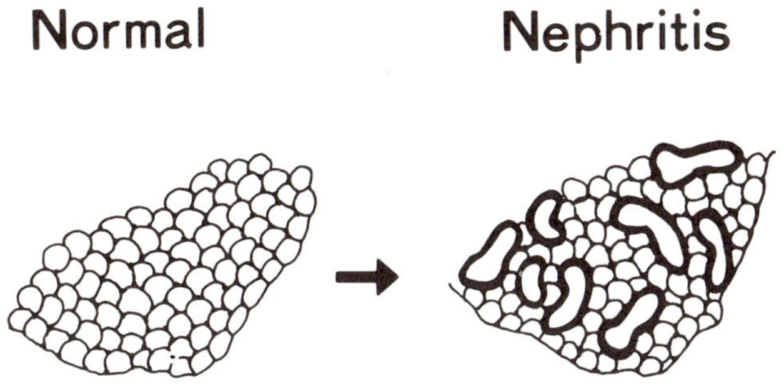

FIG. 12. Schematic representation of mechanism of proteinuria in nephrotic syndrome.

ABSTRACT

This electron microscopic study with negative staining showed that bovine and rat GBM and TBM were composed of fine strand meshes with numerous pores and molecular sieves. GBM has a role in filtration since its pore size is smaller than that of albumin. Both the observations that the structure of GBM is like a meshwork and the hypothesis that GBM acts as molecular sieve are new to the literature. Timpl et al. (1981) reported recently on a model of a continuous network of type IV collagen solubilized from a tumor basement membrane.

The main mechanism for nephrotic syndrome might be due to an enlarged GBM pore.

The "molecular sieve theory of basement membrane" in which all kinds of basement membranes consist of molecular sieves was also appraised.

REFERENCES

Arisz, L., Noble, B., Milgrom, M., Brentjens, J.R., and Andres, G.A. (1979). Experimental chronic serum sickness in rats. A model of immune complex glomerulonephritis and systemic immune complex deposition.

FIG. 9. Ultrathin section of glomerular basement membrane of a rat with CSS isolated by sonication. Note normal structure and complete absence of cell fragments. An arrow shows possible deposit on the membrane. x 71,000.

FIG. 10. Negative staining of unfixed normal rat GBM isolated by sonication with 1% PTA at higher magnification. Note meshwork structure with numerous pores (between arrows) and strands. x 646,000.

FIG. 11. Negative staining of unfixed CSS rat GBM isolated by sonication with 1% PTA at higher magnification. Note remarkable enlargement of pores (between arrow). x 264,000.

Int. Arch. Allergy Appl. Immunol. **60**, 80–88.

Brenner, B.M., Hostetter, T.H., and Humes, H.D. (1978). Molecular basis of proteinuria of glomerular origin. *N. Engl. J. Med.* **298**, 826–833.

Carlson, E.C., Brendel, K., Hjelle, J.T., and Meezan, E. (1978). Ultrastructure and biochemical analysis of isolated basement membranes from kidney glomeruli and tubules and brain and renal microvessels. *J. Ultrastruct. Res.* **62**, 26–53.

Farquhar, M.G., Wissing, S.L., and Palade, G.E. (1961). I. Ferritin transfer across the normal glomerular capillary wall. *J. Exp. Med.* **113**, 47–66.

Krisco, I., Debernardo, E., and Sato, C.S. (1977). Isolation and characterization of rat tubular basement membrane. *Kidney Int.* **12**, 238–243.

Kurtz, S.M., and McManus, J.F.A. (1960). The fine structure of the human glomerular basement membrane. *J. Ultrastruct. Res.* **4**, 81–87.

Makino, H., Ota, Z., Takaya, Y., Miyoshi, A., and Ofuji, T. (1980). Morphological changes of the molecular sieve in bovine glomerular basement membrane by protease and lysosomal enzyme digestion. *J. Electron Microsc.* **29**, 242–249.

Makino, H., Ota, Z., Takaya, Y., Miyoshi, A., and Ofuji, T. (1981). Molecular sieve in rat tubular basement membrane as revealed by negative staining. *Renal Physiol.* **4**, 180–190.

Makino, H., Toyofuku, H., Mino, Y., Takaoka, M., and Ota, Z. (1982). Molecular sieve in bovine Descemet's membrane as revealed by negative staining. *Acta Med. Okayama* **37**, 155–157.

Ota, Z., Makino, H., Miyoshi, A., Hiramatsu, M., Takahashi, K., and Ofuji, T. (1977). Electron microscopic demonstration of meshwork structure in human and bovine glomerular basement membranes. *Acta Med. Okayama* **31**, 339–342.

Ota, Z., Makino, H., Miyoshi, A., Hiramatsu, M., Takahashi, K., and Ofuji, T. (1979). Molecular sieve in glomerular basement membrane as revealed by electron microscopy. *J. Electron Microsc.* **28**, 20–28.

Ota, Z., Makino, H., Takaya, Y., and Ofuji, T. (1980). Molecular sieve in renal glomerular and tubular basement membranes as revealed by electron microscopy. *Renal Physiol.* **3**, 317–323.

Peter, Jr., T. (1975). Serum albumin. *In* "The Plasma Protein" (E.W. Putnam, ed.), Vol. 1, pp. 133–181. Academic Press, New York.

Rennke, H.G., and Venkatachalam, M.A. (1977). Structural determinations of glomerular permselectivity. *Fed. Proc., Fed. Am. Soc. Exp. Biol.* **36**, 2619–2626.

Ryan, G.B., and Karnovsky, M.J. (1976). Distribution of endogenous albumin in the rat glomerulus: role of hemodynamic factors in glomerular barrier function. *Kidney Int.* **9**, 36–45.

Spiro, R.C. (1967). Studies on the renal glomerular basement membrane: preparation and chemical composition. *J. Biol. Chem.* **242**, 1915–1922.

Timpl, R., Wiedemann, H., Van Delden, V., Furthmayer, H., and Kühn, K. (1981). A network model for the organization of type IV collagen molecules in basement membrane. *Eur. J. Biochem.* **120**, 203–211.

B. Immune Deposit Formation

The mechanisms of immune deposits in the glomeruli, particularly in the subepithelial deposits, may provide a key to open the general understanding of pathogenesis of glomerulonephritis.

The new theory of *in situ* formation has recently been subjected by several investigators with their searches by DNA-affinity to GBM, cationic antigens, the effect of lysozyme on the binding to DNA, and complement activation by cationic CIC.

Combination activities by *in situ* IC formation and complement play a significant role in the development of glomerular lesions. IC are formed in antigen excess and inducing *in situ* IC glomerulonephritis antigens should be $>$50,000 and $<$1,000,000 (MW) in size.

The third component of complement, particularly one of their breakdown products, C3d has also been found as a remaining factor to bind immune complexes producing the chronicity of the glomerulonephritis.

Discussed in this section are the mechanisms of *in situ* immune complex formations induced by cationized antigens that can bind to anionic sites of the GBM with complement activation.

Yoshihiro Hamashima

INHIBITORY EFFECT OF LYSOZYME ON THE GLOMERULAR IMMUNE COMPLEX DEPOSITION IN LUPUS MICE

Mitsumasa Nagase, Tatsuo Yamamoto and Nishio Honda

First Department of Medicine, Hamamatsu University School of Medicine
Hamamatsu

Regulating the transport of macromolecules, the glomerular basement membrane (GBM) acts as size as well as charge selective barrier, which displays a number of polyanionic surface to the circulation. Recent studies indicate that the charge of immunoreactants plays a striking role as a determinant of the glomerular deposition of immune complex (IC). The property of GBM, including electrostatical characteristics, can also be a determinant of IC deposition. Based on these facts, it has been shown lately that circulating exogenous polycations, binding to the anionic sites of GBM, alter the glomerular permeability, thus the enhancement of IC deposition in GBM can ensure (Barnes et al., 1984).

Indeed, evidence has been accumulated that alterations of anionic charge of either the GBM or immunoreactants affects the distribution as well as the amount of IC deposits in glomeruli. However, Izui et al. (1976) have in contrast raised an importance of cationic moiety of GBM collagen and negatively charged DNA in the pathogenesis of lupus nephritis.

In support of this concept, an evidence has been demonstrated quite recently that anionic protein such as anionic IgG or albumin is capable to bind to the cationic site of GBM. Therefore, we have considered it worthwhile to explore whether or not administration of cationic protein, lysozyme, may affect the deposition of IC in glomeruli of lupus mice.

MATERIALS AND METHODS

Animals: NZB/W F_1 female mice at the age of 7 lunar months were selected from our own colony. Female ICR mice were obtained from a commercial supplier (Shizuoka Jikken Doubutsu Co., Shizuoka, Japan). All animals used in this study were kept under standard laboratory conditions.

Experimental design: Under ether anesthesia, unilateral nephrectomy was performed in all animals to enhance the intraglomerular immune complex deposition (Beyer et al., 1977). The removed kidneys were fixed or frozen for the morphological examination. Then the animals were divided into 4 groups A, B, C and D: Group A, 9 NZB/W F_1 mice and group C, 10 ICR mice received intraperitoneal injection of 0.5 ml of 0.5% lysozyme saline solution per animal twice a day for 9 days. Group B, 11 NZB/W F_1 mice and group D, 10 ICR mice were treated as in groups A and C but with 0.9%

saline solution in place of lysozyme solution. On the 9th day, all animals in groups A, B, C and D were sacrificed. After sacrifice the morphological examination was performed on the remaining kidneys. In groups A and B, the sera were obtained at each sacrifice to measure the anti-DNA antibody titer using the method by Wold et al. (1968). Lysozyme was provided by Eisai Co., Tokyo, Japan.

Serum lysozyme concentration: Unilateral nephrectomy was performed in 18 ICR mice. Fifteen of them received single intraperitoneal injection of 0.5 ml of 2.5% lysozyme saline solution. The animals were sacrifiecd 1, 3, 6, 9 and 12 hr after the injection, 3 animals at one time. The remaining 3 animals were sacrificed without receiving lysozyme injection and served as controls. After sacrifice, serum lysozyme concentration was determined by spectrophotometry according to the method of Litwack (1955).

Morphological examinations: For light microscopy, the tissue pieces from each kidney were fixed in buffered 20% formalin solution, embedded in paraffin, sectioned and stained with hematoxylin-eozin and periodic-acid Schiff. Thirty glomeruli in the section from each animal were randomly chosen and the glomerular lesion were checked, classifying into 0, +1, +2 and +3 according to the severity in order; 0, almost normal; +1, proliferative changes restricted to the mesangial area; +2, proliferative changes extended moderately to the peripheral capillary walls; +3, proliferative changes extensively extended to the capillary walls. The mean value out of 30 glomeruli was recorded to represent the glomerular lesion of each animal and were used for the statistical analysis.

For immunofluorescence microscopy, the renal tissues were snap frozen in hexan, cooled by dry ice-aceton and stored at —70 ℃ until use. The section of 3 μm were made in a cryostat (Bright Instrument Co., Huntingdon, England). Then the antisera (Cappel Lab., Pennsylvania, U.S.A.) to mouse IgG and C_3 were applied, respectively. The sections were observed under an Olympus Immunofluorescence microscope (Olympus Co., Tokyo, Japan). The intraglomerular deposits were classified into 4 groups, 0, +1, +2 and +3 according to the intensity of fluorescence in order on the mesangial area and capillary wall, respectively.

For electron microscopy, the renal tissues were immersion-fixed in glutaraldehyde and postfixed in OsO_4, dehydrated through a graded series of ethanol and embedded in Quetol 812. The ultrathin sections were stained with uranyl acetate and lead citrate and observed by a JEM 100 C electron microscope (Nihondenshi Co., Tokyo, Japan).

Binding of ^{125}I-DNA to glomerular basement membrane in vitro: ^{125}I-labelled double standed DNA from HeLa cell (^{125}I-DNA) was purchased from Amersham International Plc., Buckinghamshire, England. Glomeruli were isolated from kidneys of Sprague Dowly rats by sequential sieving through graded size mesh screens. GBM was obtained from these isolated glomeruli by ultrasonic disruption. The sonicated materials were washed 4 times with 0.15 M saline solution at 1,500 *g* and the sediments were suspended in 0.15 M phosphate buffered saline solution (PBS), pH 7.4, and stored at

−70 ℃ until use. The protein concentration of GBM suspension was measured with the method described by Lowry et al. (1951). Then the binding of ^{125}I-DNA to isolated GBM was evaluated *in vitro* in the following manner.

1) *DNA binding to GBM*: 250 μg of GBM was suspended in 1 ml of 0.15 M PBS containing 10% heat inactivated (56 ℃, for 30 min) normal rat serum (NRS) and 150 μg of ^{125}I-DNA was added. Then, the suspension was incubated in a tube at 37 ℃ with constant shaking. The PBS containing ^{125}I-DNA and 10% NRS, but not GBM, was also prepared as control. The radioactivity of 175 μg of ^{125}I-DNA was counted preliminary using an automatic gamma counter (Aloka Co., Tokyo, Japan). Then, 1, 3, 6 and 12 hr after initiation of incubation, the reaction mixtures were centrifuged at 1,500 Xg for 10 min, followed by washing 3 times in PBS. The radioactivity of each tube was then counted. The specific amount of ^{125}I-DNA bound to GBM was obtained by subtracting the counts per min (cpm) of the control tubes from the cpm of the experimental tubes. The experiments were performed in duplicate and mean values were used for the calculation. The results were expressed as the percentage of GBM-bound radiolabelled preparations to the added DNA.

2) *Effect of lysozyme on the binding of DNA to GBM*: As the binding of DNA to GBM did not significantly alter during 1 to 12 hr of incubation, the incubation time was fixed to 1 hr in all experiments. Adding increasing amount of lysozyme in the medium (0, 50, 150, 300, 600, 900, 1,500 μg/ml), the incubations were done in the same processes as described above. The binding rate of ^{125}I-DNA to GBM in each tube was also calculated as just described.

RESULT

Light microscopy: The kidneys obtained by unilateral nephrectomy of lupus mice in groups A and B displayed the similar histological pictures, i.e. the lesions of glomeruli with moderate mesangial cell proliferation. By the unilateral nephrectomy, the glomerular lesions were aggravated in the contralateral kidneys. However, the aggravation of glomerular lesions were much less in those received lysozyme injections (group A) compared to the saline injected controls (group B) (Fig. 1). In contrast, the contralateral kidneys of ICR mice did not show any detectable glomerular lesions after unilateral nephrectomy and lysozyme-treatment (groups C and D) (Fig. 1).

Immunofluorescence microscopy: In the glomeruli of nephrectomized kidneys of NZB/W F_1 mice, moderate IgG deposits were found mostly in the mesangial area. After the unilateral nephrectomy, the deposition of IgG in the contralateral kidneys increased predominantly in the glomerular capillary walls. However, the IgG deposition was much less in the mice treated with lysozyme (group A) as compared to the saline treated controls (group B) (Figs. 2, 3). On the other hand, no glomerular deposition was observed in ICR mice kidneys remained after the unilateral nephrectomy as well as in those nephrectomized. It was indicated that lysozyme and saline injections did not induce any significant changes in the kidneys of these animals (groups C and D) (Fig. 3).

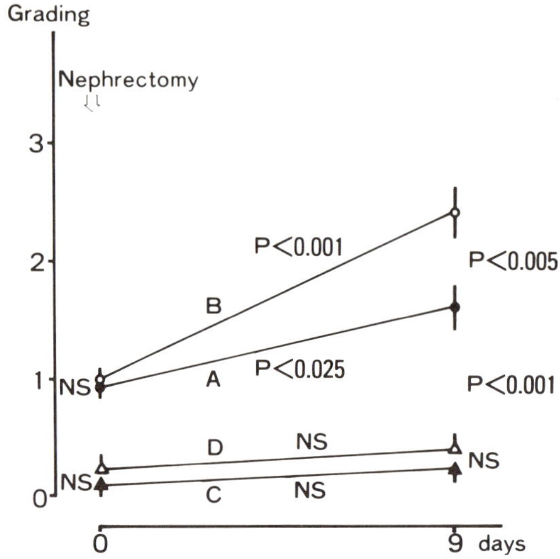

FIG. 1. Semiquantitative expression of the effect of unilateral nephrectomy with (A, C) and without (B, D) lysozyme injections on the histological changes of glomeruli in lupus mice (A, B) and ICR mice (C, D). Method: see text.

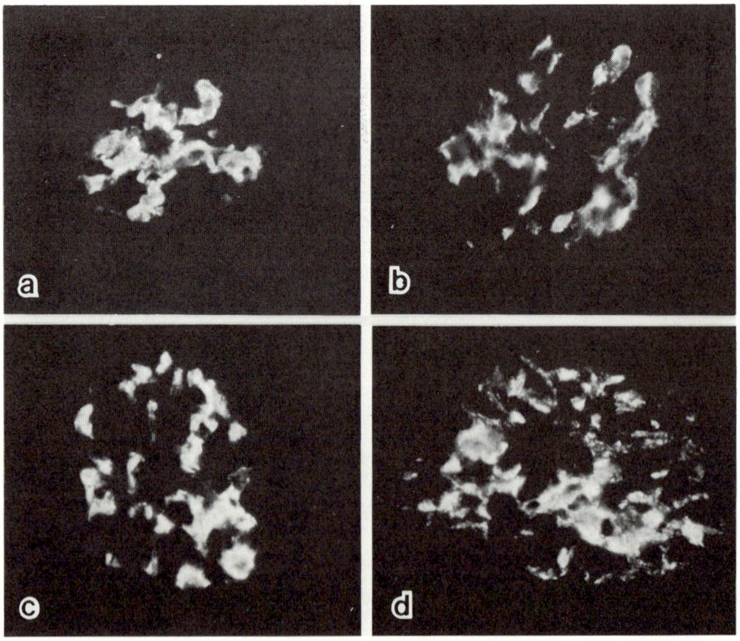

FIG. 2. Immunofluorescence pictures of glomeruli of NZB/W F_1 mice and show the localization of mouse IgG. (a) – (b) Glomeruli from the nephrectomized kidneys before

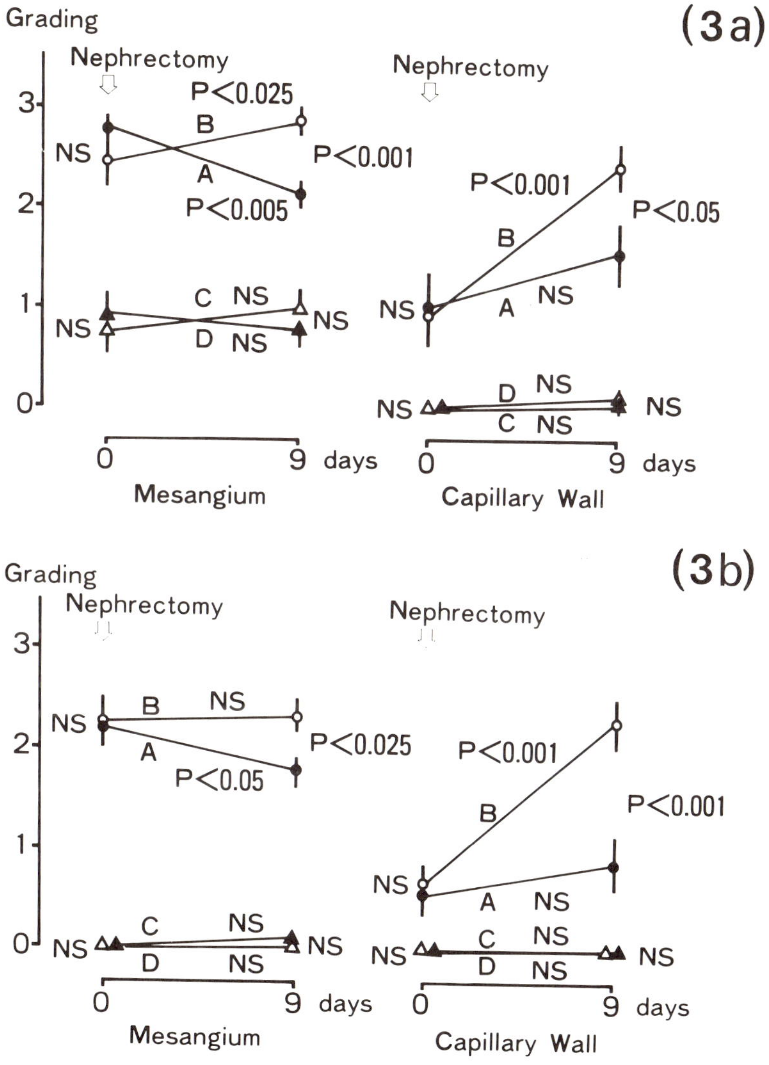

FIG. 3. Semiquantitative expression of glomerular deposition of mouse IgG (3a) and mouse C_3 (3b) in NZB/W F_1 mice. Method: see text.

---

treatment ((a) from group A and (b) from group B). (c) A glomerulus in the contralateral kidney removed after the repeated injections of lysozyme for 9 days after unilateral nephrectomy. (d) A glomerulus from the animals received the same treatment as in (c) but injected with saline in place of lysozyme solution. Method: see text.

Electron microscopy: The kidneys of lupus mice nephrectomized before treatment showed the electron dense deposits localized mostly in the mesangial areas of glomeruli, while the contralateral kidneys obtained 9 days after unilateral nephrectomy had the deposits located along the epithelial and endothelial side of GBM as well as in mesangial area. However, the subendothelial deposits were much less in both number and size in the animals treated with lysozyme than those received no lysozyme treatment (Fig. 4).

Anti-DNA antibody titer of lupus mice: Anti-DNA antibody titer of lupus mice treated with lysozyme was 34.5 ± 5.38 and those treated with saline was 29.8 ± 2.42 (mean ± SE). There was no significant difference between them.

Serum lysozyme concentration: The lysozyme concentration in the serum of the non-treated mice was 27.7 ± 5.9 μg/ml. Whereas, the values obtained 1, 3, 6, 9 and 12 hr after the intraperitoneal injection of 0.5 ml of 2.5% lysozyme saline solution were 808.8 ± 196.5, 214.0 ± 59.3, 62.4 ± 3.4, 34.4 ± 4.6

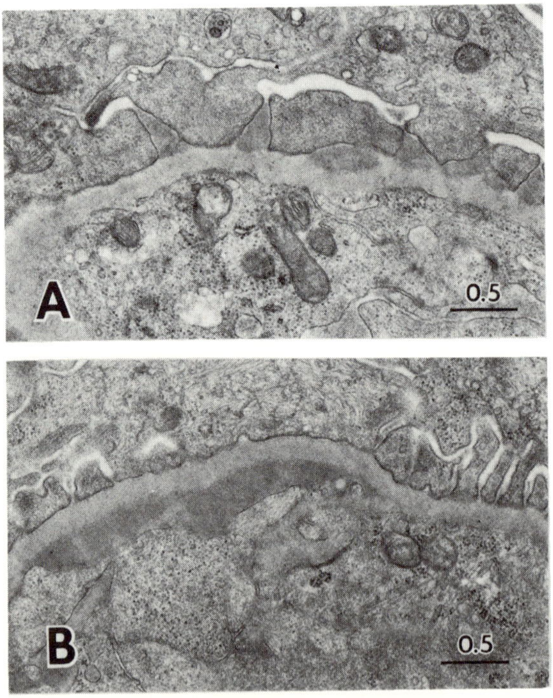

FIG. 4. Electron micrographs of glomerular walls of NZB/W F_1 mice in the kidneys remaining for 9 days after unilateral nephrectomy. (a) From the animals received lysozyme injections for 9 days after unilateral nephrectomy (group A). (b) From the animals received the same treatment as in (a) but with saline injections in place of lysozyme solution (group B). Note that the subendothelial deposits are much less in both number and size in mice treated with lysozyme as compared to those with saline. Method: see text.

and 20.7 ± 3.3 μg/ml, respectively (mean ± SE), indicating that the lysozyme concentration attains a peak 1 hr after the injections and returns to the basal level 9 to 12 hr thereafter.

Binding of ^{125}I-DNA to GBM in vitro: The binding was almost completed by 1 hr after the initiation of incubation. Approximately 40% of the added ^{125}I-DNA was bound to GBM within the first 1 hr, and the binding rate did not increase significantly thereafter until 12 hr (Fig. 5). The binding was markedly inhibited by the lysozyme in the media. The inhibitory effect increased in proportion to the increase in lysozyme concentration showing a striking dose dependency (Fig. 6).

Discussion

Recently, the evidences have been accumulated to show that the electrostatic interaction between the anionic sites of GBM and the cationic immunogens could become the first step leading the immune complex deposition in GBM. Vogt and his groups (Vogt, A. et al., 1982, Oite et al., 1982) have shown that cationized proteins were able to bind to GBM and acted as planted antigens and induced *in situ* immune complex formation in rats. Gallo et al. (1981) showed that preformed cationic immune complexes could bind to the anionic sites of GBM in a murine model of acute passive serum sickness and also they (1983) showed that cationic immunogens were more nephritogenic and had greater tendency to the formation of subepithelial deposits in a murine model of chronic active serum sickness. Madio et al. (1984) showed that the deposition of cationic anti-GBM antibody in GBM was greater than that of anionic anti-GBM antibody.

The property of the glomerulus itself, including the electrophysical characteristics of GBM, is also an important determinant for the immune complex deposition. Couser et al. (1978) injected aminonucleoside of puromycin to the early phase of autologous immune complex nephropathy rats and they observed few or no GBM deposits despite a significant increase in mesangial localization of IgG and Fx1A during the period of puromycin-induced proteinuria. The absence of GBM deposits correlated with reduced staining for polyanionic glomerular sialoprotein in proteinuric kidneys. Couser et al. (1979) also showed a similar effect of aminonucleoside of puromycin and nephrotoxic serum in passive Heymann nephritis.

The circulating exogenous polycations such as hexadimethrine (Hunsiker et al., 1981), protamine sulfate and poly-L-lysine (Vehaskari et al., 1982), polyethyleneimine (Barnes et al., 1984) are known to be able to bind to the anionic sites of GBM and cause an increase of the glomerular permeability. On the other hand, importance of cationic charge has been postulated as well. Melvin et al. (1984) demonstrated the presence of anionic IgG_4 in GBM of normal and diabetic human kidneys and suggested that circulating anionic proteins were electrostatically bound *in vivo* to the positively charged moieties in GBM. Also the anionic DNA has been indicated to bind to the cationic moiety of GBM (Izui et al., 1976).

These findings indicate clearly that the electrostatic binding of immu-

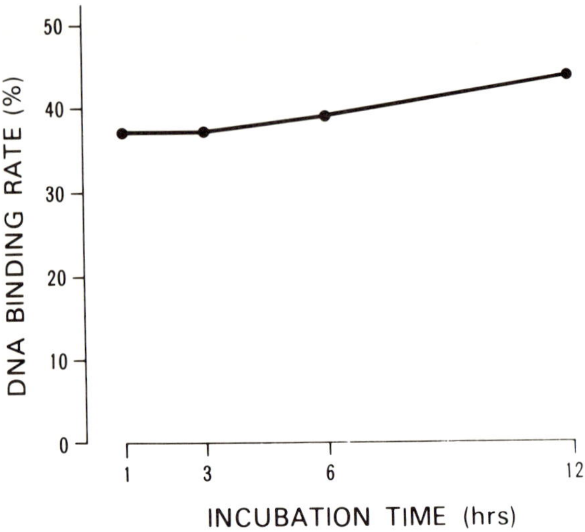

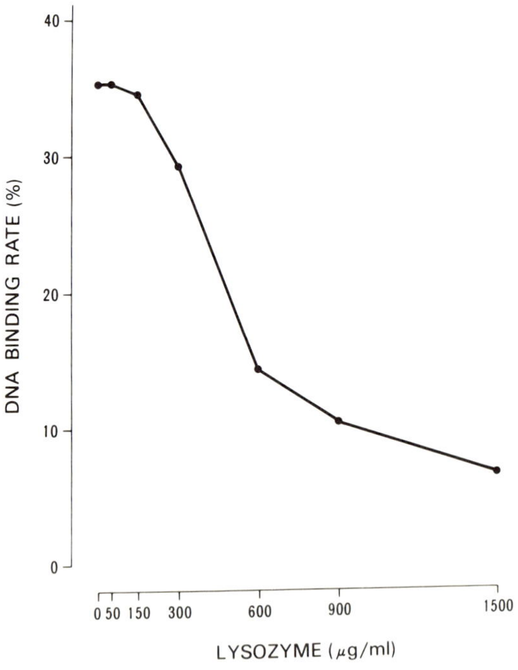

FIG. 5. *In vitro* binding test of DNA to GBM. DNA binding to GBM reached nearly 40% by 1 hr. After that the binding rates increased gradually reaching about 43% at 12 hr of incubation. Method: see text.

FIG. 6. Inhibitory effect of lysozyme on the binding of DNA to GBM. Note the marked suppression of DNA binding to GBM with the increase in lysozyme concentration. Method: see text.

nogens to the structure components of glomerular capillary wall is closely related to the glomerular immune complex deposition. We, therefore, attempted to examine the effect of the administration of lysozyme, a polycation, on the glomerular deposition of immune complex in murine lupus mice, in which DNA plays a pathogenic role as an anionic antigen.

After the unilateral nephrectomy, the glomerular lesions in the contralateral kidneys were aggravated with an increase in the immune complex deposition in NZB/W F_1 mice, but much less in those treated with repeated intraperitoneal injection of lysozyme. In contrast, ICR mice did not show any detectable glomerular lesions regardless of the unilateral nephrectomy and lysozyme treatment. This implies that the lysozyme administration does not evoke any distinguished immunologically mediated glomerular lesions.

As to the pathogenesis of murine lupus nephritis, a role of DNA-anti DNA antibody deposition has been suggested as a possible factor (Ebling et al., 1980). Izui et al. (1976) have demonstrated that the DNA bound to GBM might give rise to *in situ* immune complex formation. They also raised a possibility that the DNA binding to GBM might be due to the electrostatic force, as the binding was inhibited at low pH, low ionic strength and in the presence of anionic detergents.

As just demonstrated in the present *in vitro* study, it was revealed that the binding of DNA to GBM was strikingly inhibited by the addition of lysozyme in the media and that this inhibitory effect increased in proportion to the increasing amount of lysozyme added. It was also shown *in vivo* experiment that the serum level of lysozyme rised as high as 800 μg/mg following the lysozyme injection to mice, which was compatible to the concentration that lysozyme did suppress the DNA binding to GBM *in vitro*.

It is taken for granted that the possible enzymic action of lysozyme cannot be ignored when considering the effect of lysozyme. However, this seems unlikely because the substrate of B-l-4 glycosidase (lysozyme) has not been detected in GBM as yet. Taking these two findings together, we are inclined to propose that lysozyme can interfere electrostatically with the DNA-GBM binding by forming DNA-lysozyme complex. Adler et al. (1983) have provided a similar charge competition in the formation of glomerular immune complex deposition.

It might also be suspected that lysozyme could inhibit the glomerular immune complex deposition *via* the suppression of anti-DNA formation. However, this possibility is also unlikely, because the titers of anti-DNA antibodies did not change by the treatment of the animals with lysozyme.

It has been suggested that the formation of DNA-anti-DNA complex in GBM triggers the subsequent immune reactions in the subendothelial region, which leads to the severe proliferative glomerular lesions (Izui et al., 1976). Our qualitative observation by electron microscopy has shown a decrease of subendothelial deposits in lupus mice treated with lysozyme as compared to the non-treated animals. In view of these findings, it is concluded that the relatively mild glomerular lesions in lysozyme treated lupus mice should be due to the inhibitory effect of lysozyme on DNA binding to GBM.

Abstract

The effect of lysozyme administration on the intraglomerular deposition was studied in the unilateral nephrectomized lupus mice, NZB/W F_1. Unilateral nephrectomy enhanced the immune complex deposition with aggravation of the glomerular lesions. The lesions were much reduced in severity by the repeated intraperitoneal injection of lysozyme. In ICR mice, however, the unilateral nephrectomy and lysozyme administration did not induce any detectable glomerular lesions.

To analyze the mechanisms of this ameliorative effect of lysozyme on the glomerular lesions in lupus mice, DNA binding to the isolated glomerular basement membrane, suspected to be the pathogenic factors of lupus nephritis, was studied *in vitro*. The results indicated that the binding was markedly suppressed by lysozyme in the media. From these observations it is concluded that lysozyme injection will contribute to the suppression of *in situ* immune complex deposition by interfering the binding of DNA with the glomerular basement membrane, even partly.

References

Adler, S.G., Wang, H., Ward, H.J., Cohen, A.H., and Border, W.A. (1983). Electrical charge. Its role in the pathogenesis and prevention of experimental membranous nephropathy in the rabbit. *J. Clin. Invest.* **71**, 487–499.

Barnes, J.L., Radnik, R.A., Gilchrist, E.P., and Venkatachalam, M.A. (1984). Size and charge selective permeability defects induced in glomerular basement membrane by a polycation. *Kidney Int.* **25**, 11–19.

Beyer, M.M., Steinberg, A.D., Nicastri, A.D., and Friedman, E.A. (1977). Unilateral nephrectomy: Effect on survival in NZB/WZW mice. *Science* **198**, 511–513.

Couser, W.G., Jermanovich, N.B., Belock, S., and Stilmant, M.M. (1978). Effect of aminonucleoside nephrosis on immune complex nephropathy in rats. *J. Clin. Invest.* **61**, 561–572.

Couser, W.G., Salant, D.J., Stilmant, M.M., Arbeit, L.A., Darby, C., and Sliogeris, V.G. (1979). The effect of aminonucleoside of puromycin and nephrotoxic serum on subepithelial immune deposit formation in passive Heymann nephritis. *J. Lab. Clin. Med.* **94**, 917–932.

Ebling, F., and Hahn, B.H. (1980). Restricted subpopulations of DNA antibodies in kidneys of mice with systemic lupus. *Arthritis Rheum.* **23**, 392–403.

Gallo, G.R., Caulin-Glaser, T., and Lamm, M.E. (1981). Charge of circulating immune complexes as a factor in glomerular basement localization in mice. *J. Clin. Invest.* **67**, 1305–1311.

Gallo, G.R., Caulin-Glaser, T., Emancipator, S.N., and Lamm, M.E. (1983). Nephritogenicity and differencial distribution of glomerular immune complexes related to immunogen charge. *Lab. Invest.* **48**, 353–362.

Hunsicker L.G., Shearer, T.P., and Shaffer, S.J. (1981). Acute reversible proteinuria induced by infusion of the polycation hexadimethrine. *Kidney*

Int. **20**, 7–17.

Izui, S., Lambert, P.H., and Miesher, P.A. (1976). *In vitro* demonstration of a particular affinity of glomerular basement membrane and collagen for DNA: a possible basis for a local formation of DNA-anti-DNA complexes in systemic lupus erythematosus. *J. Exp. Med.* **144**, 428–443.

Litwack, G. (1955). Photometric determination of lysozyme activity. *Proc. Soc. Exp. Biol. Med.* **89**, 401–406.

Lowry O.H., Rosebrough, N.J., Farr, A.L., and Randall, R.J. (1951). Protein measurement with the Folin phenol reagent. *J. Biol. Chem.* **193**, 265–275.

Madio, M.P., Salant, D.J., Alder, S., Darby, C., and Couser, W.G. (1984). Effect of antibody charge and concentration on deposition of antibody to glomerular basement membrane. *Kidney Int.* **26**, 397–403.

Melvin, T., Kim, Y., and Michael, A.F. (1984). Selective binding of IgG_4 and other negatively charged plasma proteins in normal and diabetic human kidneys. *Am. J. Pathol.* **115**, 443–446.

Oite, T., Batsford, S.R., Mehatsch, M.J., Takamiya, H., and Vogt, A. (1982). Quantitative studies of *in situ* immune complex glomerulonephritis in the rat induced by planted, cationized antigen. *J. Exp. Med.* **155**, 460–474.

Vehaskari, V.M., Root, E.R., Germuth, F.G., and Robson, A.M. (1982). Glomerular charge and urinary protein excretion: Effects of systemic and intrarenal polycation infusion in the rat. *Kidney Int.* **22**, 127–135.

Vogt, A., Rohrback, R., Shimizu, F., Takamiya, H., and Batsford, S. (1982). Interaction of cationized antigen with rat glomerular basement membrane: *In situ* immune complex formation. *Kidney Int.* **22**, 27–35.

Wold, R.T., Toung, F.E., Tan, E.M., and Farr, R.S. (1968). Deoxyribonucleic acid antibody: a method to detect its primary interaction with deoxyribonucleic acid. *Science* **161**, 806–807.

SIGNIFICANCE OF COMPLEMENT BREAKDOWN PRODUCT, C3d, IN GLOMERULAR DISEASES

Yoshihiro Hamashima and Toshio Doi

Department of Pathology, Faculty of Medicine, Kyoto University, Kyoto

Most types of human glomerular injury are believed to be of immunologically mediated ones, because of the presence of granular deposits of immunoglobulin and complement in the affected glomeruli as revealed by immunofluorescence technique (Dixon, 1968; McCluskey et al., 1966). Since immunofluorescent localization of immunoglobulin and complement within glomeruli reflects directly the resultant histological changes, observation of immunofluorescence is essential for the pathological diagnosis of glomerular injury. Most of well-established glomerular diseases seem to involve the disorder of classical or alternative pathway of complement. Although immunofluorescent tests of immunoglobulin and complement are routinely made on the renal specimens, little work has been done about the complement breakdown products in various glomerular diseases.

The complement system is considered as the effector and amplification system of the humoral reaction. C3 plays a central role of the classical and the alternative pathway. C3b can be enzymatically degraded by C3bINA (I), β1H (H) and protease to be cleaved initially into iC3b and later C3c and C3d (Nagasawa and Stroud, 1977; Pangburn et al., 1977). The large fragment, C3c, is rapidly released from cell membrane into the fluid phase, while the small fragment, C3d, remains being associated with the cell membrane (Ruddy and Asten, 1971). This binding site in C3d is known to interact not only with cell membrane (Müller-Eberhard, 1975), but also with immune complexes (Czop and Nussenzweig, 1976).

In this study, we attempted to detect glomerular C3d deposits and C3d fixing circulating immune complexes (CIC) and their correlation with other clinical and histological findings in order to determine how the complement activation is significant in various glomerular diseases.

Immunoelectron Microscopy of IgA Nephropathy

IgA nephropathy reported by Berger and Hinglais (1968), is a clinical entity characterized by IgA deposits predominantly in the glomerular mesangium. Since C3 deposits are found in association with the IgA deposits in most cases, complement activation should be occurring *via* the alternative pathway of the complement system (Berger, 1969). C3 deposits, however, are not found in some cases and their immunofluorescences were generally weaker than IgA deposits.

To make clear the possible relation between IgA and C3 depositions, immunoelectron microscope observations were made on IgA nephropathy with special reference to the relationship between immune deposits including C3 degradation products and the severity of mesangial proliferation. Immunoelectron microscopic studies on antihuman γ-chain, α-chain, μ-chain, C3, and C3d in 16 patients with IgA nephropathy by the method of Nakane (McLean and Nakane, 1974; Yamada and Nakane, 1977; Wilson and Nakane, 1978) revealed the followings: The patients with minimal glomerular involvement and focal proliferative glomerulonephritis showed electron-dense reaction products of IgA in the paramesangial area, while those with diffuse proliferative glomerulonephritis showed the electron-dense deposits of IgA throughout the enlarged mesangial matrix.

C3 deposits were detected in the samples from 15 out of the 16 patients,

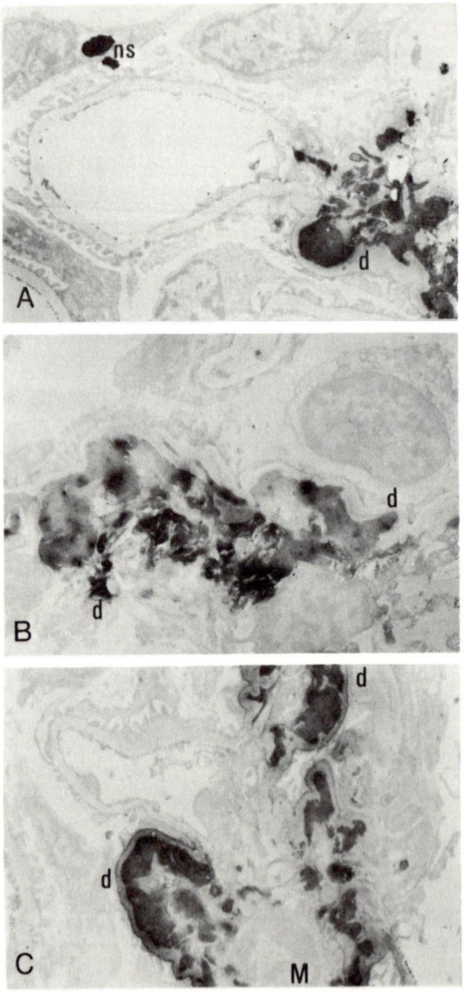

FIG. 1. Immunoelectron micrographs of IgA, C3, and C3d in typical case of diffuse mesangial proliferative glomerulonephritis.
(A). Immunoelectron microscopy reveals electron-dense reaction products of IgA deposits (d) are seen throughout the enlarged mesangial matrix. There is nonspecific staining (ns) in the epithelial cell. x 2,800
(B). Electron-dense reaction products of C3 deposits (d) are found over only a portion of the electron-dense mesangial deposits. x 2,800
(C). There are extensive electron-dense reaction products of C3d deposits (d) throughout the enlarged mesangial matrix. M, mesangial cell. x 3,500

but were less dense than IgA deposits. Distinct deposits of reaction products of C3 were observed only in some parts of the electron-dense mesangial deposits of IgA in 7 patients with IgA nephropathy. C3d deposits were found in all cases in association with IgA deposition and the intensity was much higher than that of C3 deposits and are nearly equivalent to that of IgA (Fig. 1). Our present observations indicate that extensive C3d deposits are found in association with IgA deposits. In all cases, however, C3 deposits did not show any close correlation with IgA deposits. It was impressed that heavy C3 deposits may occur at the acute phase of IgA nephropathy (Doi et al., 1984).

C3d Fixing IgA CIC in Patients with IgA Nephropathy

The mechanism of mesangial deposits of IgA in IgA nephropathy is not clear. In many patients with IgA nephropathy, however, recurrent gross hematuria is pressed by an episode of upper respiratory infection and the nephropathy recurs in the transplanted kidneys (Berger et al., 1975). An increase of IgA bearing lymphocytes in number has been also demonstrated in IgA nephropathy (Nomoto et al., 1977). An animal model for IgA immune complex nephropathy was reported by Rifai et al. (1979). These facts strongly suggest that the mesangial IgA deposits in this type of nephropathy are derived from CIC. Recently, IgA specific CIC have been detected in IgA nephropathy by several authors (Levinsky and Barratt, 1979; Kauffmann et al., 1980; Woodroffe et al., 1980; Doi et al., 1982; Lesavre et al., 1982). These assays have been based on CIC size or on the interaction of CIC with C1q, conglutinin (Kg) or cell receptors as described later. Through the fluorescent enzyme immunoassay (EIA) of $F(ab')_2$ of anti-C3d antibody in the serum of 52 patients with IgA nephropathy, we have also detected IgA class CIC fixed to C3d. The bindings assay of CIC with Kg and anti-C3d revealed that Kg binding IgA class CIC and anti-C3d binding IgA class CIC were detectable in 27% and 44% of the patients with IgA nephropathy respectively. Either one or both of the two were found in 65% of the patients, but no close correlation was found between serum IgA level and IgA class CIC detected by these methods. Although all the samples having a very high level of anti-C3d binding IgA class CIC did not always have a very high level of Kg binding IgA class CIC, there seemed to be same quantitative correlation between the two assay levels. Ultracentrifugation analysis showed that anti-C3d binding IgA class CIC were of various particles or molecules in polymeric (21 S) and monomeric IgA (7 S), whereas Kg binding IgA class CIC were mostly monomeric ones (8 S) with a minor component of heavy fractions (14 S). Both are present in IgA nephropathy. As we showed by immunoelectronmicroscopy, extensive C3d deposits are present in association with IgA deposits in all patients with IgA nephropathy (Doi et al., 1984). Anti-C3d binding assay will indicate the areas of IgA polymer deposition. Polymeric IgA is critical for renal deposition of complexes and induction of nephritic histological changes, as shown in the animal model of IgA immune complex nephritis by Rifai et al. in 1979. Lopez Trascasa et al. (1980) have noted the presence of a large amount of IgA polymers in the sera of patients with this disorder. These findings suggest that the high molecular or polymerized IgA class CIC, which can be detected by anti-C3d binding assay will be responsible for mesangial IgA deposits in IgA nephropathy (Doi et al., 1984).

C3d Deposits in Idiopathic Membranous Nephropathy

Membranous nephropathy (MN) is a well-established glomerular disease having typical electron-dense deposits in the subepithelial space along the glomerular basement membrane (GBM). Diffuse and finely granular deposits of IgG can be demonstrated invariably along the capillary loops by immunofluorescence technic, but C3 deposits are not always identified. Salant et al. (1980) reported that the complement system is an essential mediator of proteinuria in experimental MN in rats. However, it is not clear yet whether the C3 deposits is responsible for proteinuria in human MN.

In this study, observations on glomeruli from 16 patients with idiopathic MN were carried out by immunoperoxidase technic and light microscopy in order to examine the possible role of the complement system in the glomerular injury.

As the results, C3 deposits were found only in 50% of the MN patients and the C3 deposits in these patients was not so intense as that of IgG deposits. C1q and C4 deposits were seen only in a few cases. C3d, however, were deposited in all cases showing the similar location and reaction intensity as IgG deposits. The findings suggest that C3 deposits at the early stage of MN but later it is degraded and disappear. The amount of urinary protein excreted per day was significantly greater in the patients with glomerular C3 deposits than those having no C3 deposits, indicating clearly that the degree of proteinuria in MN is roughly proportionate to the glomerular C3 deposition.

Thus, the presence of C3 deposits means an active phase of MN. The finding consistents with that of Salant et al. (1980) who reported that proteinuria in the passive Heymann nephritis model of MN is complement dependent. The effect of sequential process of complement deposition on the progress of MN is the problem left to be solved.

C3d-Fixing CIC as the Parameters of Disease Activity and Prognosis in Systemic Lupus Erythematosus

At present, it is generally accepted that CIC play an essential role in various immune diseases. Numerous techniques developed for the detection of CIC contributed to clarifying the mechanisms of autoimmune diseases (Dixon, 1963; Cochrane and Köffler, 1973). But it has often been found that CIC levels detected by various assay do not always correlate with clinical activity and progress in some immune diseases. Kg binding assay, that detects iC3b-fixing CIC in human sera (Linscott et al., 1978; Brown et al., 1982) is widely used for the detection of CIC. However, iC3b, an intermediate product in C3 degradation, will have a short life span and unstable and iC3b fixing CIC is highly susceptible to proteolytic cleavage, though its fate and life span have not yet definitely been certified. C3d fixing CIC should be stable comparing to iC3b, we attempted to detect C3d fixing CIC using solid phase anti-C3d in sera from 48 patients with systemic lupus erythematosus (SLE). The size of the C3d fixing CIC was also analysed.

The results obtained with the anti-C3d assay on the sera from SLE patients are shown in Fig. 2. Compared with normal controls (mean $\pm$ s.d. = 41.0 $\pm$ 71.5 AHG μg eq/ml), SLE sera showed significantly higher ($P < 0.001$) CIC levels (420.6 $\pm$ 312.5 AHG μg eq/ml) and positivity (75%). Sera from patients

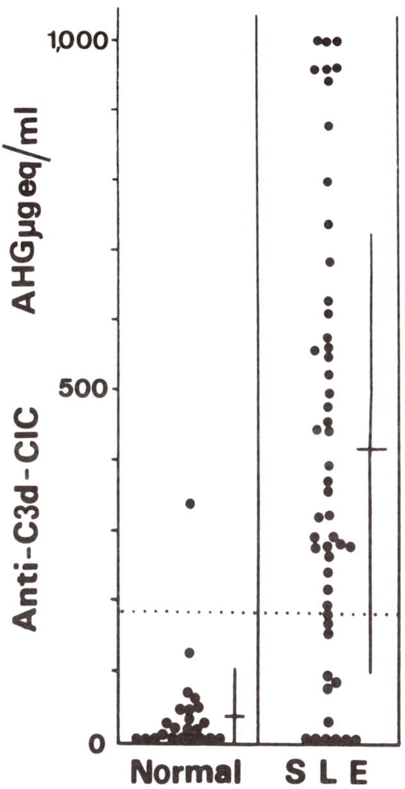

FIG. 2. CIC levels measured by the anti-C3d assay of sera from patients with SLE. The mean and s.d. are shown for each group. The upper limit of normality is indicated by a dotted line placed at 2 s.d. above the mean of the normal controls.

with rheumatoid arthritis, membranous nephropathy and IgA nephropathy also showed higher positivities compared with normal controls. In SLE sera, the anti-C3d assay showed higher positivity than the Kg assay (43%) and the C1q assay (43%), although there were few differences in positivities among the three assays in the other immune diseases tested. In SLE, CIC was detected by the C1q assay ($P < 0.01$), but not by the Kg assay. When individual values were compared quantitatively, the levels of anti-C3d-CIC were highly proportionate to those of C1q-CIC ($r_s = 0.624$, $P < 0.001$) but not to those of Kg-CIC ($r_s = 0.255$, $P > 0.05$) by Spearmen's rank correlation analysis. The results obtained by the three assays on SLE sera were analyzed in relation to clinical parameters. Examinations of sera at active stage were made on the day showing at least two positive symptoms indicated in the SLE symptom criteria of Ballou and Kushner (1979), *viz.* (1) facial erythema; (2) arthralgia; (3) Raynaud's phenomenon; (4) unexplained fever (>38.5 ℃); (5) central nerve abnormality; (6) serositis; (7) onset of oedema; (8) hypertension ($>160/90$); (9) LE cells and (10) leucopenia ($<3{,}500/mm^3$). In comparison of the CIC levels detected by the three assays on the active phases with those from inactive stages of SLE, it was found that anti-C3d-CIC were significantly higher at the active stage than those at the inactive stage ($P < 0.001$). The levels of C1q-CIC were also significantly higher in the active stage than in the inactive stage ($P < 0.01$), but Kg-CIC showed no distinct difference between them. In connection with these examinations, the sizes of anti-C3d-CIC, C1q-CIC and Kg-CIC were estimated by sucrose density gradient ultracentrifugation. Analysis on six sera from SLE and two from normal controls gave a representative pattern of the fractionation of SLE sera showing that the anti-C3d-CIC were in a broad range from 6 to 19S, including heavier (13 – 19S) reacting materials than those detected in the other two binding materials. In SLE, as just described CIC levels obtained by anti-C3d assay moved with significantly proportionate to the disease activity and the levels showed also a good correlation with some analytical data such as serum anti-dsDNA antibodies, CH_{50} and C3 levels, which are widely accepted to reflect relapses and remissions of the disease (Cameron et al., 1976; Lange, 1978). The results indicate that the anti-C3d assay is the most reliable test not only for detecting CIC but also for the prospect of progress of SLE. However, the investigations show how different types of CIC are involved in the pathogenesis of autoimmune diseases and further analysis of CIC will aid us in comprehensive understanding of SLE (Sekita et al., 1984).

Mesangial C3d and C3d-Deposition and C3d-Fixing CIC in Lupus Nephritis

As just mentioned, the severity and progress of SLE are well reflected in C3d-fixing CIC. And in this section it is demonstrated that C3d fixing CIC also reflects the level of C3d deposition in SLE glomeruli. Glomerular C3d and C3c deposition examined by direct immunofluorescent technique on the renal biopsy specimens from 50 patients with lupus nephritis showed a good correlation with the levels of C3d-fixing CIC of sera from the patients. C3d deposition was also compared with disease activity and glomerular IgG and C3c deposition as well as the levels of circulating immune complexes (CIC) measured by a solid-phase anti-C3d assay. A good correlation was also found between disease activity and the positivity of glomerular C3d deposits ($P < 0.001$), as well as C3c deposits ($P < 0.001$). Even in the patients clinically inactive or at remission C3d deposits were found in a relatively high percentage (59%) as compared with C3c deposits (17%). Mesangial C3d deposition was correlated with clinical disease activity more closely ($P < 0.005$) than capillary wall C3d deposition ($P < 0.025$). C3d deposits were detected in all of the 30 cases having positive C3c deposits, and in 15 of the 20 C3c negative cases (75%). Glomerular IgG deposits appeared being associated with C3d deposits in almost cases, both in mesangial areas and along capillary walls, with statistical significance ($P < 0.005$, $P < 0.001$, respectively). The serum levels of C3d-fixing CIC reflected exactly the intensity of mesangial C3d deposits.

As just shown C3c glomerular deposits were always accompanied by C3d deposition (30/30 cases, 100%), and 33% of the C3c negative cases (15/45) showed positive C3d deposition. The extence of positive C3d deposition without C3c deposits suggest that the affinity of C3d to the tissue components is stronger than that of C3c, though both of them are the final product of C3 activation and degradation.

The phenomenon is consistent with the fact that the C3d deposits are always positive in the renal tissue of clinically active patients and, also positive in those patients having silent symptoms at a relatively high percentage while C3c deposits are often missing even in clinical active cases. Therefore, the detection of C3d deposition without C3c means the past C3 activation in the disease history, and the detection of C3c concomitant with C3d deposition will indicate the complement-activating process and the active stage of the renal disease. Mesangial lesion of lupus nephritis will be related to the activity of the disease which is represented by a high amount of serum anti-DNA antibodies in patients (Hill et al., 1978). We have found that there was a significant correlation between mesangial lesions and CIC level detectable by solid-phase C1q-binding assay as well as anti-DNA antibody level. The excellent correlation between mesangial C3d deposition and C3d-fixing CIC and more significant correlation between clinical disease activity and mesangial C3d deposition than capillary wall C3d deposits strongly suggest the stimulated uptake of C3 fixing CIC by the mesangium at active phase of lupus nephritis (Muso et al., 1984).

REFERENCES

Ballou, S.P., and Kushner, I. (1979). Immunochemical characteristics of antibodies to DNA in patients with active systemic lupus erythematosus. *Clin. Exp. Immunol.* **37**, 58–67.

Berger, J., and Hinglais, N. (1968). Les dépôts intercapillaries d'IgA-IgG. *J. Urol. Néphrol.* **74**, 694–695.

Berger, J. (1969). IgA glomerular deposits in renal disease. *Transplant. Proc.* **1**, 939–944.

Berger, J., Yaneva, H., Nabarra, B., and Barbanel, C. (1975). Recurrcnce of mesangial deposition of IgA after renal transplantation. *Kidney Int.* **7**, 232–241.

Brown, E.J., Gaither, T.A., Hammer, C.H., Hosea, S.W., and Frank, M.M. (1982). The use of conglutinin in a quantitative assay for the presence of cell-bound C3bi and evidence that a single molecule of C3bi is capable of binding conglutinin. *J. Immunol.* **128**, 860–865.

Cameron, J.S., Lessof, H.H., Ogg, C.S., Williams, B.D., and Williams, D.G. (1976). Disease activity in the nephritis of systemic lupus erythematosus in relation to serum complement concentrations. DNA binding capacity and precipitating anti-DNA antibody. *Clin. Exp. Immunol.*

25, 418–427.

Cochrane, C.G., and Koffler, D. (1973). Immune complex disease in experimental animals and man. *Adv. Immunol.* **16**, 185–264.

Czop, J., and Nussenzweig, V. (1976). Studies on the mechanism of solubilization of immune precipitates by serum. *J. Exp. Med.* **143**, 615–630.

Dixon, F.J. (1963). The role of antigen-antibody complexes in disease. *Harvey Lect.* **58**, 21–52.

Dixon, F.J. (1968). The pathogenesis of glomerulonephritis. *Am. J. Med.* **44**, 493–498.

Doi, T., Kanatsu, K., Sekita, K., Yoshida, H., Nagai, H., and Hamashima, Y. (1982). Circulating immune complexes of IgG, IgA, and IgM classes in various glomerular diseases. *Nephron* **32**, 335–341.

Doi, T., Kanatsu, K., Nagai, H., Kohrogi, N., Kuwahara, T., and Hamashima, Y. (1984). Immunoelectron microscopic studies of IgA nephropathy. *Nephron* **36**, 246–251.

Doi, T., Kanatsu, K., Nagai, H., Suehiro, F., Kuwahara, T., and Hamashima, Y. (1984). Demonstration of C3d deposits in membranous nephropathy. *Nephron* **37**, 232–235.

Doi, T., Kanatsu, K., Sekita, K., Yoshida, H., Nagai, H., and Hamashima, Y. (1984). Detection of IgA class circulating immune complexes bound to anti-C3d antibody in patients with IgA nephropathy. *J. Immunol. Methods* **69**, 95–104.

Hill, G.S., Hinglais, N., Tron, F., and Bach, J.F. (1984). Systemic lupus erythematosus morphologic correlation with immunologic and clinical data at the time of biopsy. *Am. J. Med.* **64**, 61–79.

Kauffmann, R.H., Herrmann, W.A., Meijer, C.J.L.M., Daha, M.R., and Van Es, L.A. (1980). Circulating IgA-immune complexes in Henoch-Schönlein purpura. *Am. J. Med.* **69**, 859–866.

Lange, A., (1978). Evaluation of the simultaneous estimation of anti-dsDNA and anti-ssDNA antibodies for clinical purposes. *Clin. Exp. Immunol.* **31**, 472–481.

Lesavre, P.H., Digeon, M., and Bach, J.F. (1982). Analysis of circulating IgA and detection of immune complexes in primary IgA nephropathy. *Clin. Exp. Immunol.* **48**, 61–69.

Levinsky, R.J., and Barratt, T.M. (1979). IgA immune complexes in Henoch-Schönlein purpura. *Lancet* ii, 1100–1103.

Linscott, W.D., Ranken, R., and Trigria, R.P. (1978). Evidence that bovine conglutinin reacts with an early product of C3b degradation, and an improved conglutinin assay. *J. Immunol.* **121**, 658–664.

Lopez Trascasa, M., Egindo, J., Sancho, J., and Hernando, L. (1980). IgA glomerulonephritis (Berger's disease): evidence of high serum levels of polymeric IgA. *Clin. Exp. Immunol.* **42**, 247–254.

McCluskey, R.T., Vassali, P., Gallo, G., and Baldwin, D.S. (1966). An immunofluorescent study of pathogenic mechanisms in glomerular diseases. *N. Engl. J. Med.* **272**, 695–701.

McLean, I.W., and Nakane, P.K. (1974). Periodate-lysine-paraformaldehyde fixative. A new fixative for immunoelectron microscopy. *J. Histochem. Cytochem.* **122**, 1077–1083.

Müller-Eberhard, H.J. (1975). Complement. *Annu. Rev. Biochem.* **44**, 697–

724.

Muso, E., Sekita, K., Doi, T., Kuwahara, T., Yoshida, H., Tamura, T., Kawai, C., and Hamashima, Y. (1984). Immunopathological correlation between mesangial C3d-deposition and C3d-fixing circulating immune complexes in lupus nephritis. *Clin. Immunol. Immunopathol.* **32**, 351–358.

Nagasawa, S., and Stroud, R.M. (1977). Mechanism of action of the C3b inactivator: requirement for a high molecular weight cofactor (C3b-C4b INA-cofactor) and production of a new C3b derivative (C3b'). *Immunochemistry* **14**, 749–756.

Nomoto, Y., Sakai, H., and Arimori, S. (1979). Increase of IgA-bearing lymphocytes in peripheral blood from patients with IgA nephropathy. *Am. J. Clin. Pathol.* **71**, 158–160.

Pangburn, M.K., Schreiber, R.D., and Müller-Eberhard, H.J. (1977). Human complement C3b inactivator: isolation characterization, and demonstration of an absolute requirement for the serum protein β1H for cleavage of C3b and C4b in solution. *J. Exp. Med.* **146**, 257–270.

Rifai, A., Small, Jr., P.A., Teague, P.O., and Ayoub, E.M. (1979). Experimental IgA nephropathy. *J. Exp. Med.* **150**, 1161–1173.

Ruddy, S., and Austen, K.F. (1971). C3b inactivator of man. II. Fragments produced by C3b inactivator cleavage of cell-bound or fluid phase C3b. *J. Immunol.* **107**, 742–750.

Salant, D.J., Belok, S., Madaio, M.P., and Couser, W.G. (1980). A new role for complement in experimental membranous nephropathy in rats. *J. Clin. Invest.* **66**, 1339–1350.

Sekita, K., Doi, T., Muso, E., Yoshida, H., Kanatsu, K., and Hamashima, Y. (1984). Correlation of C3d fixing circulating immune complexes with disease activity and clinical parameters in patients with systemic lupus erythematosus. *Clin. Exp. Immunol.* **55**, 487–494.

Wilson, M.B., and Nakane, P.K. (1978). Recent development in the periodate method of conjugating horseradish peroxidase to antibodies. *In* "Immunofluorescence and Related Staining Techniques" (W. Knapp, K. Holubar and G. Wick, eds.), pp. 215–224. Elsevier, Amsterdam.

Woodroffe, A.J., Gormly, A.A., McKenzie, P.E., Wootton, A.M., Thompson, A.J., Seymour, A.E., and Clarkson, A.R. (1980). Immunologic studies in IgA nephropathy. *Kidney Int.* **18**, 366–374.

Yamada, G., and Nakane, P.K. (1977). Hepatitis B core and surface antigens in liver tissue light and electron microscopic localization by the peroxidase-labeled antibody method. *Lab. Invest.* **136**, 649–659.

ULTRAMICROSCOPIC LOCALIZATION OF CATIONIZED ANTIGEN ON THE GLOMERULAR BASEMENT MEMBRANE (GBM) IN THE COURSE OF ACTIVE *IN SITU* IMMUNE COMPLEX GLOMERULONEPHRITIS

Takashi Oite[1] and Fujio Shimizu

Department of Immunology, Institute of Nephrology
Niigata University School of Medicine, Niigata

Cationic substances are considered to play an important role for the induction of immune complex glomerulonephritis (GN). If nephritogenic antigens are cationic, they possess affinity for negatively charged glomerular basement membrane (GBM) and can act as a target for circulating antibody, resulting in *in situ* immune complex formation (Vogt et al., 1980; Batsford et al., 1980). Quantitative studies in a passive model of *in situ* immune complex GN using cationized human IgG revealed that a very small amount of antigen reaching the kidney would be sufficient to cause GN with heavy proteinuria (Oite et al., 1982).

Recently, we reported that a severe unilateral immune complex GN could be induced by injection of cationized proteins in immunized rats (Oite et al., 1983; Oite et al., in press).

Here, we report on the histological changes and the sequence of antigen localization in this active model of *in situ* immune complex GN. This morphological study provides insight into the fate of immune deposits and the mechanism of injury to the GBM in the immune complex GN.

Materials and Methods

Rats: All experiments were performed in 6 – 8-week old Wistar and Wistar-King-Aptakeman rats.

Preparation of cationized human IgG and ferritin: Cationization was done as described previously (Oite et al., 1982; Vogt et al., 1982). The degree of cationization was estimated from isoelectric focusing in a slab gel system. Cationized human IgG and ferritin used in this study had a isoelectric point exceeding 9.5.

Histologic examination: For light microscopic examination renal tissue was fixed in buffered formalin, embedded in paraffin, and 4 μm sections were stained with hematoxylin-eosin (HE), periodic acid-Schiff (PAS) or periodic acid silver methenamine (PAM).

[1]Supported by research grant (59570145) from the Ministry of Education of Japan.

For immunofluorescence kidney specimens were snap-frozen in n-hexane cooled to −70 ℃. Frozen sections were stained with monospecific fluorescence isothiocyanate (FITC)-conjugated anti-human IgG (Behringwerke), anti-rat IgG and anti-rat C3 (Nordic Immunochemicals). Rabbit antiserum to horse spleen ferritin was prepared and labeled with FITC, as described previously (Batsford et al., 1983).

Conventional electron microscopy and staining anionic sites: Tissue fixed with 2.5% glutaraldehyde in 0.1 M phosphate buffer (pH 7.4) was processed for electron microscopy. Electron microscopic demonstration of glomerular anionic sites using a cationic probe, polyethyleneimine (PEI) (Polyscience Inc.) was performed according to the method of Schurer et al. (1977). As described previously (Suzuki et al., 1983), rats were injected intravenously with 0.3 ml of 0.5% PEI (MW. 40,000 − 60,000) solution and sacrificed 15 min later. Renal cortical tissue specimens were immersed in 0.2 M cacodylate buffer, pH 7.4, 400 mOsm, postfixed with 1% osmic acid and processed for embedding in Epon. Unstained sections or sections stained with lead citrate for a few seconds were examined in a model HS9 Hitachi electron microscope.

Results and Discussion

Immunofluorescent findings: The distribution of cationized proteins (human IgG and ferritin) 1 hr after renal perfusion was examined. Positive fluorescence along the glomerular capillary wall was confined to the left, perfused kidney (Fig. 1a). Rat IgG was also localized in a homogenous pattern similar to that of cationized antigens (Fig. 1b). These deposits became more granular during the course of the disease (Fig. 1c), as described previously in a passive model (Oite et al., 1982). The development into a typical granular-staining pattern following *in situ* immune complex formation is of the same nature as that in passive Heymann nephritis (Couser et al., 1978).

Immunofluorescent intensity of staining for cationized antigens decreased faster than that of rat IgG. Cationized antigens and rat C3 were usually undetectable along the glomerular capillary walls from day 28 onwards, while staining for rat IgG remained moderately positive in a mesangial pattern (Fig. 1d).

Light microscopy: Histologic findings are described only in the left kidneys in an active model using cationized human IgG because there were no abnormalities in the right kidneys in any experimental group.

There were no apparent changes 1 hr after renal perfusion. From 12 to 24 hr a diffuse infiltration of polymorphonuclear leukocytes (PMN), exudation of proteinaceous substances into the Bowman's space and urinary casts in the tubular lumen were found (Fig. 2).

In addition to the endocapillary proliferation, adhesion of the glomerular capillary walls to Bowman's capsules and infiltration of cellular elements such as PMN and mononuclear cells into Bowman's space were observed from days 3 to 7.

Distinctive histologic features on day 7 were crescent formation and periglomerular cell infiltration, consisting chiefly of mononuclear cells; 10 to 20% of all glomeruli were affected by these morphological changes (Fig. 3).

The histological changes and immunofluorescent findings in the glomeruli in an active model using cationized ferritin were substantially equal to those described above.

Electron microscopy: Recently, we reported that the injection of small quantities of cationized human IgG into the left renal artery of preimmunized rat could lead to a severe unilateral immune complex GN (Oite et al., 1983). Electron microscopy in this study revealed subepithelial dense deposits which

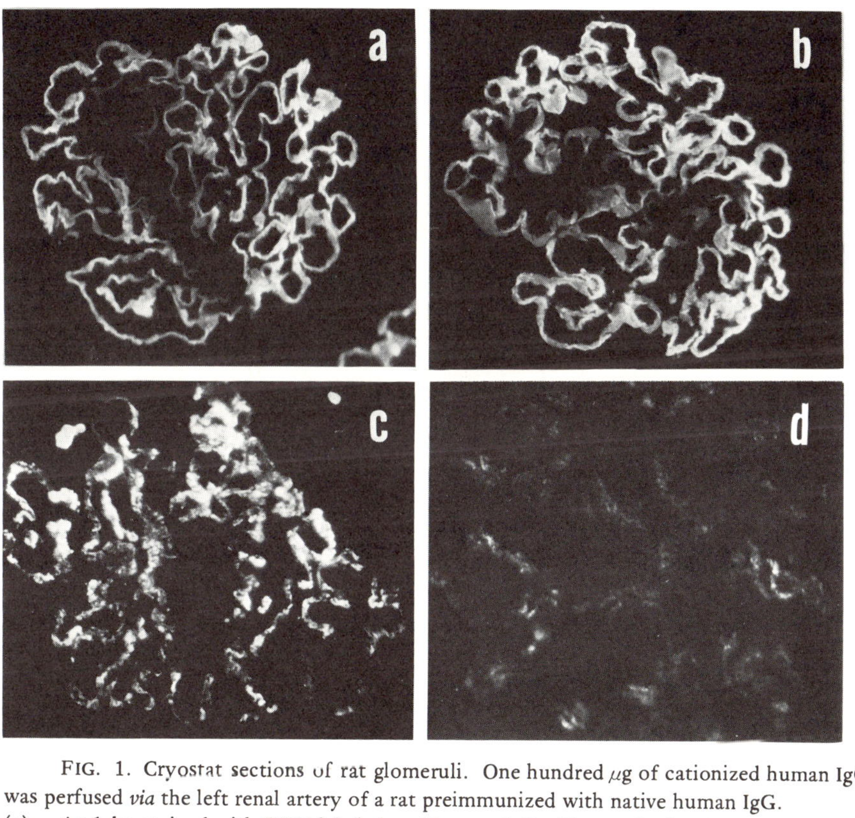

FIG. 1. Cryostat sections of rat glomeruli. One hundred μg of cationized human IgG was perfused *via* the left renal artery of a rat preimmunized with native human IgG.
(a) At 1 hr, stained with FITC labeled anti-human IgG. Glomerular localization of human IgG was seen along the capillary wall (x 250).
(b) At 1 hr, rat IgG was found along the capillary wall in a pattern similar to that of human IgG (x 250).
(c) On day 7, stained with FITC labeled anti-rat IgG. Discrete granular deposition of rat IgG was seen along the glomerular capillary wall (x 250).
(d) On day 28, stained with FITC labeled anti-rat IgG. A chief localization of rat IgG was found in the mesangial region (x 250).

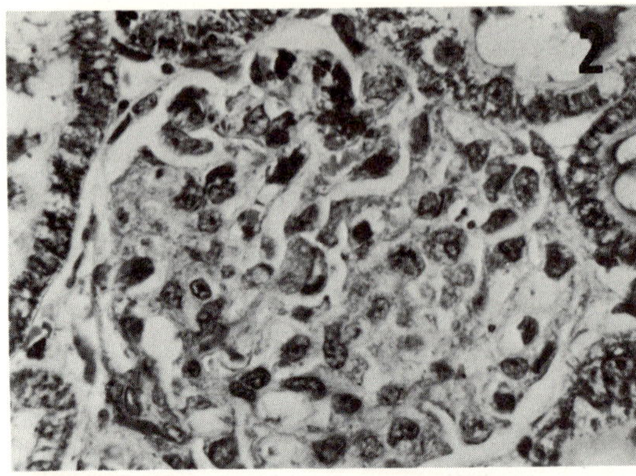
2

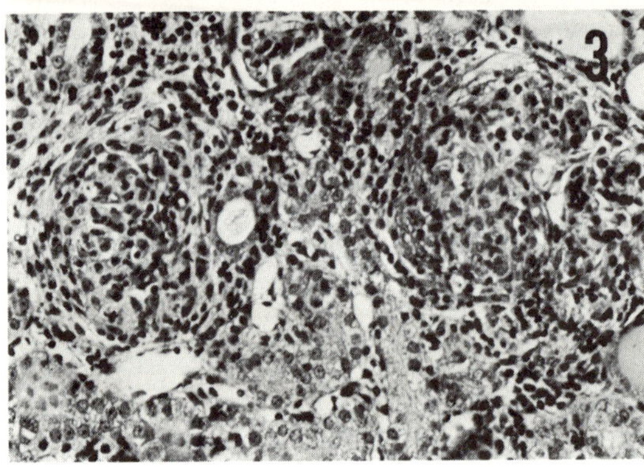
3

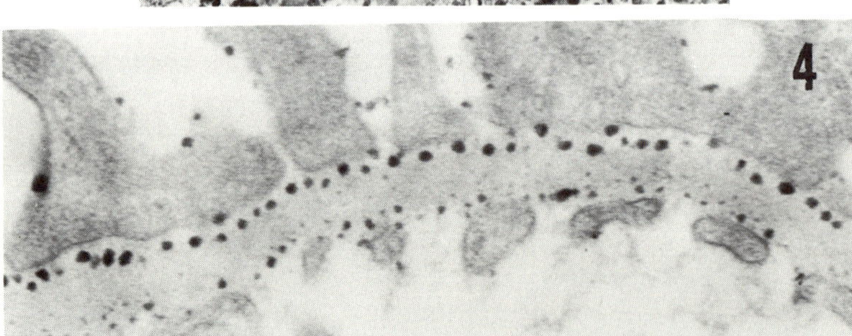
4

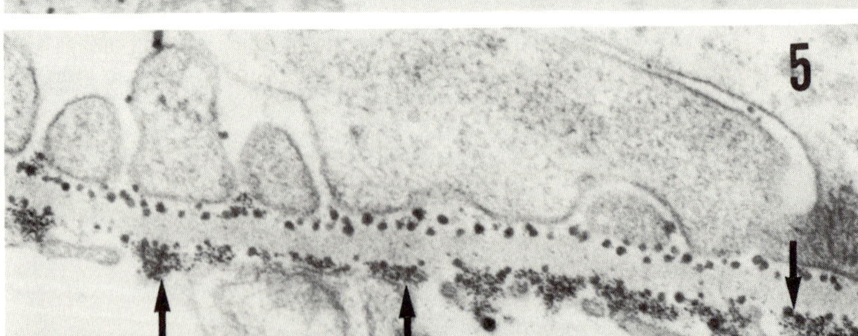
5

became larger and formed regularly distributed humps with time of disease course. However, in this study little was known about the correlation between the initial binding of cationic antigen to the anionic sites on the GBM, endocapillary cell proliferation and the disappearance of antigen from the glomerular capillary wall. Here, we wish to focus on the sequence of antigen localization and interaction of immune deposits with anionic sites on the GBM, by using cationized ferritin as an electron microscopically visible antigen, in combination with PEI-stain.

PEI is a suitable cationic probe to demonstrate the anionic sites of the glomerular capillary wall when injected intravenously (Suzuki et al., 1983). Fig. 4 shows the distribution of anionic sites detected with PEI-staining on the GBM in the normal rat kidney.

One hr after renal perfusion in the preimmunized rat, most of the ferritin aggregates were localized subendothelially, corresponded to the anionic sites of the *lamina rara interna* (Fig. 5). There were infiltrating PMN and monocytes in the capillary loops. As shown in Fig. 6a, monocytes were often in direct contact with the immune complexes associated with anionic sites of the *lamina rara interna*, and phagocytized ferritin aggregates and PEI particles. Monocytes were also in intimate contact with a section of the GBM, denuded of endothelium, where ferritin aggregates were invisible (Fig. 6b). The initial sites of local immune complex formation were at the subendothelial side of the GBM. This finding is important to understand the mechanism of the GBM injury because representatives of the inflammatory mediators system including complement, coagulation and cellular factors (PMN, monocytes, platelets) are able to reach the immune deposits through the fenestrated endothelium. PEI-stain revealed that only a very few ferritin aggregates were seen in the vicinity of the anionic sites of the *lamina rara externa* and the mesangium at 1 hr (Fig. 7).

At 24 hr, numerous ferritin aggregates were localized subepithelially and intramembranously. Ferritin aggregates were preferentially observed directly beneath the slit membrane and in contact with cell membrane of the foot process (Fig. 8a). In the subepithelial hump-like deposits, ferritin molecules were present only rarely (Fig. 8b). Ferritin aggregates were also observed in the mesangial matrix (Fig. 8a). The amount of ferritin aggregates located in the mesangial area appeared to increase with time. This finding

---

FIG. 2. Light microscopic changes of the glomerulus. At 12 hr, there is a diffuse infiltration of PMN and a urinary cast in the tubular lumen was found (PAM, x 300).

FIG. 3. Cellular crescent on day 7. Extracellular cell proliferation and periglomerular cell infiltration were seen (HE, x 120).

FIG. 4. A section of the glomerulus from a normal rat injected with PEI. PEI particles were distributed along the *lamina rara* of the GBM and on the surface of epithelial foot processes (stained with lead citrate, x 40,000).

FIG. 5. A section of the glomerulus from a preimmunized rat 1 hr after renal perfusion with 500 μg of cationized ferritin. Most of ferritin aggregates were associated with the anionic sites of the *lamina rara interna*, detected with PEI (arrows) (stained with lead citrate, x 40,000).

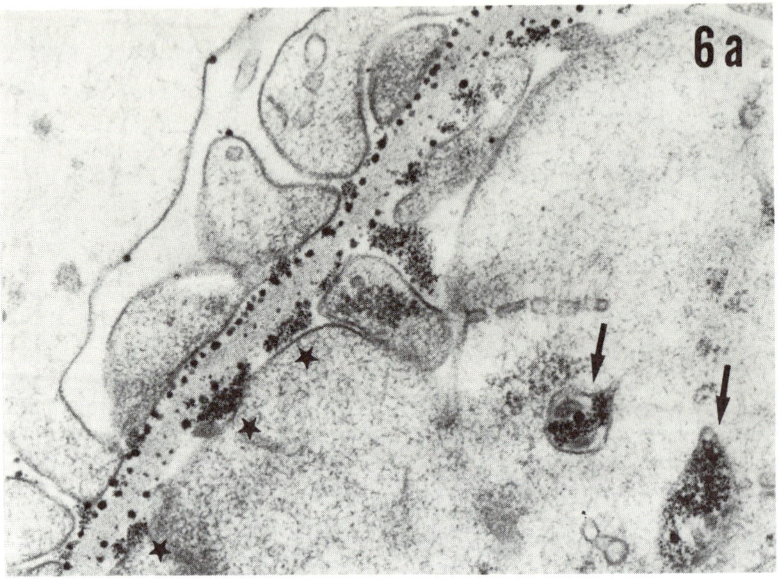

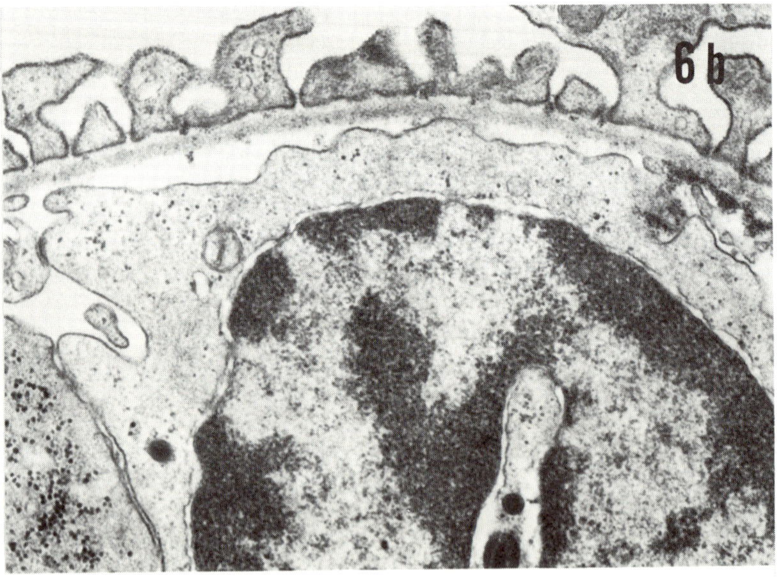

FIG. 6. Electron micrographs of the glomeruli from the rat 1 hr after renal perfusion.
(a) In combination with PEI-stain. A monocyte was in direct contact with ferritin aggregates associated with anionic sites of the *lamina rara interna* (asterisks). Ferritin aggregates and PEI particles were found in the cytoplasm of the monocyte (arrows) (stained with lead citrate, x 40,000).
(b) A monocyte was in intimate contact with a section of the GBM, denuded of endothelium, where ferritin particles were lost (x 26,000).

suggested that some of cationized ferritin molecules localized subendothelially were taken up into the mesangium as its clearing function.

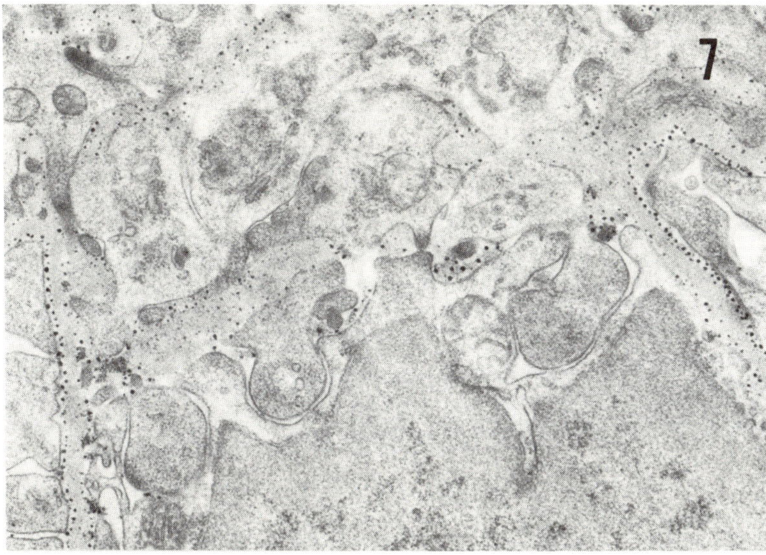

FIG. 7. Electron micrograph of the glomerulus, in combination with PEI-stain 1 hr after renal perfusion. Only a very few ferritin particles were present in the vicinity of the anionic sites of the *lamina rara externa* and the mesangium (stained with lead citrate, x 30,000).

ABSTRACT

The injection of microgram quantities of cationized human IgG or ferritin into the left renal artery of a preimmunized rat could result in a severe unilateral immune complex glomerulonephritis. Cationized antigens and rat IgG were distributed along the glomerular capillary wall in a pattern that became increasingly granular with time. Electron microscopic studies in combination with the staining of anionic sites on the glomerular basement membrane (GBM) revealed that the initial site of *in situ* immune complex formation was mainly on the subendothelial side of the GBM, corresponding to the anionic sites in the *lamina rara interna*. The local immune complex formation was followed by accumulation of blood born cells such as polymorphonuclear leukocytes and monocytes.

In the model using cationized ferritin, numerous ferritin aggregates were present subepithelially and intramembranously 24 hr after renal perfusion. In the subepithelial hump-like dense deposits, ferritin molecules were seen only rarely. Ferritin aggregates were also observed in the mesangial area. The amount of ferritin aggregates located there appeared to increase with time. This finding suggested that some of cationized antigens localized subendothelially were transported into the mesangium as its clearing function.

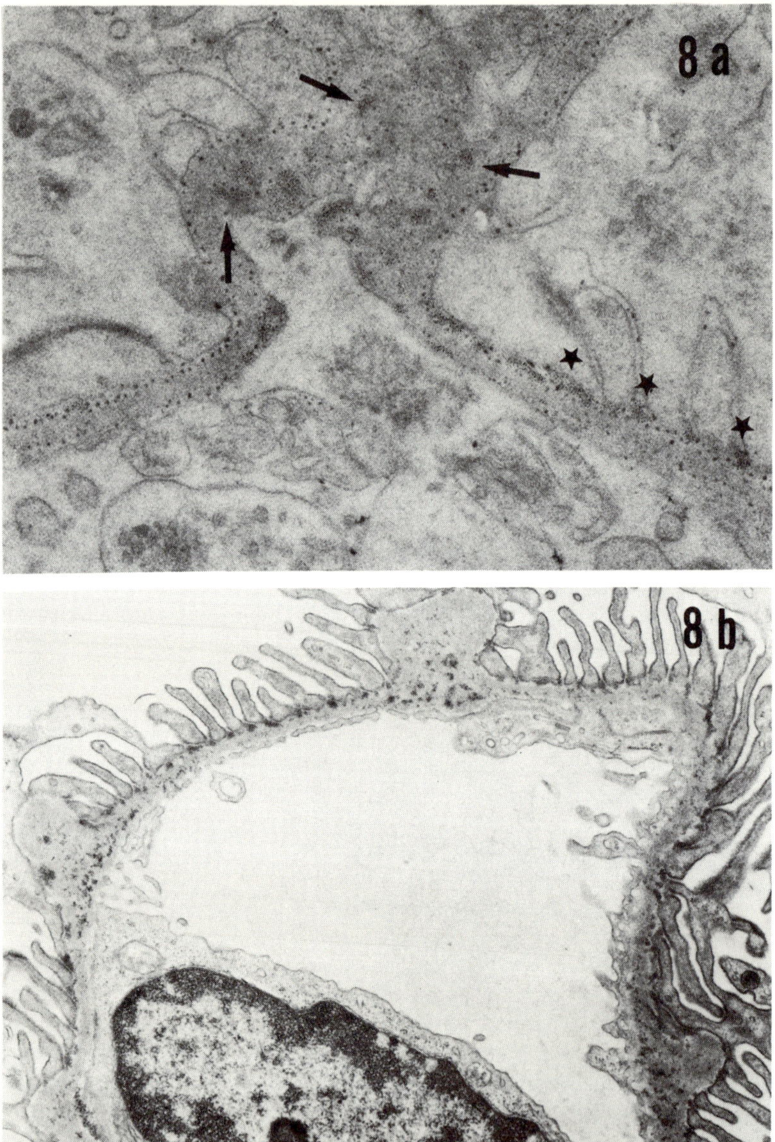

FIG. 8. Electron micrographs of the glomeruli from the rat 24 hr after renal perfusion.

(a) In combination with PEI-stain. Most of ferritin particles were observed subepithelially, particularly direct beneath the slit membrane and in contact with the cell membrane of the foot process (asterisks). Ferritin aggragates were also seen in the mesangial matrix (arrows) (stained with lead citrate, x 30,000).

(b) Ferritin aggregates were found subepithelially and intramembranously. In the subepithelial hump-like deposits, ferritin molecules were seen only sparsely (x 13,000).

References

Batsford, S.R., Oite, T., Takamiya, H., and Vogt, A. (1980). Anionic binding sites in the glomerular basement membrane: Possible role on the pathogenesis of immune complex glomerulonephritis. *Renal Physiol.* **3**, 336–340.

Batsford, S.R., Sasaki, M., Takamiya, H., and Vogt, A. (1983). Cationic molecule-induced nephrotic syndrome in rabbits. Lack of immune complex involvement. *Lab. Invest.* **49**, 260–269.

Couser, W.G., Steinmuller, D.R., Stilmant, M.M., Salant, D.J., and Lowenstein, L.M. (1978). Experimental glomerulonephritis in the isolated perfused rat kidney. *J. Clin. Invest.* **62**, 1275–1287.

Oite, T., Batsford, S.R., Mihatsch, M.J., Takamiya, H., and Vogt, A. (1982). Quantitative studies of *in situ* immune complex glomerulonephritis in the rat induced by planted, cationized antigen. *J. Exp. Med.* **155**, 460–474.

Oite, T., Shimizu, F., Kihara, I., Batsford, S.R., and Vogt, A. (1983). An active model of immune complex glomerulonephritis in the rat employing cationized antigen. *Am. J. Pathol.* **112**, 185–194.

Oite, T., Shimizu, F., Suzuki, Y., and Vogt, A. (1985). Ultramicroscopic localization of cationized antigen in the glomerular basement membrane in the course of active, *in situ* immune complex glomerulonephritis. *Virchows Arch. (Cell Pathol.).* (in press)

Schurer, J.W., Hoedemaeker, Ph.J., and Molenaar, I. (1977). Polyethyleneimine as tracer particle for (immuno)electron-microscopy. *J. Histochem. Cytochem.* **25**, 384–387.

Suzuki, Y., Maezawa, A., Matsui, K., Oite, T., Koda, Y., and Arakawa, M. (1983). Alteration of glomerular anionic sites by the development of subepithelial deposits in experimental glomerulonephritis in the rat. *Virchows Arch. (Cell Pathol.)*, **44**, 209–222.

Vogt, A., Schmidt, U., Takamiya, H., and Batsford, S.R. (1980). *In situ* immune complex nephritis and basic proteins. *In* "Proceedings of European Dialysis and Transplantation Association" (B. Robinson and J. Hawkins, eds.), Vol. 17, pp. 613–620. Pitman Medical Publishing, Tumbridge Wells, Kent.

Vogt, A., Rohrbach, R., Shimizu, F., Takamiya, H., and Batsford, S.R. (1982). Interaction of cationized antigen with rat glomerular basement membrane: *In situ* immune complex formation. *Kidney Int.* **22**, 27–35.

IN SITU IMMUNE COMPLEX FORMATION VERSUS CIRCULATING IMMUNE COMPLEX DEPOSITION: *IN SITU* IMMUNE COMPLEX GLOMERULONEPHRITIS INDUCED BY CATIONIC IMMUNE COMPLEX AS PLANTED ANTIGEN

Haruo Takamiya[1]

Department of Internal Medicine, Shigei Medical Research Hospital, Okayama

Stephen Batsford and Arnold Vogt

Institut für Immunologie im Zentrum für Hygiene, Klinikum der Albert-Ludwigs-Universität, Freiburg im Breisgau

Two concepts of the pathomechanism of immune complex (IC) mediated glomerulonephritis (GN), i.e. deposition and *in situ* formation of IC in the glomerular basement membrane (GBM), have been subjects of much interest and controversy for several years. Based on the comprehensive studies of Germuth et al. (1953, 1973, 1979) and Dixon et al. (1958, 1961) on acute and chronic models of serum sickness GN, it was generally believed that IC mediated GN initiates by deposition of soluble circulating immune complexes (CIC) in glomeruli, because they observed that experimental GN arised coincidently with the immune elimination of antigen, the appearance of CIC as well as the presence of both antigen and antibody in the lesion, resembling the spectrum of human GN. However, most studies by intravenous injection of preformed soluble IC's into animals have failed to demonstrate subepithelial localization (Couser and Salant, 1980).

The traditional concept has been recently challenged by the second mechanism of granular immune deposit formation in glomeruli, namely, *in situ* immune complex formation (Couser and Salant, 1980), in which the reaction of free circulating antibody with antigen fixed or already present in the glomerulus results. While anti-GBM nephritis may be regarded as a prototype of *in situ* immune complex glomerulonephritis (ICGN), a typical one of granular immune deposit formation was shown in passive Heymann nephritis of the rat (Van Damme et al., 1978; Couser et al., 1978) and its responsible antigen was confirmed to be an intrinsic constituent of the GBM (Kerjaschki and Farquhar, 1983).

It has been recently observed that the GBM is a filtration barrier not only for size as thought in the past but also for charge as an effect of glomerular polyanion (Rennke et al., 1975; Chang et al., 1975; Latta et al.,

[1] Supported by the Deutsche Forschungsgemeinschaft in part.

1975; Caulfield and Farquhar, 1976; Venkatachalam et al., 1978; Kanwar and Farquhar, 1979). Cationized proteins could be readily planted at the anionic sites of the GBM as target antigens to induce *in situ* ICGN in animals quite similar to the membranous nephropathy in man (Vogt et al., 1980, 1982, 1985; Batsford et al., 1980a, 1980b; Fleuren et al., 1980; Border et al., 1982; Oite et al., 1982, 1983; Vogt and Batsford, 1982; Vogt, 1984).

Thus, recent studies provided many evidences for *in situ* IC formation. It should be reasonable, however, to expect that injection of soluble cationic IC would bind to the anionic sites of the GBM like cationized proteins. Gallo et al. (1981) showed actually that preformed soluble cationic IC localized in the subepithelial and subendothelial sites of the GBM after intravenous injection into mice.

In the present study, we have investigated whether a preformed cationic IC could act as a target for circulating antibody and cause *in situ* ICGN.

Materials and Methods

Experiments were performed in male Wistar rats of body weight between 80 and 120 g.

Ferritin was prepared from horse spleens by the method of Vogt et al. (1968), human IgG was obtained from Beriglobin (Behringwerke, FRG) and rabbit IgG fraction was prepared by repeated precipitation with 33% saturated ammonium sulfate.

Antisera to ferritin and human IgG were raised in rabbits and antiserum to rabbit IgG was produced in sheep by repeated injections of respective antigen in Freund's complete adjuvant. Antisera were inactivated at 56 ℃ for 30 min and stored at −20 ℃. The IgG fractions of high titer antisera were labeled with fluorescein isothiocyanate (FITC) or with tetramethyl rhodamine isothiocyanate (TRITC) by the method of Hijmans et al. (1969) for immunofluorescent staining.

Cationization of ferritin and human IgG was done as described previously (Batsford et al., 1980a), based on the method of Danon et al. (1972). The degree of cationization was determined by isoelectric focussing in a slab gel system (Desaga, Heidelberg, FRG). Both ferritin and human IgG were highly cationized to yield isoelectric point (pI) over 10.0.

Four types of soluble IC were prepared *in vitro* by slowly adding appropriate antibody to the amount of sevenfold antigen excess while gently stirring at room temperature: (1) native ferritin (pI 4.0 − 5.0) reacted with rabbit anti-ferritin IgG (pI 5.0 − 8.0) yielded pI 5.0 − 7.5, (2) cationized ferritin (pI $>$10.0) with rabbit anti-ferritin IgG (pI 5.0 − 8.0) yielded pI 8.0 − 10.0, (3) native human IgG (pI 5.5 − 7.5) with rabbit anti-human IgG (pI 5.5 − 7.5) yielded pI 5.5 − 7.5, (4) cationized human IgG (pI $>$ 10.0) with rabbit anti-human IgG (pI 5.5 − 7.5) yielded pI 8.0 − 10.0.

Both native and cationic ferritin IC's were simultaneously run by pevicon electrophoresis as shown in Fig. 1 and soluble IC fractions of small size were isolated from the enclosed zones by centrifugation at 3,000 rpm for 10 min. The IC solutions were dialysed against phosphate buffered saline (PBS) pH 7.2. Native and cationic IC's of human IgG were fractionated by sucrose gradient sedimentation and soluble IC's of small size were collected to be thoroughly dialysed against PBS pH 7.2.

Preliminary experiments were performed to investigate interaction of the native and cationic ferritin IC's with the GBM. Seventeen mg of crude unpurified IC's in 1.0 ml of warm (37 ℃) PBS were injected directly into the left renal arteries of rats, as the method previously described (Batsford et al., 1980a) and the animals were sacrificed 1 hr later for examination. Controls included were 1) cationized ferritin plus normal rabbit IgG 2) buffer plus rabbit anti-ferritin IgG 3) cationized ferritin alone. As it was proven that native ferritin IC didn't bind with the GBM, further experiments were carried out merely with isolated cationic IC's of both ferritin and human IgG.

Twenty to 150 μg of isolated soluble fractions from cationic ferritin IC and cationic human IgG IC were injected directly into the left renal arteries. Both groups included 12 rats. Three rats of both groups became intravenous injection of 1 ml sheep anti-rabbit IgG antiserum and another 3 rats from every group got that of 1 ml rabbit anti-ferritin antiserum or 1 ml rabbit anti-human IgG antiserum respectively 1 hr after perfusion of the kidney. Rats were sacrificed for examination 1 hr to 4 weeks after the perfusion.

Immunofluorescent microscopy was carried out on 4 μm frozen sections which were air dried and fixed in acetone before stained with FITC or TRITC-labeled anti-ferritin, anti-rabbit IgG, FITC-labeled anti-sheep IgG, anti-rat IgG and anti-rat C3. FITC-labeled anti-rat IgG and C3 were purchased from Nordic Immunochemicals, Tilberg, Netherlands.

Electron microscopy was performed on material fixed immediately with

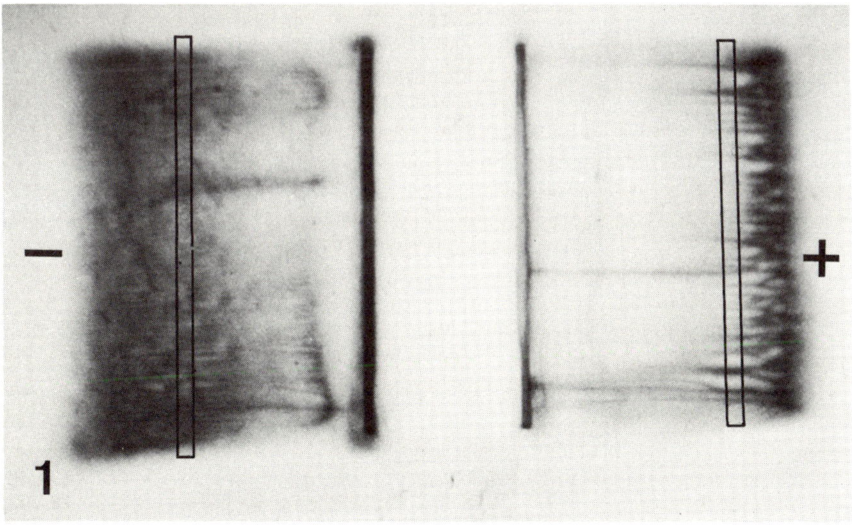

FIG. 1. Simultaneous preparative pevicon electrophoresis of native, on the right, and cationic ferritin IC on the left side. Pure IC fractions of small size were isolated from the enclosed zones.

glutaraldehyde after removal of the kidney, as described by Zollinger and Mihatsch (1978).

Urine samples were collected in metabolic cages to be examined for the presence of blood cells and protein.

RESULTS

One hr after perfusion of crude IC native ferritin IC was observed in a mesangial pattern by immunofluorescence but never seen along the glomerular capillary wall (Fig. 2a). In contrast, cationic IC bound abundantly to the capillary wall (Fig. 2b). Double staining with FITC-labeled anti-ferritin antibody and TRITC-labeled anti-rabbit IgG antibody both from goat yielded identical localization to prove the presence of antigen antibody complex, because the antibody alone perfused to control revealed no staining along the glomerular capillary loop. Ultrastructural finding of the same kidney perfused with cationic IC showed that many ferritin molecules accumulated under the slit diaphragm, beneath the foot process as well as in the subendothelial area (Fig. 3). While subendothelially grouped ferritin seemed to be aggregated IC, that in the subepithelial space could comprise not only IC of small size but also free ferritin.

Isolated cationic ferritin IC was localized in a granular pattern by immunofluorescence on the periphery of the glomerular capillary wall or of flocculus 1 hr after perfusion (Fig. 4a), partially disappeared in 24 hr (Fig. 4b) and was least but still clearly observed on the 11th day in a characteristic granular pattern as shown in Fig. 4c. Electron microscopic investigation of the same specimen with Fig. 4a disclosed that a large quantity of ferritin molecules were taken in the cytoplasm especially in the lysosomes of the podocytes. In addition, many molecules were accumulated beneath the slit diaphragm and some small or larger complexes were located in all three layers of the GBM, presumably according to charge and size of IC's 1 hr after perfusion of the kidney as shown in Fig. 5. The number of ferritin molecules which were distributed not only in the cytoplasm of the podocytes but also in the GBM remarkably decreased in 24 hr, except that those enclosed in the lysosomes of the podocytes seemed to be little changed. Eleven days after perfusion, ferritin molecules were seen but in the lysosomes of the podocytes as rather amorphous material than individual molecules.

The characteristic form of immunofluorescence in Fig. 4 might be designated as "epithelial granular pattern" on the basis of above mentioned findings by electron microscopy.

Neither electron dense deposits nor effacement of foot processes with proteinuria were formed and complement activation was not observed by mere deposition of preformed cationic ferritin IC in the GBM.

However, an intravenous injection of either sheep antiserum to the rabbit IgG, present in the planted IC, or rabbit antibody to ferritin 1 hr after perfusion formed dense deposits in all three layers of the GBM.

In the rat kidneys 1 hr after perfusion with isolated cationic human IgG IC, rabbit IgG was clearly localized along the capillary wall of the glomerulus by immunofluorescence. The same tissue revealed no remarkable changes of

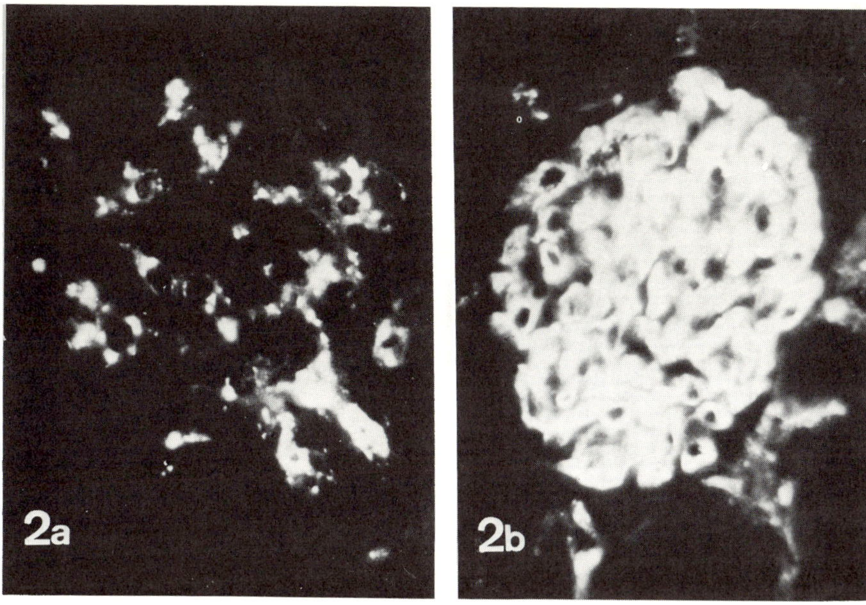

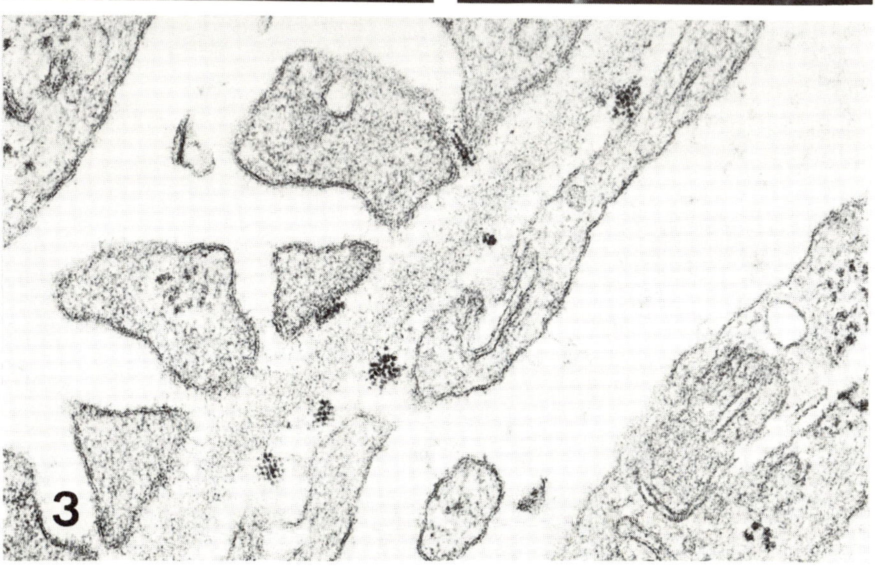

FIG. 2. Rat kidneys, 1 hr after perfusion of crude IC (17 mg), stained with TRITC labeled anti-rabbit IgG. x 400. (a) Native ferritin IC didn't bind to the GBM but to the mesangium. (b) Cationic ferritin IC was localized preferably along the glomerular capillary wall.

FIG. 3. The same kidney as Fig. 2b, perfused with crude cationic ferritin IC. Marked accumulation of ferritin molecules, presumably aggregated IC in the subendothelial area. In addition, some ferritin molecules can be seen between and beneath the foot processes. x 75,600.

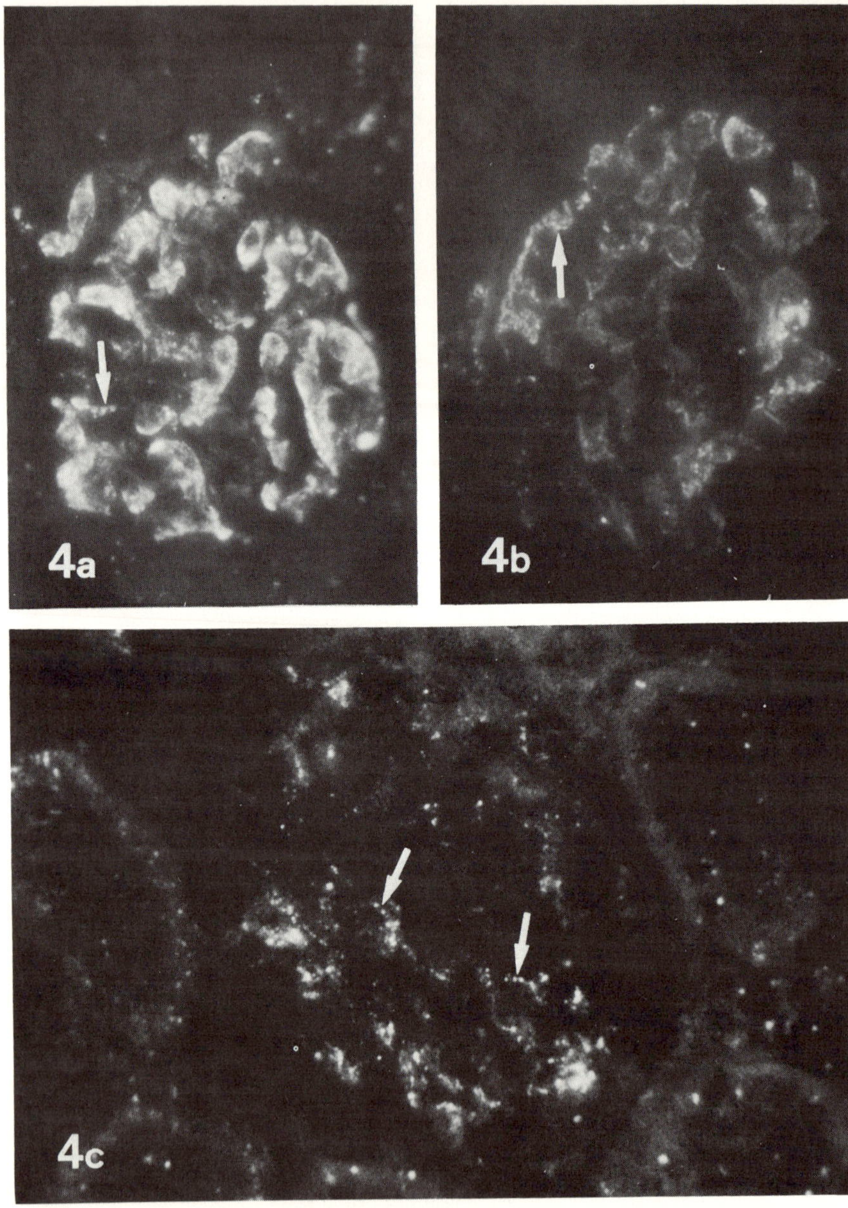

FIG. 4. Rat kidneys after perfusion of purified cationic ferritin IC (150 μg), stained with TRITC labeled anti-rabbit IgG. x 400.
Cationic IC of small size appeared rapidly in the cytoplasm of podocytes already 1 hr after perfusion (a), decreasing by 24 hr (b) and weak but distinctly granular localization was still observed on the 11th day (c). The immunofluorescence is granular in nature (arrows) and this characteristic form of staining might be designated as "epithelial granular pattern" on the basis of electron microscopic observation (see Fig. 5).

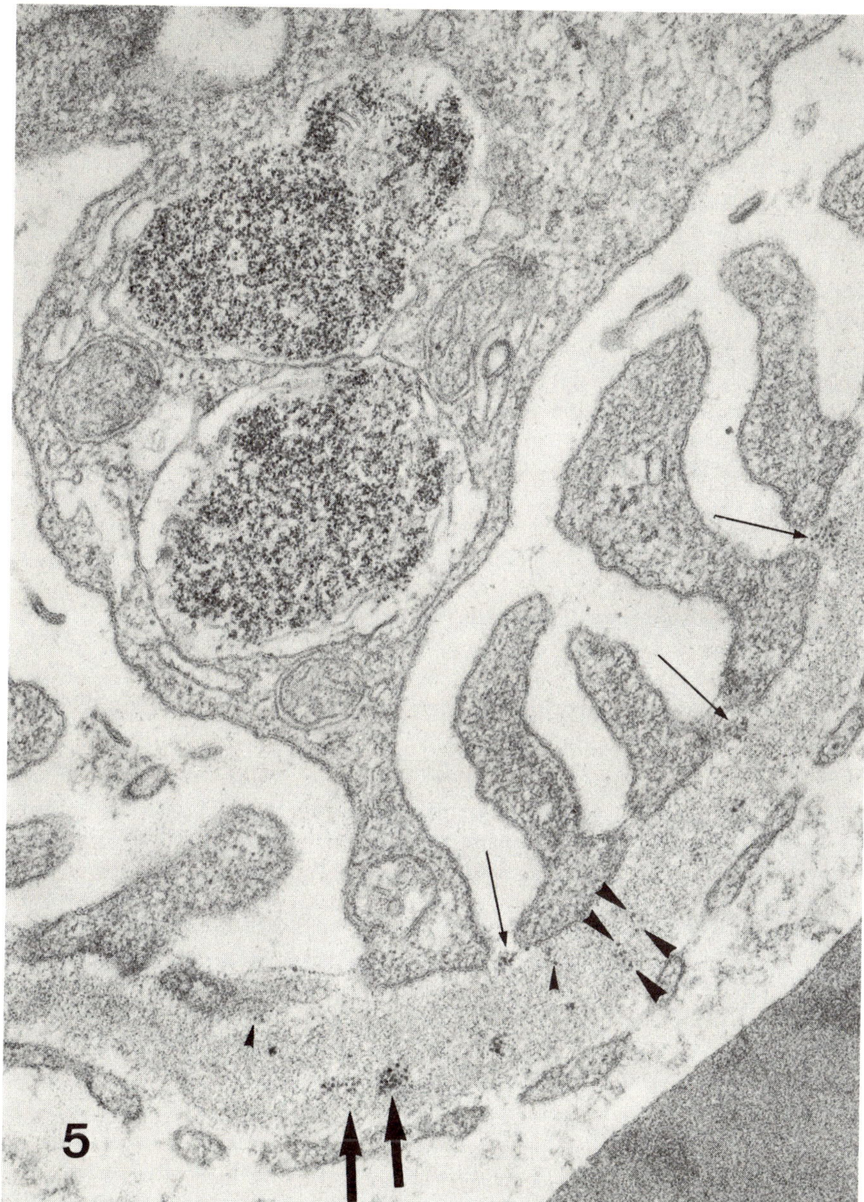

FIG. 5. The same kidney as Fig. 4a, a large quantity of ferritin molecules are engulfed by the podocyte, especially in the lysosomes. Many molecules are accumulated under the slit diaphragm (thin arrows), some are seen beneath the foot processes (small arrowheads), some small complexes are located in the *lamina densa* (large allowheads) and some larger ones are present in the endothelial side (thick arrows) of the GBM, however, formation of typical dense deposits have never occurred. x 70,000.

the glomerular capillary wall by electron microscopy as shown in Fig. 6. If antibody to the antibody which was a constituent of the planted IC was injected, massive electron dense deposits were formed not only in the subepithelial area but also in the subendothelium (Fig. 7) as well as intramembranously accompanied with effacement of foot processes and mild proteinuria (Fig. 8).

Persistence of planted cationic ferritin IC was, as shown in the Table 1, remarkably prolonged by subsequent binding of either sheep antibody to the rabbit IgG or rabbit anti-ferritin antibody accompanying activation of C3 and following reaction of autologous IgG in the lesion.

DISCUSSION

The presented results confirm that cationic but not anionic soluble IC is able to bind to the GBM in agreement with repeated studies those were performed by intravenous injection of preformed native IC (Mellors and

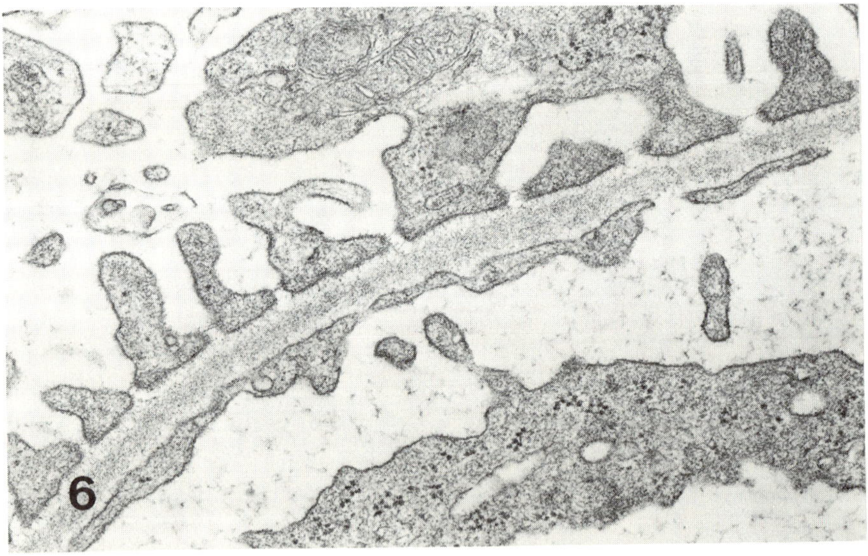

FIG. 6. Rat kidney, 1 hr after perfusion of purified cationic human IgG IC (20 μg). Neither immune formation nor any change of podocyte was noticed. x 36,000.

FIG. 7. Rat kidney, 28 days after injection of antiserum to rabbit IgG following the perfusion of isolated cationic human IgG IC (20 μg) 1 hr later. Note the remarkable formation of dense deposits in the subepithelial as well as subendothelial (arrowheads) areas, accentuated in the former and the thickening of the GBM with swollen foot processes in comparison to Fig. 6. x 36,000.

FIG. 8. The same kidney as Fig. 7. In addition to the numerous subepithelial dense deposits some is formed intramembranously, accompanied with effacement of foot processes. x 34,000.

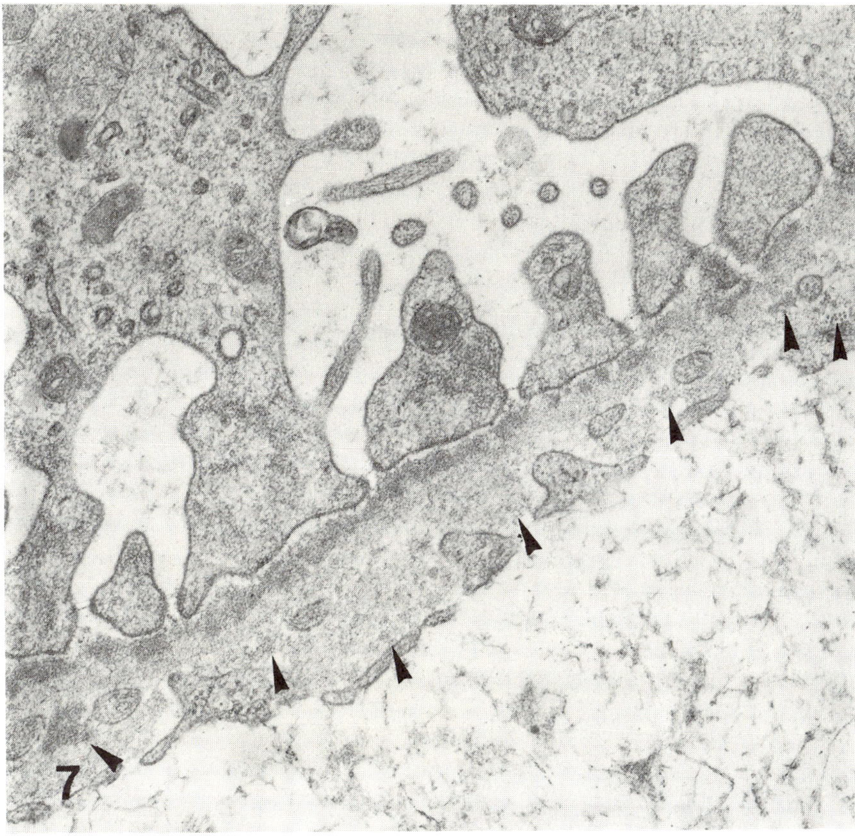

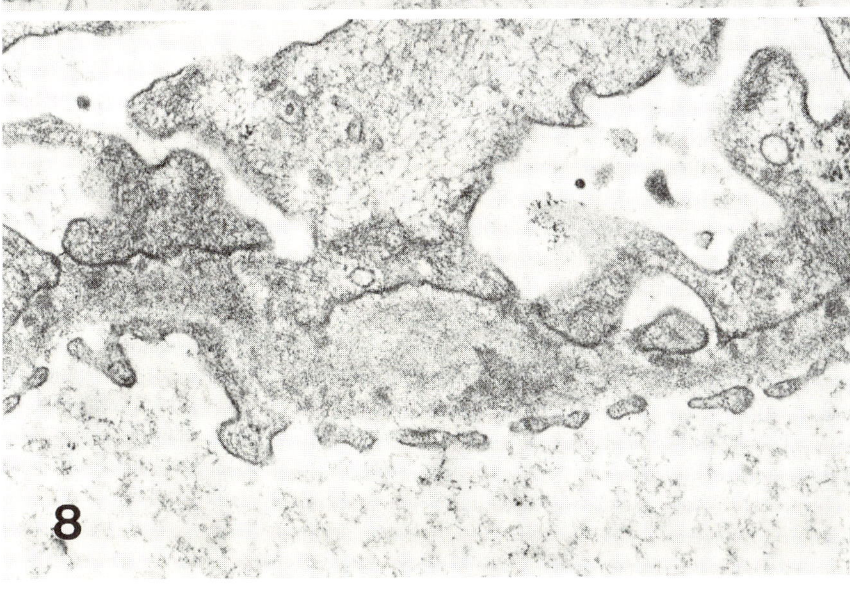

TABLE 1

PERSISTENCE OF PLANTED CATIONIC FERRITIN–ANTIFERRITIN IC IN THE GBM

Renal perfusion (IC 150 μg)	Yes	Yes	Yes	Yes
Sheep anti-rabbit IgG, 1 hr later	No	No	Yes	No
Rabbit anti-ferritin, 1 hr later	No	No	No	Yes
Time after renal perfusion	1 h	11 d	11 d	11 d
Immunofluorescence				
ferritin	++	±	±	±
rabbit IgG	++	+	++	++++
rat C3	±	±	++	++
rat IgG	±	±	+	+
sheep IgG	−	−	++++	−

Brzosko, 1962; McCluskey et al., 1962; Weiser and Laxon, 1962; Okumura et al., 1971; Wright et al., 1973; Ford, 1975; Haakenstad et al., 1975, 1976; Van Damme et al., 1978; Koyama et al., 1978; Germuth et al., 1979; Kijlstra et al., 1979; Couser and Salant, 1980) and with more recent ones by Gallo et al. (1981) or by Gauthier et al. (1982) who used both cationized antigen and antibody or cationized antibody alone respectively to get cationic IC. Gallo et al. (1981) found that soluble preformed cationic IC bound to discrete sites in both *lamina rarae* 1 hr after intravenous administration into mice. Gauthier et al. (1982) showed also by mice that large-latticed cationic IC formed with cationized antibody fixed to both *lamina rarae*, predominantly to the subendothelial area after intravenous injection and persisted in the GBM through 14 days developing large subepithelial deposits with autologous response of IgG as well as C3 to the planted IC. Now a poor correlation between the presence of IC in the circulation and in glomeruli especially in patients with membranous nephropathy (Couser and Salant, 1980) could be accounted for, because cationic macromolecules which satisfied the critical minimum charge and size requirements of about pI 9.0 and size 40,000 daltons for accumulation in the glomerular subepithelial area (Vogt et al., 1985) were removed from the circulation within 5 min (Vogt et al., 1982).

It should be especially noted that mere deposition of cationic soluble IC didn't result in GN, as Couser (1981) described that trapped CIC in glomeruli wouldn't be particularly nephritogenic, however, subsequent *in situ* reaction of antibody to either of the constituents prolonged persistence of the planted IC with activation of C3 and developed GN accompanied by formation of electron dense immune deposits in all three layers of the GBM, predominantly in the subepithelial area.

Planted cationic ferritin IC localized rapidly throughout the GBM and some larger complexes consisting of 2 to 3 ferritin molecules were observed even in the middle layer of the GBM 1 hr after administration, as can be seen in Fig. 5, in contrast to the model of *in situ* ICGN employing cationized ferritin (Batsford et al., 1980a, b; Vogt et al., 1982; Vogt and Batsford,

1982) which was never found in aggregated form within the *lamina densa* at any time (Vogt et al., 1982). The presented localization of cationic IC and lack of host reaction to the planted IC antigen are consistent with findings of Caulin-Glaser et al. (1983) who showed that covalently linked non-dissociating cationic IC with average sedimentation coefficient of 28S could deposit in both *lamina rarae* as well as in the *lamina densa* and none of mice revealed staining for C3 or IgG of mouse 1 hr after injection.

Whether the planted cationic IC antigens could persist in the GBM long enough to be precipitated by autologus immune response, as Gauthier et al. (1982) observed, should be elucidated, because the lattice of IC has a significant role in glomerular deposition of complexes (Mannik, 1982) and the formation of electron dense deposits in the subepithelial area require a precipitating antigen-antibody system (Agodoa et al., 1983).

In general, accumulation of macromolecules including CIC in the GBM is a function of charge (Gallo et al., 1983) and size (Vogt et al., 1982). Requirements for binding of cationic molecules with the GBM seem to be higher pI than 9.0 and in the range of 40,000 to 1,000,000 daltons of size (Vogt, 1984). Naturally occurring antigens can vary in charge and size, while responsive antibodies are usually in broad spectrum of charge. In a such situation it can be expected that cationic IC of net surface charge which gratify the above requisites would be formed in the circulation, even if in a small amount and directly planted in the GBM to be precipitated *in situ* by subsequent reaction of antibodies to the IC antigens.

It is to be pointed out that cationic antibody could play a role in *in situ* ICGN, because not only cationic antigen but also cationic antibody contribute to building up of cationic IC which persists longer than cationic antibody alone in the GBM, as Gauthier et al. (1982) confirmed. In 1980, Ebling and Hahn had already described that they had eluted more cationic antibody with anti-DNA specificity than that in the circulation from NZB/W MRL/l mouse kidneys. Furthermore, Kawaguchi et al. found recently that chemically cationized antibody to ferritin with reduced but maintained antigen-binding activity bound to anionic sites of the GBM by renal perfusion and combined subsequently injected ferritin antigen *in situ*, leading to immune deposit GN with mild proteinuria (to be published) and these findings could support our hypothesis previously described elsewhere (Batsford et al., 1980b).

Cationic IC as well as cationic antigen will be rapidly taken by podocytes after accumulation in the subepithelial area and stay in the lysosome for a long time undergoing enzymatic digestion to show rather amorphous structure than individual molecules, as far as ferritin IC and ferritin antigen are concerned. Such dynamic appearance of cationic antigen and antibody or their complex will be reflected on the proposed "epithelial granular pattern" by immunofluorescence, which has never been described so far as we are informed. It is of notice that human IgG can be localized in the cytoplasm and lysosomes of podocytes by immunoperoxidase method combined with hemotoxylin-eosin staining on biopsy material of the kidney with membranous nephropathy and other glomerular immune deposit diseases (Takamiya et al., in press) after embedding in plastic (Takamiya et al., 1979) suggesting the significance of cationic IC and cationic antibody for the pathomechanism of human ICGN.

Thus, it is considerable that not all but a limited IC with required positive net surface charge and size will be planted in the GBM, if it will appear in the circulation probably amongst cationic antigen and free antibody in nature, to form precipitating IC by subsequent reaction of antibody with activation of complement factors as well as cellular mediators (Thaiss et al., 1983) developing *in situ* ICGN which reveals immune deposits not only subepithelially but also subendothelially as well as intramembranously, different from *in situ* ICGN induced by homogenous cationic antigen characterized by formation of immune deposits exclusively in the subepithelial area similar to membranous nephropathy in man.

CONCLUSIONS

1. No localization of native IC in the GBM was observed by immunofluorescence and electron microscopy.
2. Preformed circulating IC localized in the GBM, when they were cationic.
3. A large quantity of cationic IC was trapped by the glomerular epithelial cells yielding immunofluorescence of "epithelial granular pattern" proposed.
4. The cationic IC localized in all three layers of the GBM, presumably depending on their net positive surface charge and size.
5. Subepithelial, intramembranous as well as subendothelial immune deposits were formed *in situ* simultaneously according to the location of IC antigen by subsequent administration of antibody to either of the constituents.
6. The binding of cationic IC in the GBM may not result in GN, however, GN can develop when the IC acts as planted antigen with further *in situ* binding of antibody.

ABSTRACT

The present investigation studied whether preformed, cationic immune complex (IC) could act as a target for circulating antibody and cause *in situ* IC glomerulonephritis. IC were formed in antigen excess, native and cationized (pI $>$10.0) horse ferritin and human IgG were used and small IC were separated by pevicon electrophoresis and sucrose gradient sedimentation respectively.

Twenty to 150 μg of these preparations were perfused directly into the left renal artery of male Wistar rats. No localization of anionic IC (pI 5.0 — 7.5) was seen by immunofluorescence and electron microscopy. Cationic ferritin IC (pI 8.0 — 10.0) localized in all three layers of the GBM, however, formation of electron dense deposits along the GBM, complement activation and proteinuria were not observed.

In further experiment perfusion of cationic IC was followed by antiserum to either of the constituents intravenously 1 hr later. Under these conditions massive subepithelial, intramembranous and subendothelial immune deposits were formed *in situ* accompanying activation of complement and mild proteinuria.

REFERENCES

Agodoa, L.Y.C., Gauthier, V.J., and Mannik, M. (1983). Precipitating antigen-antibody systems are required for the formation of subepithelial electron-dense immune deposits in rat glomeruli. *J. Exp. Med.* **158**, 1259–1271.

Batsford, S.R., Takamiya, H., and Vogt, A. (1980a). A model of *in situ* immune complex glomerulonephritis in the rat employing cationized ferritin. *Clin. Nephrol.* **14**, 211–216.

Batsford, S., Oite, T., Takamiya, H., and Vogt, A. (1980b). Anionic binding sites in the glomerular basement membrane: possible role in the pathogenesis of immune complex glomerulonephritis. *Renal Physiol.* **3**, 336–340.

Border, W.A., Ward, H.J., Kamil, E.S., and Coben, A.H. (1982). Induction of membranous nephropathy in rabbits by administration of an exogenous cationic antigen. *J. Clin. Invest.* **69**, 451–461.

Caulfield, J.P., and Farquhar, M.G. (1976). Distribution of anionic sites in glomerular basement membranes: Their possible role in filtration and attachment. *Proc. Natl. Acad. Sci. U.S.A.* **73**, 1646–1650.

Caulin-Glaser, T., Gallo, G.R., and Lamm, M.E. (1983). Nondissociating cationic immune complexes can deposit in glomerular basement membrane. *J. Exp. Med.* **158**, 1561–1572.

Chang, R.L.S., Deen, W.M., Robertson, C.R., and Brenner, B.M. (1975). Permselectivity of the glomerular capillary wall. III. Restricted transport of polyanions. *Kidney Int.* **8**, 212–218.

Couser, W.G., Steinmuller, D.R., Stilmant, M.M., Salant, D.J., and Lowenstein, L.M. (1978). Experimental glomerulonephritis in the isolated perfused rat kidney. *J. Clin. Invest.* **62**, 1275–1287.

Couser, W.G., and Salant, D.J. (1980). *In situ* immune complex formation and glomerular injury. *Kidney Int.* **17**, 1–13.

Couser, W.G. (1981). What are circulating immune complex doing in glomerulonephritis? *N. Engl. J. Med.* **304**, 1230–1232.

Danon, D., Goldstein, L., Marikovsky, Y., and Skutelsky, E. (1972). Use of cationized ferritin as a label of negative charges on cell surfaces. *J. Ultrastruct. Res.* **38**, 500–510.

Dixon, F.J., Vazquez, J.J., Weigle, W.V., and Cochrane, C.G. (1958). Pathogenesis of serum sickness. *Arch. Pathol.* **65**, 18–28.

Dixon, F.J., Feldman, J.D., and Vazquez, J.J. (1961). Experimental nephritis. The pathogenesis of a laboratory model resembling the spectrum of human glomerulonephritis. *J. Exp. Med.* **113**, 899–920.

Ebling, F., and Hahn, B.H. (1980). Restricted subpopulations of DNA antibodies in kidneys of mice with systemic lupus. Comparison of antibodies in serum and renal eluates. *Arthritis Rheum.* **23**, 392–403.

Fleuren, G., Grond, J., and Hoedemaeker, P.J. (1980). *In situ* formation of subepithelial glomerular immune complexes in passive serum sickness. *Kidney Int.* **17**, 631–637.

Ford, P.M. (1975). The effect of manipulation of reticuloendothelial system activity of glomerular deposition of aggregated protein and immune complexes in two different strains of mice. *Br. J. Exp. Pathol.* **56**,

523–529.

Gallo, G.R., Caulin-Glaser, T., and Lamm, M.E. (1981). Charge of circulating immune complexes as a factor in glomerular basement membrane localization in mice. *J. Clin. Invest.* **67**, 1305–1311.

Gallo, G.R., Caulin-Glaser, T., Emancipator, S.N., and Lamm, M.E. (1983). Nephritogenicity and differential distribution of glomerular immune complexes related to immunogen charge. *Lab. Invest.* **48**, 353–362.

Gauthier, V.J., Mannik, M., and Striker, G.E. (1982). Effect of cationized antibodies in preformed immune complexes on deposition and persistence in renal glomeruli. *J. Exp. Med.* **156**, 766–777.

Germuth, Jr., F.G. (1953). Comparative histologic and immunologic study in rabbits of induced hypersensitivity of serum sickness type. *J. Exp. Med.* **97**, 257–282.

Germuth, Jr., F.G., and Rodriguez, E. (1973). Immunopathology of the renal glomerulus. Little Brown, Boston.

Germuth, Jr., F.G., Rodriguez, E., Lorelle, C.A., Trump, E.I., Milano, L.L., and Wise, O'L. (1979). Passive immune complex glomerulonephritis in mice: models for various lesions found in human disease. II. Low avidity complexes and diffuse proliferative glomerulonephritis with subepithelial deposits. *Lab. Invest.* **41**, 366–371.

Haakenstad, A.O., Case, J.B., and Mannik, M. (1975). Effect of cortisone on the disappearance kinetics and tissue localization of soluble immune complexes. *J. Immunol.* **114**, 1153–1160.

Haakenstad, A.O., Striker, G.E., and Mannik, M. (1976). The glomerular deposition of soluble immune complexes prepared with reduced and alkylated antibodies and with intact antibodies in mice. *Lab. Invest.* **35**, 293–301.

Hijmans, W., Schuit, H.R.E., and Klein, F. (1969). An immunofluorescence procedure for the detection of intracellular immunoglobulins. *Clin. Exp. Immunol.* **4**, 457–472.

Kanwar, Y.S., and Farquhar, M.G. (1979). Anionic sites in the glomerular basement membrane. *J. Cell Biol.* **81**, 137–153.

Kerjaschki, D., and Farquhar, M.G. (1983). Immunocytochemical localization of the Heymann nephritis antigen (GP330) in glomerular epithelial cells of normal Lewis rats. *J. Exp. Med.* **157**, 667–686.

Kijlstra, A., Daha, M.R., and van Es, L.A. (1979). Immune complexes in experimental glomerulonephritis. *Behring Inst. Mitt.* No. 64, 45–53.

Koyama, A., Niwa, Y., Shigematsu, H., Taniguchi, M., and Tada, T. (1978). Studies on passive serum sickness. II. Factors determining the localization of antigen-antibody complexes in the murine renal glomerulus. *Lab. Invest.* **38**, 253–262.

Latta, H., Johnson, W.H., and Standley, T.M. (1975). Sialoglycoproteins and filtration barriers in the glomerular capillary wall. *J. Ultrastruct. Res.* **51**, 354–376.

Mannik, M. (1982). Pathophysiology of circulating immune complexes. *Arthritis Rheum.* **25**, 783–787.

McCluskey, R.T., Benacerraf, B., and Miller, F. (1962). Passive acute glomerulonephritis induced by antigen-antibody complexes solubilized in hapten excess. *Proc. Soc. Exp. Biol. Med.* **111**, 764–768.

Mellors, R.C., and Brzosko, W.J. (1962). Studies in molecular pathology: I. Localization and pathogenetic role of heterologous immune complexes. *J. Exp. Med.* **115**, 891–903.

Oite, T., Batsford, S.R., Mihatsch, M.J., Takamiya, H., and Vogt, A. (1982). Quantitative studies of *in situ* immune complex glomerulonephritis in the rat induced by planted, cationized antigen. *J. Exp. Med.* **155**, 460–473.

Oite, T., Shimizu, F., Kihara, I., Batsford, S.R., and Vogt, A. (1983). An active model of immune complex glomerulonephritis in the rat employing cationized ferritin. *Am. J. Pathol.* **112**, 185–194.

Okumura, K., Kondo, Y., and Tada, T. (1971). Studies on passive serum sickness. I. The glomerular fine structure of serum sickness nephritis induced by preformed antigen-antibody complexes in the mouse. *Lab. Invest.* **24**, 383–391.

Rennke, H.G., Cotran, R.S., and Venkatachalam, M.A. (1975). Role of molecular charge in glomerular permeability: Tracer studies with cationized ferritins. *J. Cell. Biol.* **67**, 638–646.

Takamiya, H., Kawaguchi, M., Ohmori, H., Yagisawa, M., Kosaka, K., and Vogt, A. Routine application of immunohistochemical staining on renal biopsy material embedded in plastic. *In* "Proceedings of the VIth Asian Colloquium in Nephrology" Kuala Lumpur. (in press)

Takamiya, H., Batsford, S.R., Tokunaga, J., and Vogt, A. (1979). Immunohistological staining of antigens on semithin sections of specimens embedded in plastic (GMA-Quetol 523). *J. Immunol. Methods* **30**, 277–288.

Thaiss, F., Batsford, S., Mihatsch, M., Bittersuermann, D., and Vogt, A. (1983). Mediator systems in *in situ* immune complex glomerulonephritis. *Kidney Int.* **23**, 199.

Van Damme, B.J.C., Fleuren, G.J., Bakker, W.W., Vernier, R.L., and Hoedemaeker, P.J. (1978). Experimental glomerulonephritis in the rat induced by antibodies directed against tubular antigens: V. Fixed glomerular antigens in the pathogenesis of heterologous immune complex glomerulonephritis. *Lab. Invest.* **38**, 502–510.

Venkatachalam, M.A., Rennke, H.G., Seiler, M.W., and Cotran, R.S. (1978). Structural and functional effect of glomerular polyanion. *In* "Biology and Chemistry of Basement Membranes" (N.A. Kefalides, ed.), pp. 149–164. Academic Press, New York.

Vogt, A., Bockhorn, H., Kozima, K., and Sasaki, M. (1968). Electron microscopic localization of the nephrotoxic antibody in the glomeruli of the rat after intravenous application of purified nephritogenic antibody-ferritin conjugates. *J. Exp. Med.* **127**, 867–878.

Vogt, A., Schmidt, H.U., Takamiya, H., and Batsford, S. (1980). '*In situ*' immune complex nephritis and basic proteins. *In* "Proc. Eur. Dial. Transplant Assoc., Vol. 17" (B. Robinson and J. Hawkins, eds.), pp. 613–619. Pitman Medical Publishing, Tumbridge Wells, Kent.

Vogt, A., Rohrbach, R., Shimizu, F., Takamiya, H., and Batsford, S. (1982). Interaction of cationized antigen with rat glomerular basement membrane. *In situ* immune complex formation. *Kidney Int.* **22**, 27–35.

Vogt, A., and Batsford, S.R. (1982). Eine neue Vorstellung zur Pathogenese der Imunkomplexnephritis. *Klin. Wochenschr.* **60**, 1095–1101.

Vogt, A., (1984). New aspects of the pathogenesis of immune complex glomerulonephritis: formation of subepithelial deposits. *Clin. Nephrol.* **21**, 15–20.

Vogt, A., Batsford, S., and Takamiya, H. (1985). Factors influencing the formation of subepithelial immune deposits in the renal glomerulus. *In* "Glomerular Dysfunction and Biopathology of Vascular Wall" (S. Seno, A.L. Copley, M.A. Venkatachalam and Y. Hamashima, eds.), pp. 225–235. Academic Press, Tokyo.

Weiser, R.S., and Laxon, C. (1962). The fate of fluorescein-labelled soluble antigen-antibody complex in the mouse. *J. Infect Dis.* **111**, 55–58.

Wright, N.G., Morrison, W.I., Thompson, H., and Cornwell, H.J.C. (1973). Experimental adenovirus immune complex glomerulonephritis. *Br. J. Exp. Pathol.* **54**, 628–633.

Zollinger, H.U., and Mihatsch, M.J. (1978). *In* "Renal Pathology in Biopsy" Springer Verlag, Berlin, Heidelberg, New York.

FACTORS INFLUENCING THE FORMATION OF SUBEPITHELIAL IMMUNE DEPOSITS IN THE RENAL GLOMERULUS

Arnold Vogt[1] and Stephen Batsford

Institut für Immunologie im Zentrum für Hygiene, Klinikum der Albert-Ludwigs-Universität, Freiburg im Breisgau

Haruo Takamiya

Department of Internal Medicine, Shigei Medical Research Hospital, Okayama

General Considerations on Formation of Subepithelial Immune Deposits

All theories pertaining to the formation of glomerular subepithelial deposits are required to explain how macromolecules, which under physiological conditions are excluded from the filtration process, can reach the region beyond the *lamina densa*. The question does this hold true for circulating, soluble immune complexes is especially intriguing. We shall concern ourselves here mainly with extraglomerular antigens that may be of endogenous or exogenous origin. Of course the antigen involved can be either an antigenic constituent of a glomerular structure or an extrinsic molecule (Dixon and Wilson, 1979). A further important aspect is the distinction between *in situ* formation of deposits and the deposition of immune complexes as preformed units (Couser and Salant, 1980). Current opinions concerning the above points are summarized in Table 1.

TABLE 1

CURRENT OPINIONS ON MECHANISMS OF SUBEPITHELIAL DEPOSIT FORMATION IN THE RENAL GLOMERULUS

Antigen	*In situ* formation	Deposition of preformed IC
Intrinsic Constituent of the glomerulus	Yes	Not relevant
Extrinsic* anionic	No (?)	No (?)
Extrinsic* cationic	Yes	Yes

*This can be of autologous (for example DNA) or exogenous (for example antigens from infectious agents) origin.

[1] Supported by the Deutsche Forschungsgemeinschaft.

Heymann Nephritis – A Special Case

The best studied model demonstrating *in situ* formation of subepithelial deposits is Heymann nephritis. This is one of the special cases where the target antigen is probably a structural component of the glomerular capillary wall (Couser and Salant, 1980) and problems of penetration are restricted to antibody and mediators of inflammation. On the basis of their size one expects permeation of antibody molecules through the *lamina densa* to be slow. In agreement with this, in passive Heymann nephritis, it takes about 4 to 5 days till a sufficient number of antibody molecules reach the target antigen beyond the *lamina densa* and form subepithelial deposits in a quantity sufficient to cause kidney damage resulting in proteinuria (Salant et al., 1980).

Glomerular Filtration – A Size and Charge Dependent Phenomena

In the case of extrinsic antigen it is important to know whether the antigen in question is negatively or positively charged (Batsford et al., 1980; Vogt, 1984; Vogt and Batsford, 1982, 1984).

Findings gathered in the past 10 years have shown that glomerular filtration is a function not only of size but also of charge (Bohrer et al., 1978; Chang et al., 1975; Kanwar, 1984; Rennke et al., 1975, 1978). Both *laminae rarae* contain a filamentous network of proteoglycans conferring a highly negative overall net charge to the GBM (Kanwar and Farquhar, 1979; Rennke et al., 1983). Anionic molecules reaching the glomerular filter are hindered from entering the GBM by electrostatic repulsion. Only molecules with a size smaller than that of albumin (69,000 daltons) are allowed to pass in any quantity and can reach the urinary space (Fig. 1). In contrast cationic molecules, even of the size of ferritin (480,000 daltons, effective molecular radius 61 Å), can easily penetrate all three layers of the GBM (Rennke et al., 1975).

Subepithelial Immune Deposits and Anionic Moieties – Antigen Overloading or Charge Neutralization

By what means do anionic macromolecules and anionic immune complexes gain access to the subepithelial space? In the chronic serum sickness model of nephritis anionic proteins, like BSA, are often used. Such antigens have difficulty in penetrating the GBM, nevertheless development of subepithelial deposits can be observed. Two mechanisms of subepithelial deposit formation in this type of nephritis model warrant consideration at present. One is *in situ* formation due to antigen overloading. To induce immune complex nephritis in the serum sickness model huge amounts of antigen have to be administered. Kidney damage is caused preferentially in those animals with a

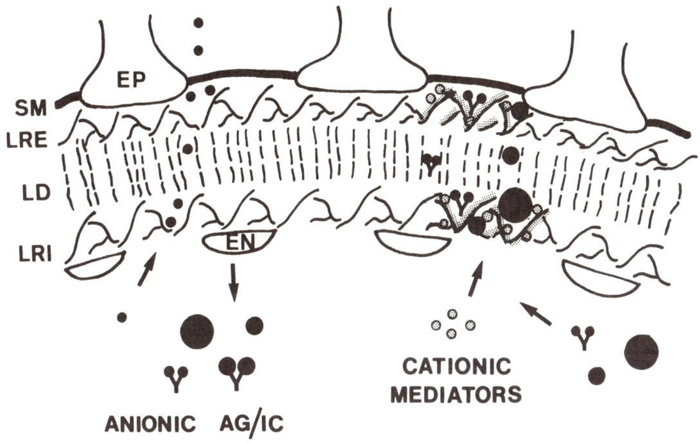

FIG. 1. HANDLING OF ANIONIC ANTIGENS (AG) AND IMMUNE COMPLEXES (IC) BY THE GBM. Macromolecules are repulsed by the fixed negative charges, only small antigens (effective radius < 40 Å) can reach the subepithelial space (see left hand side of diagram). Neutralization of the negative charges in the filtration barrier may permit penetration of larger anionic moieties. This could be achieved by cationic mediators released during inflammatory processes (see right hand side of diagram).
ABBREVIATIONS: EN, Endothelial cell; EP, Epithelial cell; LD, *Lamina densa*; LRE, *Lamina rara externa*; LRI, *Lamina rara interna*; SM, Slit membrane; thin and thick solid lines and filled circles, negatively charged; dotted structures, positively charged; broken lines, neutral; Y, antibody.

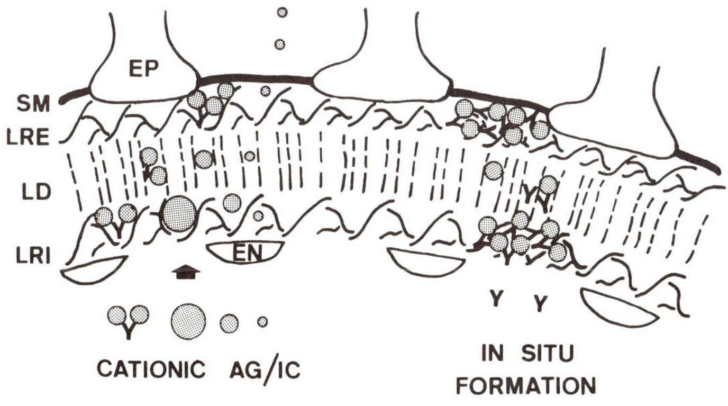

FIG. 2. HANDLING OF CATIONIC ANTIGENS AND IMMUNE COMPLEXES BY THE GBM. Cationic macromolecules and immune complexes are not repulsed electrostatically and can reach the subepithelial space. The *lamina densa* appears to act as a size selective barrier, with an effective cut-off of about 10^6 daltons (see left hand side of diagram). The right hand side depicts how subepithelial IC may be formed following binding of antibody to planted cationic antigen. ABBREVIATIONS, see FIG. 1.

moderate antibody response and exhibiting alternating modest excess of antigen followed by antibody excess (Dixon et al., 1961; Germuth and Rodriguez, 1973). Under these conditions it is not unwarranted to assume that a low but significant number of antigen and antibody molecules succeed in permeating the *lamina densa* and meet beyond this filtration barrier to form subepithelial immune complexes. Another possibility is that subepithelial deposition of anionic immune complexes, formed in the circulation, is brought about by local release of mediators. If cationic, these mediators could pave the way for anionic moieties (Fig. 1). It is known that injection of polycations such as polyethyleneimine (PEI) and protamine sulfate can neutralize the fixed anionic sites in the glomerular wall (charge neutralization or inversion) enabling anionic molecules to penetrate into the deeper layers of the basement membrane. In kidneys perfused with protamine Kelley and Cavallo (1978) observed a three to six fold increase in the number of ferritin molecules found beyond the inner aspect of the GBM, relative to unperfused controls. A more impressive effect was seen after pretreatment with the polycation PEI (Barnes et al., 1984). This latter polycation even permits the glomerular deposition of preformed, soluble immune complexes, although most of the deposits were found subendothelially (Barnes and Venkatachalam, 1984).

The effect of charge neutralization on the handling of macromolecules by the GBM is not totally understood at the moment. Whether local release of cationic mediators from inflammatory cells or platelets (e.g. during infections) can facilitate glomerular immune complex deposition has to be clarified. Even if a local release of cationic mediators does indeed cause a transitory increase in permeability, theoretical considerations relegate the chance for subepithelial deposition of anionic immune complexes to a very low level of likelyhood. The immune complexes will comprise only a very small proportion of the total anionic material in the blood. Not only this but being of large size, one would predict that the smaller serum proteins will win the race to the outer part of the basement membrane. This assumption is in line with the experimental data obtained. Subepithelial deposition of anionic tracer molecules and soluble immune complexes can be observed only under extreme conditions. Pretreatment with excessive (non-physiologic) doses of polycations and application of huge amounts of the tracer molecules does enable significant numbers of anionic moieties to reach the subepithelial area, although in comparison to cationized molecules the number is still very small. Whether this is due to inadequate charge neutralization or to the 'clogging' effect described by Kanwar and Rosenzweig (1982) or to an as yet unknown mechanism(s) has still to be elucidated.

Cationic Antigens and Subepithelial Immune Deposit Formation

The situation with cationic antigens is simpler. Positively charged molecules have free access to the filtration barrier (Fig. 2), they are not hindered by electrostatic repulsion forces and molecules of the size of ferritin (480,000 daltons, effective radius 61 Å) can easily permeate the *lamina densa* and reach the subepithelial area in large numbers (when highly cationized) (Vogt et al.,

1982). As with polycations the cationic or cationized antigen molecules interact with and bind to anionic structures in the *laminae rarae*. The binding forces are apparently not as strong as those between antigen and antibody or those between PEI and the fixed anionic sites. The filtration pressure and thermic movement seems to be sufficient to transport cationic macromolecules across the filtration barrier.

Accumulation of Cationic Antigens in the GBM is a Function of Charge and Size

It may take an appreciable time for highly cationic molecules of large size to permeate all three layers of the GBM. The affinity of cationic antigens for anionic sites should depend not only on charge differences but also on size. Larger molecules have the chance to interact with more anionic sites than smaller ones, i.e. they can behave like multivalent moieties.

The experimental data (Fig. 3) fits in with these considerations. The following findings were obtained by direct immunofluorescence after intra-

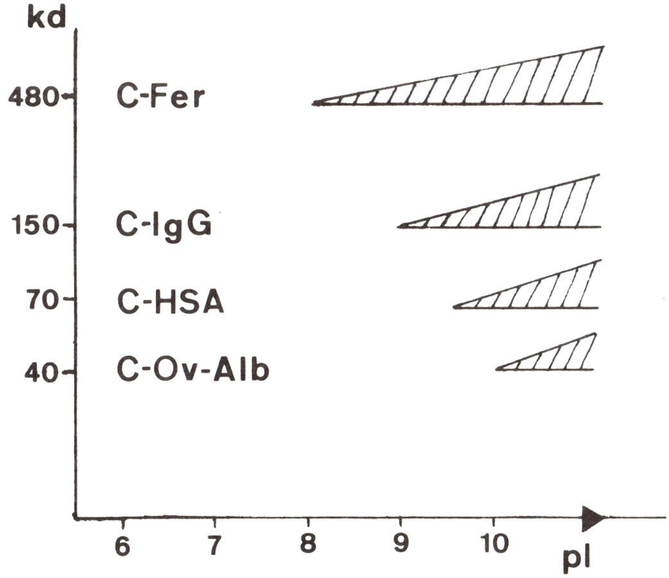

FIG. 3. Interaction of chemically cationized proteins with the GBM as a function of charge and size. 1 – 5 mg of each probe (Ov-albumin, human-serum-albumin, human-IgG, horse spleen ferritin), cationized (C-) to various degrees, was injected i.v. into rats. Kidneys were removed 30 min. later and stained with the appropriate FITC labeled antibody. Intensity of staining in a capillary pattern is indicated by the shaded areas. Data compiled from the references of Vogt et al., 1980; 1982.

venous injection of 1 to 5 mg of the cationic (cationized) probes into rats. Relatively small cationic molecules like monomeric lysozyme (13,400 daltons, pI 11.0) are not detectable within glomerular structures by immunofluorescence after intravenous injection. Small molecules like lysozyme rapidly pass the glomerular filter. Ovalbumin (40,000 daltons) accumulates unequivocally in a capillary pattern only when highly cationized i.e. its pI exceeds 10.0. HSA (69,000 daltons) and HuIgG (150,000 daltons) became detectable along the glomerular capillary wall when cationized fractions with a pI of about 9.0 and higher were injected. The critical minimum charge and size requirements of a molecule for glomerular accumulation seem to be a pI of about 9.0 and a size of about 40,000 daltons.

Detection of antigen affinity for the GBM can be made more sensitive when — as we have noted — subsequent to the cationic probe specific antibody is injected and immunofluorescence staining to detect accumulation of antibody globulin is performed. Using this experimental design and polymers of the natural cationic molecules lysozyme, ribonuclease and myoglobin, the critical parameters controlling glomerular affinity (accumulation along the glomerular capillary wall) could be further delineated. Crosslinking of the above cationic proteins allowed us to vary the size of probes of uniform charge. Trimeric lysozyme (42,000 daltons, pI 11.0) and trimeric ribonuclease (41,100 daltons, pI 9.45) (but not monomer or dimer) could be planted in the glomerular capillaries and complexed by the subsequently injected antibody while polymers (including pentamers) of myoglobin (pI 8.3) did not show any affinity for the GBM (unpublished). Thus the size and charge requirements for binding with chemically cationized proteins (size 40,000 daltons, pI 9.0) delineated above, were confirmed using natural cationic proteins.

Subendothelial – Subepithelial Transfer of Cationic Antigen-Complexes; Ultrastructural Studies

In the type of studies mentioned above electron microscopy revealed a predominant or — when highly cationic antigens were applied — an exclusively subepithelial localization of the glomerular deposits. Kinetic studies with electron dense, cationized ferritin as a marker showed that some molecules reach the subepithelial area after only a few minutes. Two hours after intravenous injection of 5 mg of cationized ferritin about the same number of ferritin molecules were present on both sides of the *lamina densa*. By 8 hours virtually all the remaining molecules were seen in the subepithelial area, (disregarding ferritin taken up by glomerular cells). When not latticed by specific antibody the molecules disappeared from the glomerulus within 12 to 36 hours and no subepithelial deposits developed. This sequence is illustrated in Fig. 4. In contrast cationic antigen which had reacted with antibody remained within glomerular structures for a prolonged period (weeks to months). Under the experimental conditions used — time interval between injection of cationized antigen and injection of antibody of 30 to 120 min — the immune complexes were formed *in situ*, most of them initially at an endothelial site. The number of ferritin-antibody complexes on the inner side of the capillary wall decreased with time while a parallel increase in the amount of ferritin

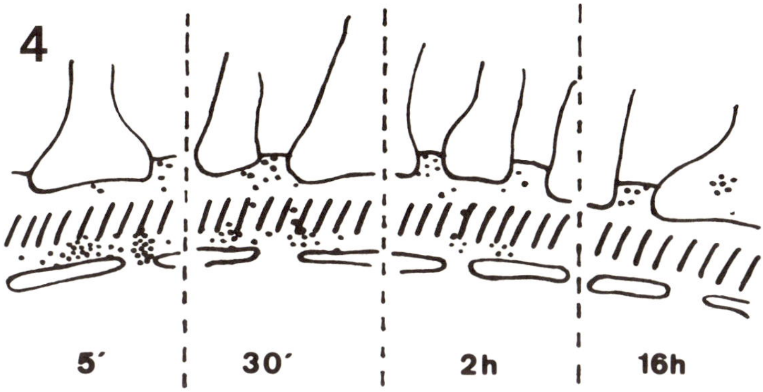

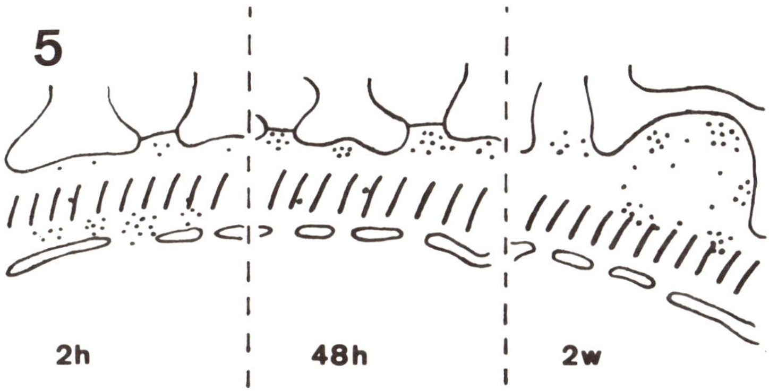

FIG. 4. Passage of highly cationized monomeric ferritin across the glomerular capillary wall. Transfer of ferritin from the inner to the outer aspects of the GBM is rapid, with some molecules reaching the subepithelial space within minutes. By 16 – 32 hr all molecules have left the GBM. Illustrations based on data from the reference of Vogt et al., 1982.

FIG. 5. Retention of cationized ferritin in the GBM when complexed with antibody. Initial site of complex formation is the inner side of the GBM. By 48 h the complexes have been transferred to the outer side, where they persist for weeks. Extensive hump formation can be seen. Illustrations based on data from the reference of Vogt et al., 1982.

containing deposits at the subepithelial site occured. By 24 – 48 hr the remaining ferritin deposits were all located subepithelially. At no timepoint investigated could larger aggregates be seen to permeate the *lamina densa*. We assume that only dissociated (free) ferritin and antibody molecules, or perhaps small antigen-antibody complexes (1:1 or 1:2 complexes) can pass the *lamina densa*. Having reached the subepithelial area they may recombine to larger aggregates and persist for a long time. These events are shown in Fig. 5. To traverse the GBM cationic antigens/immune complexes may not require the help of mediators that increase the permeability of the GBM since, in animals depleted of complement, neutrophils and/or macrophages formation of subepithelial deposits was not impaired (Thaiss et al., 1983).

In contrast to anionic complexes, soluble immune complexes formed with cationic antigens can localize in all three layers of the GBM. Isolated soluble immune complexes (pI 8 — 10) comprising cationized ferritin and specific antibody only persisted for long periods when antibody to either of the constituents was given subsequently to trap and enlarge the permeating complexes (Takamiya, 1985). Persistence of subepithelial deposits depends on lattice formation (Mannik et al., 1983). The patterns of glomerular deposition of soluble immune complexes are largely dependent on charge. The more cationic the complex the greater is the chance that subepithelial localization will occur (Gallo et al., 1981, 1983). Working with covalently linked antigen-antibody complexes it has been shown that complexes of size up to 28S may pass the *lamina densa* and reach the subepithelial region (Caulin-Glaser et al., 1983). That small units of dissociated immune complexes are able to pass the *lamina densa* was shown in experiments with cationized, dimeric ferritin which is in respect of size comparable to immune complexes consisting of one ferritin and up to three antibody molecules. Though considerably reduced in comparison to monomer, a significant number of dimeric ferritin molecules reached the subepithelial area; cationized trimeric ferritins were only exceptionally seen within the *lamina densa* (unpublished).

Nephritogenic Potential of Cationic Antigens

When cationized antigen is directly perfused into the left renal artery and specific antibody is administered intravenously 60 min later acute unilateral immune complex nephritis, with massive proteinuria can be induced in rats (Batsford et al., 1980). Immune complexes were deposited or located almost exclusively subepithelially. Quantitative studies with radio-labeled antigen and antibody showed that in rats as little as 10 μg antigen (cationized human IgG) and 30 μg antibody globulin is sufficient to cause nephritis (Oite et al., 1982).

In contrast to subepithelial deposit formation, which probably occurs without the help of mediators, induction of glomerular injury and proteinuria is only seen when complement, granulocytes and monocytes can participate (Thaiss et al., 1983). Recently an active variant of this model has been developed with a much more pronounced involvement of inflammatory cells (Oite et al., 1983).

Cationic Extracellular Streptococcal Antigens

Of interest for our understanding of the pathogenesis of postinfectious immune complex nephritis is the recent finding that cationic, extracellular products of a nephritogenic group A streptococcal strain were present in glomerular deposits in biopsy specimens obtained from cases of acute post-streptococcal glomerulonephritis (Vogt et al., 1983).

These cationic products showed a significant affinity for the GBM when injected intravenously into the rat followed by the specific antibody (Vogt et al., 1985). The molecular weight and the pI of these cationic fractions were determined to be 35,000 daltons and higher than pH 9.0 respectively. By electron microscopy mesangial, subendothelial and subepithelial deposits were seen (unpublished observations).

Conclusions

From the foregoing analysis it is reasonable to assume that cationized antigens may play a causative role in those human nephritides where subepithelial deposits are prominent, as in membranous nephropathy, postinfectious glomerulonephritis and lupus nephritis.

Regarding the question as to whether anionic or cationic macromolecules are more likely to act as nephritogenic antigens, at least in the above mentioned types of nephritis most of the known data are in favour of the latter.

Abstract

Evidence obtained in recent years clearly points to the key role of electrical charge in the formation of subepithelial immune deposits. Detailed experimental studies with cationized or naturally cationic proteins have demonstrated the affinity of these antigens for the GBM. Positively charged molecules are capable of reaching the subepithelial space even when of large size, without the aid of mediators. Experimentally cationic antigens can be employed as targets to induce *in situ* immune complex GN that resembles membranous nephropathy. Preformed, circulating immune complexes can also reach the subepithelial space, provided they are highly cationic; their persistence is dependent on lattice formation.

References

Barnes, J.L., Radnik, R.A., Gilchrist, E.P., and Venkatachalam, M.A. (1984). Size and charge selective permeability defects induced in glomerular basement membrane by a polycation. *Kidney Int.* **25**, 11–19.

Barnes, J.L., and Venkatachalam, M.A. (1984). Enhancement of glomerular immune complex deposition by a circulating polycation. *J. Exp. Med.* **160**, 286–293.

Batsford, S., Oite, T., Takamiya, H., and Vogt, A. (1980). Anionic binding sites in the glomerular basement membrane: possible role in the pathogenesis of immune complex glomerulonephritis. *Renal Physiol.* **3**, 336–340.

Batsford, S.R., Takamiya, H., and Vogt, A. (1980). A model of *in situ* immune complex glomerulonephritis in the rat employing cationized ferritin. *Clin. Nephrol.* **14**, 211–216.

Bohrer, M.P., Baylis, C., Humes, H.D., Glassock, R.J., Robertson, C.R., and Brenner, B.M. (1978). Permselectivity of the glomerular capillary walls: facilitated filtration of circulating polycations. *J. Clin. Invest.* **61**, 72–78.

Caulin-Glaser, T., Gallo, G.R., and Lamm, M.E. (1983). Nondissociating cationic immune complexes can deposit in glomerular basement membrane. *J. Exp. Med.* **158**, 1561–1572.

Chang, R.L.S., Deen, W.M., Robertson, C.R., and Brenner, B.M. (1975). Permselectivity of the glomerular capillary wall. III. Restricted transport of polyanions. *Kidney Int.* **8**, 212–218.

Couser, W.G., and Salant, D.J. (1980). *In situ* immune complex formation and glomerular injury. *Kidney Int.* **17**, 1–13.

Dixon, F.J., Feldman, J.D., and Vazquez, J.J. (1961). Experimental nephritis. The pathogenesis of a laboratory model resembling the spectrum of human glomerulonephritis. *J. Exp. Med.* **113**, 899–920.

Dixon, F.J., and Wilson, C.B. (1979). Immunological renal injury produced by formation and deposition of immune complexes. *In* "Contemporary Issues on Nephropathy Vol. 2. Immunological Mechanisms of Renal Disease" (C.B. Wilson, B.M. Brenner and J.H. Stein, eds.), pp. 1–34. Churchill Livingstone, New York.

Gallo, G.R., Caulin-Glaser, T., Emancipator, S.N., and Lamm, M.E. (1983). Nephritogenicity and differential distribution of glomerular immune complexes related to immunogen charge. *Lab. Invest.* **48**, 353–362.

Gallo, G.R., Caulin-Glaser, T., and Lamm, M.E. (1981). Charge of circulating immune complexes as a factor in glomerular basement membrane localization in mice. *J. Clin. Invest.* **67**, 1305–1311.

Germuth, Jr., F.G., and Rodriguez, E. (1973). Immunopathology of the Renal Glomerulus. Little Brown, Boston.

Kanwar, Y.S. (1984). Biology of Disease. Biophysiology of glomerular filtration and proteinuria. *Lab. Invest.* **51**, 7–21.

Kanwar, Y.S., and Farquhar, M.G. (1979). Anionic sites in the glomerular basement membrane: in vivo and in vitro localization to the lamina rarae by cationic probes. *J. Cell. Biol.* **81**, 137–153.

Kanwar, Y.S., and Rosenzweig, L.J. (1982). Clogging of the glomerular basement membrane. *J. Cell. Biol.* **93**, 489–494.

Kelley, V.E., and Cavallo, T. (1978). Glomerular permeability. Transfer of native ferritin in glomeruli with decreased anionic sites. *Lab. Invest.* **39**, 547–553.

Mannik, M., Agodoa, L.Y.C., and David, K.A. (1983). Rearrangement of immune complexes in glomeruli leads to persistence and development of electron dense deposits. *J. Exp. Med.* **157**, 1516–1528.

Oite, T., Batsford, S.R., Mihatsch, M.J., Takamiya, H., and Vogt, A. (1982). Quantitative studies of *in situ* immune complex glomerulonephritis in the rat induced by planted, cationized antigen. *J. Exp. Med.* **155**, 460–473.

Oite, T., Shimizu, F., Kihara, I., Batsford, S.R., and Vogt, A. (1983). An active model of immune complex glomerulonephritis in the rat employing cationized ferritin. *Am. J. Path.* **112**, 185–194.

Reale, E., Luciano, L., and Kühn, K.W. (1983). Ultrastructural architecture of proteoglycans in the glomerular basement membrane. *J. Histochem. Cytochem.* **31**, 662–668.

Rennke, H.G., Cotran, R.S., and Venkatachalam, M.A. (1975). Role of molecular charge in glomerular permeability: Tracer studies with cationized ferritins. *J. Cell. Biol.* **67**, 638–646.

Rennke, H.G., Patel, Y., and Venkatachalam, M.A. (1978). Glomerular filtration of proteins: clearance of anionic, neutral and cationic horseradish peroxidase in the rat. *Kidney Int.* **13**, 278–288.

Salant, D.J., Darby, C., and Couser, W.G. (1980). Experimental membranous nephropathy in rats. Quantitative studies of glomerular immune deposit formation in isolated glomeruli and whole animals. *J. Clin. Invest.* **66**, 71–81.

Takamiya, H., Batsford, S., and Vogt, A. (1985). *In situ* immune complex formation versus circulating immune complex deposition: *In situ* immune complex glomerulonephritis induced by cationic immune complex as planted antigen. *In* "Glomerular Dysfunction and Biopathology of Vascular Wall" (S. Seno, A.L. Copley, M.A. Venkatachalam and Y. Hamashima, eds.), pp. 209–224. Academic Press, Tokyo.

Thaiss, F., Batsford, S., Mihatsch, M., Bittersuermann, D., and Vogt, A. (1983). Mediator systems in *in situ* immune complex glomerulonephritis. *Kidney Int.* **23**, 199.

Vogt, A. (1984). New aspects of the pathogenesis of immune complex glomerulonephritis: formation of subepithelial deposits. *Clin. Nephrol.* **21**, 15–20.

Vogt, A., and Batsford, S.R. (1982). Eine neue Vorstellung zur Pathogenese der Imunkomplexnephritis. *Klin. Wochenschr.* **60**, 1095–1101.

Vogt, A., and Batsford, S. (1984). Local immune complex formation and pathogenesis of glomerulonephritis. *Contrib. Nephrol.* **43**, 51–63.

Vogt, A., Batsford, S., Rodriguez-Iturbe, B., and Garcia, R. (1983). Cationic antigens in poststreptococcal glomerulonephritis. *Clin. Nephrol.* **20**, 271–279.

Vogt, A., Mertz, A., Batsford, S., and Rodriguez-Iturbe, B. (1985). Cationic, extracellular streptococcal antigen; affinity for the renal glomerulus. Recent Advances in Streptococci and Streptococcal Diseases, Reedbooks, in Press.

Vogt, A., Rohrbach, R., Shimizu, F., Takamiya, H., and Batsford, S. (1982). Interaction of cationized antigen with rat glomerular basement membrane: *In situ* immune complex formation. *Kidney Int.* **22**, 27–35.

Vogt, A., Schmidt, H.U., Takamiya, H., and Batsford, S. (1980). '*In situ*' immune complex nephritis and basic proteins. *In* "Proc. Eur. Dial. Transplant Assoc., Vol. 17" (B. Robinson and J. Hawkins), pp. 613–619. *Pitman Medical Publishing*, Tumbridge Wells, Kent.

Index